P9-DIA-537

Encountering the Sacred in Psychotherapy

Encountering the Sacred in Psychotherapy

How to Talk with People about Their Spiritual Lives

JAMES L. GRIFFITH
MELISSA ELLIOTT GRIFFITH

THE GUILFORD PRESS
New York   London

© 2002 The Guilford Press
A Division of Guilford Publications, Inc.
72 Spring Street, New York, NY 10012
www.guilford.com

Printed in the United States of America

This book is printed on acid-free paper.

Last digit is print number: 9 8 7 6 5 4 3 2 1

Library of Congress Cataloging-in-Publication Data

Griffith, James L., 1950–
    Encountering the sacred in psychotherapy : how to talk with people
about their spiritual lives / by James L. Griffith, Melissa Elliott Griffith.
      p.   cm.
    Includes bibliographical references and index.
    ISBN 1-57230-701-3 (hardcover)
    1. Psychotherapy—Religious aspects. 2. Psychotherapy patients—
Religious life. I. Griffith, Melissa Elliott, 1952– II. Title.

RC455.4.R4 G75 2002
616.89'14—dc21
                                      2001040474

Of those who have shared their stories with us,

Some live in the perpetual shadow of medical or
    psychiatric illness,
Others have survived political torture and exile from
    their homelands,
Many people of Kosovë, with our colleagues at the
    University of Prishtina,
Toil to keep alive the spirit of a people without turning
    to hatred.

To these who must live alongside problems that can
    be neither solved nor ended,
Whose spirituality has sustained hope, purpose,
    and community,
We dedicate this book.

About the Authors

James L. Griffith, MD, is Professor of Psychiatry and Neurology at The George Washington University Medical Center, where he directs the psychiatry residency training program and the consultation–liaison psychiatry service. **Melissa Elliott Griffith, CNS, LMFT,** serves on the psychiatry clinical faculty at The George Washington University Medical Center and practices psychotherapy in Vienna, Virginia. They are both affiliated with the Center for Multicultural Human Services in Falls Church, Virginia. They are also coauthors of *The Body Speaks: Therapeutic Dialogues for Mind Body Problems* (Basic Books, 1994).

Preface

"Blest be the tie that binds . . ."

The singing of the blessing begins, all the voices of my kin, all who can come to the Christmas reunion of the descendants of Mose and Minnie Rivers Elliott. We are crowded together, hands joined in a circle in Aunt Sue's den in Water Valley, Mississippi. I am not often in this circle now. Geography and schedules have recently kept me and my family away more years than not, but being at the gathering in the days of my child-hood was as constant as Christmas itself. I don't know how old I was when I noticed my daddy's eyes glistening on the last verse:

"When we asunder part, it gives us inward pain;
But we shall still be joined in heart, And hope to meet again."

At some point, I came to know that all together my family held the memory of those who had passed on, held them in the circle still, with longing and with gratitude.

In the moments of fear and despair in my life, this hymn sings to me and I can know that I am not alone. It is the knowledge that I am not only connected to the Water Valley circle, but to other circles, broken and repaired, past and future, seen and unseen, which allows me to be in a posture of relatedness, arms outstretched, hopeful that circles can be made and trusted.

Before this writing, I had never put words to what the circle, and the singing of this blessing, has come to mean to me. I did not realize the depth and fullness of its significance in my life until now, and because I have described it to another, it will be even more sustaining and available to me. This is the gift of telling our spiritual stories. Griff and I choose to call a story like this a spiritual story because it is one of connection that transcends time and space. It is one that can inspire hope within me in hard times. When those times come again, and I feel myself to be unraveling, I may do as I have done before and consult a therapist. If so, I would like to be able to speak this story, so that it can be woven in as a strong and shining thread alongside the loose and frayed ones.

When people consult with us as therapists, we want them, too, to be able to tell spiritual and religious stories that inspire hope and connection for them, as well as any that bring despair and isolation. We are each passionately interested in how we can make this possible, how we as therapists may both encourage and inadvertently thwart the meaning making of these experiences. With the help of others who have participated with us in research, therapy, and training, we have been exploring these interests. We offer in this book our work in progress.

We searched for language that would not make unwanted distinctions, and still we struggle with the words we have chosen. We speak of opening therapy to sacred conversations when we talk with persons about their experiences of the spiritual, yet we believe that whenever we hold with care the trust of those who consult with us, our therapeutic conversations are *sacred encounters*. Whenever we listen to or host a conversation in which people listen to one another with open hearts, *the spiritual* is within that connection.

There are myriad ways of expressing spirituality and many traditions. Our greatest concern about this book is that some of those go unmentioned or are discussed only briefly and are rarely illustrated in the therapy vignettes. Stories of therapies that invoke the Eastern traditions and spiritualities that are not God-centered are few in this text in comparison to the many that include Western traditions, especially those of Protestant Christianity. Our colleagues who have been our readers have been concerned for us, that we might be perceived to be too narrow, and have generously offered to share some of their stories with us to increase the breadth of this text. We were tempted, but have decided to tell only the stories that we have heard in therapy and that we have lived. Surely, then, we have not addressed many spiritual expressions or dilemmas that can arise in therapy. Sometimes, acutely aware of our limitations, we have longed to collaborate in this writing with a group of therapists that would include, at the least, a Buddhist, a Hindu, a Muslim, and a Jew. Because it would stray from our purpose, and because we needed to bring closure to this project, we chose not to do so. To our relief and delight, Froma Walsh has recently edited just such a book, *Spiritual Resources in Family Therapy* (1999), which we recommend as an excellent complement to this text. Indeed, since this project's inception, much has been published about psychotherapy and spirituality. Again, in order to keep focus and to bring closure, we have not attempted to review that literature here, but this burgeoning body of exciting research and clinical articles will be even larger by the time this book is published.

We have sought to understand when to open therapy to a dialogue about spirituality and how to do that in culturally appropriate ways. We are reminded of a conversation with Charles Waldegrave of the Family Center in New Zealand, a collaboration of Maori, Pacific Island, and European workers who have been a fount of spirituality in therapy for us and so many in North America. We asked Charles, "It's been said that you honor the Maori spirituality by praying together before a session. Is it true? Do you pray before all your sessions at the center?"

"Ah, well, life is a prayer, isn't it?" he said. "Sometimes, if it is culturally appropriate, we speak it together, sometimes not."

This is our hope, that we speak about spirituality with those persons for whom it is culturally appropriate and relevant, and do not speak about it when it is not appropriate or not their desire. Because the gift people give those listening to their stories is a sacred trust, we must always try to be attuned to when and how we can most helpfully receive and respond. This book is the story of the ways we have learned, so far, to be attuned to these gifts, to be receptive to the varied presentations of spiritual and religious life, to be discerning of those times when it becomes a destructive force, and to be responsive in ways that honor and strengthen the circles of community, tradition, and faith that sustain and connect.

Acknowledgments

The people to whom we are most indebted for the writing of this book, of course, cannot be named here. They have spoken with us in therapy sessions, in family meetings, at the hospital bedside, and in research projects. They have both inspired us with their spiritual stories and informed us about ways to usefully participate with them in story making. When we sent out the vignettes of this book drawn from our experiences with these individuals, they responded with edits and permission to publish. Most of them participated in choosing pseudonyms and disguises to render their stories true and still protect their privacy, while some requested that we not alter names or particulars and tell the story just as it was. Many sent meaningful letters, thoughtful reflections on our time together, and on developments in their lives since our series of meetings. Receiving these letters was the best part of writing this book. Though the format of this book does not allow for their publication, these letters have improved our rendering of the vignettes and influenced our thinking about therapy and about life.

    I (*Griff*) began working in earnest to open my clinical work to the spiritual lives of my patients in the early 1980s, during my psychiatry residency at Massachusetts General Hospital (MGH). For generations of MGH residents, Ned Cassem—Jesuit priest, Harvard professor, and Chairman of the Massachusetts General Hospital Department of Psychiatry—has modeled a clinical seamlessness that addresses in one movement both symptoms of mental illness and dilemmas of the human spirit. The discipline and focus that Ned and his faculty colleague, George Murray, exacted from MGH psychiatry residents led us to suspect that our clinical training was heavily laced with the rigor of Jesuit training. Nearly 20 years later I was startled to realize just how much I had absorbed from Ned when I listened at a national conference to his invited lecture on spirituality in medical illness. I heard him illustrate in that lecture so many of the kinds of questions I thought I had originated. Under his supervision and mentorship, I learned even more than I had realized.

A second inspiration in the early 1980s was the "Psychology and Theology Luncheon Group," a mixed group of psychiatrists, psychologists, and theologians who met monthly over a long lunch in Cambridge to discuss an extraordinary range of topics, from religious visions in temporal lobe epilepsy to the confrontation of evil in a psychotherapy session. A guiding spirit for this group was Boston psychoanalyst Ana-Maria Rizzuto, whose seminal work, *The Birth of the Living God* (University of Chicago Press, 1979), had given to clinicians the idea of object relations for understanding the power of a person's felt presence of a God and its meaning in his or her psychological world. During five years in Boston, these discussions with John McDargh, Reb McMichael, David Bear, Steve Nisenbaum, Bob Weber, and other group members kept raising practical questions about the beliefs and practices of spirituality and their meaning for mental illness and mental health.

Our friend Reb McMichael returned to Mississippi and formed such a group there, inviting us to join in lively conversations with him and other therapists and clerics, Ruth Black, Ruth Woodliff-Stanley, and Mark and Lisa McLain among them. One outgrowth of these conversations was the creation in the 1990s of a research group with psychologist Jeanetta Rains and psychiatry residents Carol Tingle, Alexis Polles, Nancy Krejmas, Dinesh Mittal, and Mark McLain that produced a series of research reports on the significance for clinical work of people's relationships to a personal God (Griffith et al., 1992, 1995; Polles et al., 1993; Tingle et al., 1993). Mississippians Priscilla Pearson, Gloria Howard Martin, and Julie Propst joined our discussions and shared our excitement about applying narrative ideas to the multiple and contradictory experiences people had of God. We found these notions to closely fit and to usefully loosen therapy conversations in our culture.

But could these ideas also be useful *outside* our culture? Griff had begun to write about this work, and wanted me (*Melissa*) to join him in spreading the ideas we were developing, but I was hesitant. Taking these concepts into the wider world was fraught with difficulties for me. How could I talk about opening to many different expressions of spirituality when 95% of my experience, professional and personal, was with Protestant Christianity? Imposing our culture on others was the last thing either of us wanted to do. Sallyann Roth came to the rescue and joined us as a co-presenter the first time we put forth these ideas at a national meeting. Her presence and stories dispelled any notions of narrowness. Later, Kaethe Weingarten invited me to contribute to an issue on cultural resistance that she was composing for the *Journal of Feminist Family Therapy*. She said that what we were doing was "radical" in the context of secular psychotherapy, and, though I would not have presumed to call it that, I was heartened that she understood that we wanted to encourage curiosity and openness toward an aspect of people's lives that our field had often regarded as boring, irrelevant, and ignorant. With trembling confidence, I did write and Sallyann penned a gracious response.

Griff and I then offered a series of workshops. Jill Freedman could not have known that she finally teased me out of my mire of concerns with a jovial phone call after one of these workshops. "What is this?" she said. "It seems like everyone who enters my office is wanting to talk about God now!" Had it not been for the encouraging acts of these three women of Jewish lineage, each vastly different from me and from one another in our expressions of spirituality, all therapists I trusted and admired, I might never have been able to believe Griff's arguments, that what we were developing could have wide applicability and that I should join him in writing this book.

A book as many years in the making as this one has scores of friends and colleagues to whom we owe gratitude. We have been blessed with a community of therapists who have a commitment to social justice and an interest in narrative ideas. Though several of them have experienced the oppressive effects of religion, they nonetheless have created forums so that we could engage with them and others in understanding and honoring people's religious and spiritual lives in psychotherapy. Among these, particularly Sallie Motch, Rachel Dash, Michael Dixon, Vicki Dickerson, Gene Combs, Glenda Fredman, Susan Shaw, Janet Adams-Westcott, Bill Madsen, Margarita Tarragona, Jo Ellen Patterson, Craig Smith, Jerry Gale, Delane Kinney, Ann Madigan, Zoy Kazan, Peggy Sax, Linda Terry-Guyer, Bill Lax, and Steve Madigan have responded with interest and honesty to our work. We have been privileged

xiv   Acknowledgments

to learn from other narrative teachers, Trevor Hudson, Kiwi Tammassee, Charles Waldegrave, Wally McKenzie, and Sue Boardman-McKissack, who have long honored people's spirituality in therapy.

Some colleagues' influence is so pervasive that it is impossible to adequately cite them. Peggy Penn's graceful and creative therapy and writing has for many years inspired us to see our own work anew and to continue to write. We are grateful to Harry Goolishian, Harlene Anderson, Tom Andersen, Lynn Hoffman, John Shotter, Karl Tomm, Michael White, Cheryl White, and David Epston, whose work continues to shape and challenge ours. Jack Lannamann, Betsy Wood, John Rolland, Froma Walsh, Frank Fernandez, and Lois Slovik have influenced us both clinically and philosophically.

We have been sustained by Washington colleagues who both befriended and believed in us—David and Joann Reiss, Steve and Sybil Wolin, Jeff Akman, Jane McGoldrick, Eric McCollum, Sandi Stith, Margie Stohner, Georgeanne Schopp, Ann Womack, and Karen Weihs. Lynne Gaby and Judy Okawa have extended this work, seeking with us to understand how spirituality aids the resilience of severely traumatized refugees.

Friends and family have gathered us up when we could not pull things together. Our parents, Van and Helen and Lamont and Louise, taught us not to give up, and our children, Marianna and Van, would not let us. Janet Cavett, our family theologian, aided us with her biblical knowledge. Judith Landau informed us with her cultural knowledge. Carole Samworth, Martha Jurchak, and Jane Bise maternally monitored our progress. They still asked about the book when we said, "Don't ask." We are forever grateful to Kaethe Weingarten, who gave her attention to every paragraph and improved almost every page.

If every person were surrounded by friends like ours and supported by a professional who gave them the patience, understanding, and encouragement that our editor, Kitty Moore, has given to us, we therapists would have much less work to do. In addition to her considerable editorial skills, Kitty's persistence and forgiveness have made it possible, when it seemed impossible, for us to complete this project. Near the end, when our spirits were flagging, Kitty enlisted the aid of Denise Leto, whose enthusiastic e-mails and exquisitely attentive editing gave us a second wind and enabled us to stay the course. The entire team at The Guilford Press has assumed a precise, practical, and hopeful stance toward this project. Their partnering with us has made us better writing partners to each other.

Contents

Chapter One

New Ways of
Hearing Sacred Stories

In these pages we hope to show ways to open therapy to the spiritual lives of people who consult us; to listen for and to their experiences; to learn about their religious beliefs, spiritual practices, and sustaining faith communities; and to recognize and respond when these powers are used destructively. We begin with Devi's story because it is about the heart of this work, which is the practice of wonder. The practice of wonder— being available to what is not yet known or expected—is a therapeutic practice for the life of conversations, for the people who consult with us, and for us.

When Devi first arrived, she had to check to see if her pager was on. She explained that we might be interrupted because her husband required that she respond immediately if he called to ask her whereabouts. Her request was for help in leaving this marriage. While she had not married for immigration reasons, her pending citizenship would be at risk if she divorced. Though she was successful in her studies and her work and fluent in three languages, Devi had come to believe her husband's insults that she was stupid and inept. She said she had lost her appetite for eating, and almost for living. "I feel that I am disappearing," she said, and this was reflected in the thinness of her body and the

1

vagueness in her eyes. I (Melissa) was the third therapist she had seen. The couple had attempted marital therapy, and Devi had tried to change herself in many ways to please her husband, but she could no longer endure his degradation and threats.

Devi and her mother had journeyed from their homeland of India to the United States to obtain an American education for Devi. She had excelled in school and spoke nearly flawless English. Midway through one of her sentences she paused, apologizing for a minor linguistic mistake. I had not noticed. I marveled at her fluency, but I wondered what our conversation might be like if she were able to speak about the entrapment in her marriage in her native tongue. It was then that she told me that her husband would not permit her to speak in her own language, not even when talking with her mother on the phone. He considered her to be culturally and racially inferior and wanted her to disguise as much as possible of her ethnicity. I offered to search for a therapist who could communicate with her in Hindi. Devi did not want to see a different therapist. She didn't mind speaking English in therapy, but she did long to speak Hindi with her mother on the telephone in her own home.

Two weeks later Devi came to see me again. She still felt trapped. Although her situation had worsened at home, she was still unable to leave. She had secured a safe place in case of an emergency, but insisted that she presently was in no physical danger. The danger, she said, was that she might give up. She was sustained only by her friends and her mother. They were worried about her and called daily, begging her to leave.

I asked that she invite her mother to our next meeting. Her mother, Ms. Chowdry, arrived dressed in a sari with her head lowered, and, after a long period of silence, made only one pleading comment in a soft and deferential tone. I could not understand all of her words, a mixture of Hindi and English, but I needed no translation for the intense love, helplessness, and fear in her voice as she entreated her daughter to leave her husband, to come home with her that very day. "My mother is saying that she doesn't want me to become another Nicole Brown Simpson," Devi explained. Ms. Chowdry nodded and again addressed her daughter in Hindi. Devi gently reprimanded, "Speak English." At this moment, I became acutely aware of Devi's earlier description of her husband requiring that she and her mother converse in English.

"Please," I said, "speak in your own language. You don't need to translate for me unless you want to. I will ask questions that may be helpful, and the two of you can use them as you wish. I have confidence that you will find a way to talk with each other about what is most important, and that your talk will be more comfortable and fruitful if you talk in your own language."

The conversation seemed to flow well and I became optimistic that Devi was unified with Ms. Chowdry in the decision to put her safety first. I was surprised and worried when, near the end of the session, Devi confessed that she was still confused. She said she would stay in the marriage a bit longer until she achieved more financial and immigration security. Ms. Chowdry bent down, hiding her face in her hands. I inquired about her sadness and her worries, expecting her to speak of her sorrow for her daughter. She spoke plaintively in Hindi and Devi translated: "My mother says to tell you that she is sad because she is homesick."

"What would she do with such a serious problem if she were at home?" I asked.

"If she had a serious problem, she would go to the temple," replied Ms. Chowdry. They conversed a bit more in Hindi. Then Devi turned to me and said, "My mother says the temple is what she misses most about home. She went to pray there every day."

I asked Ms. Chowdry to describe the temple and what it was like to be there. "Peaceful," she answered. I wondered aloud what it would be like to be in the temple together now: "Would the peacefulness bring answers to Devi?" Ms. Chowdry and Devi became quiet. I sensed the sacredness of this moment and felt that more questions would be an intrusion. Then I thought that even my presence might be an intrusion, much like it might be if I were a guest at their temple, present when their need was to pray, undistracted by attention to their guest. I slipped out my office door, telling them I would give them privacy for a while, and requesting that they open the door when they had finished talking.

In about 10 minutes, they invited me back. Devi and her mother seemed peaceful, and her mother no longer looked sad. Devi had resolved to leave her husband. We set up our next appointment. Devi called the next day to let me know that she had left my office with her mother, never to sleep in her husband's home again. She expressed gratitude to me for holding the meeting, for encouraging them to speak in Hindi, and for leaving the room so that she and her mother could pray. She identified these acts as different from anything that had happened in her previous therapies. It was different for me, too, I thought to myself.

We chatted a while about our shared admiration for the gentleness and wisdom of her mother.

Relatively quickly, with the help of Indian and American friends and immigration lawyers, Devi was able to obtain a divorce. When I last spoke with her, she was interested in starting a group for immigrant women trapped in abusive relationships.

Devi had many strengths—intelligence and insight, a good job, a safe place to go, a concerned, supportive friendship network, and the love of a wise and persistent mother. Surely all these contributed to the courageous step she took. However, she was finally able to see clearly and to act when she and her mother entered the peacefulness offered by their spirituality.

What did the therapy have to do with the entry into this spirituality? For us, this is the crucial question. It seemed to "just happen," a moment of mystery that cannot be fully understood, and certainly could not have been orchestrated. Nevertheless, we want to understand as much as possible about it. Devi's reflections after the session may point the way: "It is good that we spoke in our own language," she said, "and good that my mother and I could pray."

Urging Ms. Chowdry and Devi to speak in a language unknown to me was, in that particular instance, prompted by my wishing the therapy atmosphere to be radically different from the home atmosphere of Devi's marriage. But that specific act is reflective of the general way we aspire to work with people's spiritual experiences in therapy. The two of us are often urging them to speak in languages with which we are unfamiliar. Stepping out of the room, trusting Devi and her mother to determine when to invite me back in, illustrates what often seems to be the choreography of our conversations with people about their spiritual experiences.

SPIRITUALITY CHALLENGES THERAPISTS

The two of us can tell many similar stories in which a person in crisis who is constrained by assumptions, beliefs, and customs seems to have no options. However, shifting the site of negotiations from the psychological or physical world into the person's spiritual world opens new possibilities that we can never fully fathom. Perhaps this is no surprise, given how widespread is the influence of spirituality in the lives of people. In 1996 the freethinking quarterly *Free Enquiry* commissioned its own poll, doubting prior reports about the pervasiveness of religious beliefs in American society (Goldhaber Research Associations, 1996). To its surprise, almost 90% of those interviewed expressed belief in a personal God who can answer prayer. Given its bias toward agnosticism, the *Free Enquiry* poll appeared to settle definitively any questions as to the pervasiveness of religious beliefs among Americans. When those who practice spiritualities that are not God-centered are added to these numbers, it seems that some form of spiritual life is important for most of those who come for psychotherapy.

Nevertheless, the majority of mental health professionals, with the notable exception of pastoral counselors, have struggled during the past century to find a proper place for people's spiritual lives. This was brought home to me (Griff) a couple of years ago by two psychiatry residents who were waiting for me after our morning hospital rounds on a surgical floor, hesitant but wanting to discuss the way I had spoken with a patient awaiting surgery. Puzzled and disturbed, the residents said that they had never mixed religion and psychotherapy because they had always thought of the latter as a scientific endeavor. Furthermore, they wondered, "How can you talk about a relationship with God when there is just one person there?" An internist had asked us to evaluate his patient, a man with kidney disease, whom the internist believed to be depressed. During the interview, the patient mentioned that he had been praying. I asked if he were comfortable speaking with me about it. Would he tell me what words he had prayed? He did so. How had he sensed that God had received the prayer? What seemed to be God's response? He seemed quite interested in speaking about these things, so I inquired further. What did God know about his problems that others did not understand? What did he most hope that God could understand? After we left his bedside, I had talked briefly with the medical students and psychiatry residents about the ongoing conversations that many patients have with a personal God, and the decisions toward healing or dying that are often made therein, depending on the turns such hidden conversations take. The two residents felt troubled over how they were to fit what they had witnessed into the rest of what they were learning about psychiatry.

The mental health professions generally have held an ambivalent and distant relationship with spirituality and religion. The reasons for this are multiple and complex. Like the two residents, some feel that psychotherapy is about science and that talk of religion or spirituality can only bring irrational contaminants that might be detrimental. Others feel incompetent, aware of their lack of expertise in theological matters. Still others are concerned about intruding into private areas, offending by their ignorance or difference, or imposing their own religious beliefs upon their patients. They may remember only too well personal memories or culturewide accounts of oppression in the name of religion—the coercing, silencing, censoring, and constraining operations by the more powerful upon the less. We, along with many therapists, are keenly aware of the myriad ways that institutionalized religions have been and are still used in the service of maintaining the status quo; consolidating power, centralizing wealth, perpetuating gender oppression, prescribing roles and rules, and punishing dissenters. Even spiritual practices that are not God-centered can be used for harm, encouraging escape from the world, detaching people from the realities in which they and those who need them live, and disabling processes that could lead to change.

For two decades, the two of us have interviewed individuals and their families in clinical settings: those seeking psychotherapy and those in the hospital who are medically or psychiatrically ill. Alongside the usual physical, psychological, and relational inquiries—not always, but when there seemed to be an opening—we have asked questions about how spirituality and religion mattered in their lives. Particularly when human relationships were absent, distant, or inaccessible, relationships with a personal God could provide a primary avenue for therapeutic change. This power was little different among those whose spirituality was grounded not in relationship with a transcendent, personified God, but in an immanent connectedness and attunement with the surrounding world and the beings in it.

This book will present ways we have developed for opening therapy to the creative and healing possibilities inherent in the spirituality of those who consult us, while countering ways in which it can destroy or cripple. First, though, we will each tell the aspects of our own stories that shaped and tinted the lens through which we see spirituality, community, and culture. We try always to stand alongside others, to see and learn from their vantage points, but this, too, is through our own vision, with its special acuities and blind spots. Just as our stories differ from each other and we can each see possibilities and pitfalls that the other cannot so easily see, we imagine that anyone reading this is bringing yet more differences, and can see and will hear what we cannot. We hope you will stop to consider your own story—which aspects are relevant to how you listen and speak and wonder about spirituality with those who bring their stories to you.

GRIFF'S STORY

I came from families of Mississippi dirt farmers who carved small farms out of virgin pine forests and swamplands. My mother had been the first in four generations of Mississippi forebears to attend a college. William Faulkner (1978, p. 87) wrote about my people: "Hill farmers—at once frail and work-worn, yet curiously imperishable—who seem to become old men at fifty and invincible to time." It is through his words that I now think about the Griffiths, Harveys, Greenes, and Hembys who enabled my birth: "The lowly and invincible of the earth—to endure and endure and then endure, tomorrow and tomorrow and tomorrow" (p. 104). One could not understand these farming families who lived so close to the earth without understanding the force of their religion. More than anything else, it was their faith that enabled endurance, that provided hope, if not for this life then for the one to come. I recognized the power of this faith and knew intuitively that it need be included within whatever medical or psychiatric treatment would be offered them, whether for a medical illness, depressed mood, or troubled marriage, if that treatment were to be worthwhile.

My childhood family and culture were so thoroughly Southern Baptist that anything not Baptist—the Presbyterians, the Methodists, certainly the Catholics—seemed peculiar and inappropriate. I knew no Jewish people and everything north of Memphis merged into the darkness of "The North" that was "New York." This of course made it impossible to distinguish the meaning of religion, because there was no background to distinguish it against. I sensed from an early age that I would spend my life among people—university academics, strangers from outside the South, a "godless people"—who would not know the faith or the culture from which I came. This turned out to be my fate in ways more complex than the stark dichotomies I knew from my childhood.

I was 30 years old when I entered psychiatric training in Boston. By this time I had completed training as a neurologist and had turned away from a career as a laboratory neurophysiologist. I slowly had realized that even a complete elucidation of the circuitry of the brain would still fail to answer the questions in which I was most interested: I wanted to deal with meaning and purpose in persons' lives, not just lengthen a life or rid it of disease. As I entered psychiatry and studied the different psychological theories of human behavior, I puzzled over what distinguished the physiological, psychological, and spiritual domains, and I wondered whether they were simply different ways of looking at the same thing. I was baffled in my efforts to understand pain—biologically, it was known to be trains of electrochemical impulses coursing up the spinal cord to the brain through C and A-delta nerve fibers. Psychologically, pain was understood in terms of its qualities—sharp, burning, aching, throbbing—as they appeared in conscious awareness. Spiritually, the language of pain was that of suffering, hope, endurance, and despair. I gradually realized that I had engaged in a quest for the Rosetta stone—a tool that could translate back and forth among the languages of biology, psychology, and spirituality, in order to grasp the whole that they were addressing. Speaking explicitly about the spiritual dimension, however, was not part of the psychiatric Zeitgeist. In 1986, when I wrote my first article about working in therapy with religious experience, I feared it would meet with such a hostile response that it might end my academic career.

As a psychiatrist and neurologist in the 1980s, I was working with patients who were medically ill and suffering from symptoms affecting moods, thoughts, or actions. These were often patients for whom survival entailed a deliberate choice to live: patients with head injuries, chronic pain, end-stage kidney disease, or metastatic cancer, whose lives contained too much pain and sorrow to take it for granted that life would be worth living. Questions that healthy people could ignore instead demanded immediate answers: What is the purpose of my life? To whom does it matter that I live? Who understands my experience? What can be hoped for? No treatment would move forward unless a way could be found to incorporate this spiritual dimension into the patient's care.

My patients and their families taught me the practical significance of spirituality and religion. Medical illnesses display the dirty laundry of religion. It is not just that an ill person's faith is challenged—Can he or she keep faith alive in the face of disease, pain, and disability?—but that the wisdom of following a religious tradition can become uncertain. There are many ill persons who find comfort, understanding, and meaning in their relationship with their God, but others feel abandoned by God, feel guilty for having become ill, or neglect their health by adhering to religious beliefs or practices. Clearly, religion can both heal and harm.

This dual face of religion was not a new discovery as I entered medicine. At an age before I could grasp the political arguments, I understood that the words "white Christian" stood for hatred in the tracts of paper scattered through my community by the Citizens Councils, Ku Klux Klan, and such groups. Simultaneously, I knew many white Christians who were warm, loving, accepting people. I noticed the latter did not feel a need to point out their skin color. A kerosene-drenched burning cross placed at a crossroad outside my town by Ku Klux Klansmen best captured this duality of loving acceptance/hateful exclusion that has plagued Christianity. I have never been able to idealize religion. I have always respected and sometimes feared its power to enact both good and evil.

Throughout much of my life I had been accustomed to distinguishing between *spirituality* as something generic, personal, and "of the heart" and *religion* as an outward expression in which one joined with others in the collective worship of God. As I talked with medically ill and psychiatrically ill people, however, differences between spirituality and religion became more blurred than distinct. What was affirmed as "spirituality" for one person would be similarly described as "religion" by another, and vice versa. Sometimes a person seemed to embrace the dichotomy mainly to support a political stance that rejected acts of oppression committed in the name of religious traditions while protecting a personal commitment to spirituality. Many people would use the words synonymously, or would regard traditional religious practices as the best method for entering the domain of spirituality. I felt muddled and labeled my computer disk with its notes on spirituality in psychotherapy, "Dark Forest," remembering my childhood spent wandering in the swamps of southern Mississippi. It seemed so easy for those who entered to lose their way.

Such a book as this invariably elicits certain questions: But what do *you* believe now? What do *you* believe is the truth about God? About spirituality? About religion? While I think I understand the press for answers to these questions, the questions themselves no longer make sense to me at the personal level that is requested. That is, I don't live my daily life under the underlying assumptions embedded in these questions about the existence of objective truths. I also object to a common cultural assumption in the United States that the best way to get to know another person's spirituality is ask about beliefs. An important reason we have written this book is to illuminate ways in which spirituality is expressed in addition to beliefs. However, I can respond to this query if I change the question to What do you experience as real about God, religion, and spirituality?

I had to confront this question midway through my psychiatry residency in Boston, when I was mired in such anguish that I could not see life beyond the pain. Some of this sorrow had to do with a dilemma in my life to which I had no answer. Much of it was due to a recognition that came through my personal psychotherapy that I did not know how to live beyond a sorrow that had always been in the background and seemed to flow in inexhaustible quantities. I became aware how all the protective structures in my life were not working, including the Christian faith and practices of my upbringing. Then one night, sinking in despair, it was as though my foot stepped on something solid. It was the realization that through all my years of formal religious practice—attending church, speaking the blessings at mealtime, working in a church-basement free health clinic—there always had existed in the shadows a separate, parallel track of spiritual experience that seemed formless, free, and flowing like a wild river. I did not understand what I had encountered but knew that I could trust it. I began sitting through Sunday church services at Old South Church on Copley Square, letting myself be bathed in this river, my mind empty of words, not hearing the sermon, feeling the reverberating sounds of the choir but unable to hear its music. For months these moments on Sunday morning at Old South were my only respite. I struggled through each week waiting impatiently for this time on Sunday morning when, however briefly, I could feel touched by this river, my pain quieted, replaced by moments of ecstasy in this Presence.

I could not then or now say more in words than what is said here about this time of my life. Slowly I became more robust. I learned ways to fill life with meaning, to find each day exciting and exuberant. My relationship with this river has become more of an ongoing dialogue, but still a conversation that never has known words. I have become reconciled to Wittgenstein's (1922, p. 189) admonition: "Whereof one cannot speak, thereof one must remain silent." In its silence, I listen, as this stream flows through conversations and relationships I have with other people. It is of course an irony that this book, so much focused on bringing spiritual experience into the language of psychotherapy should be written by one whose spirituality knows so few words.

MELISSA'S STORY

As compared to the life and legacy Griff describes in the Mississippi hill country, life in the Mississippi Delta was much gentler. At least it certainly seemed so in the neighborhood, church, and family into which I was born. Many years would pass before I would glimpse that harsher side of Delta life, and understand the labors by which the Delta came to gain its fame as the Birthplace of the Blues. As the third of three daughters, I grew up protected by my family and my community, and we, in turn, protected by our middle-class and white privileges. Many of our family friends, though not all, were part of our Methodist church. Most of the others were Protestant Christians, although my parents also had Jewish and Catholic friends. I think that everyone I knew went to church somewhere. I learned the subtleties of cordiality, what one should talk about with whom, by observing my parents with their friends. I recall my mother planning menus, serving no alcohol if our Baptist friends were coming, but having wine with dinner when the Episcopalian friends came. At first, I thought this was hypocrisy. In time, I understood it as thoughtful hospitality. Years later, as a therapist, when I first ventured into speaking with people about spiritual matters, I would sometimes wish I had the sensitivities in hosting those conversations that my mother had in serving her guests.

Church, more than anything to me, meant a caring community, people who gladly donated their time, cooking, and blood, when you were ill. It was a place for singing, sermons, and fellowship on Sunday mornings, and for quiet meditation on Sunday evenings. Religion and spirituality merged there for me, as it served as a center of open connectedness to God and others, a place where kids who were marginalized at school could come and be treated with respect. The wider view provided by time, distance, and inclusion of others' perspectives would reveal that our connectedness was not so open. Our church in many ways benefited from, and too rarely questioned, the segregated and unjust society of which it was a part. Paradoxically though, it simultaneously nourished an ethic in a few who would come to challenge and change the culture. Across our town, in the bosom of the churches of the African American community, the civil rights movement was being planned and prayed through. Then and now, I experience the church as an institution capable of both oppression and liberation.

The week that we were working on a final revision of this chapter,

Griff and I attended a *Kristallnacht* service, an annual tradition joining three congregations—Jewish, Roman Catholic, and Episcopal—who gather to commemorate the Night of the Broken Glass, November 9 and 10, 1938, when the Nazi regime made its first organized assault on the Jewish people in towns and cities throughout Germany. As I understand the story of the commemoration, it was begun by a beloved rabbi in Washington, DC, who invited his neighboring clergy to join their congregations in a recognition that this event affected us all. The site of the service rotates each year, and this year brought our Episcopal church the honor of hosting it. The packed sanctuary was silent as the survivors of the Holocaust led the procession, followed by the Jewish, then Catholic, then Episcopal clergy and choirs. After singing, passages were read from the Gospel—"Love your God with all your heart, all your might, and all your soul" and "Love your neighbor as yourself." Then, in a gentle clear voice, Mrs. Regina Spiegel told us how it had been for her family in the time of *Kristallnacht*. She had been 13 years old when it all began. Before the Holocaust ended, her mother, father, three sisters, a nephew, and a brother had perished in the death camp Treblinka. She herself had done slave labor, imprisoned in both Bergen-Belsen and Auschwitz. Of all she and her family had endured, she said, "The hardest thing was that our neighbors turned on us. If we had only had neighbors like you, whose churches exhort you to care and speak up for your neighbors, these terrible things could not have happened." Her words remain with me, prompting a hope and a question. How I hope Mrs. Spiegel is right, but I wonder, would we choose to know? To act? To love our neighbors as ourselves? Are we choosing that now?

All the major religious traditions, and many of the newer spiritualities, urge their followers to compassion and justice. If our religion serves only to bind us to those who are similar, and does not open our eyes and ears and hearts to those who are different, it does harm to us and to others. If our private spirituality does not lead us in public to be the neighbors Mrs. Spiegel could count on, of what use is it? So, when I converse with someone in therapy about his or her spiritual practices, when I inquire about their religious community, beliefs, or personal God, it is with the hope of fostering that which connects the person to hope and justice, to loved ones and to neighbors yet unknown.

That spiritual convictions do not always lead to greater connection but sometimes to greater alienation was first made real to me one college summer when I worked as a nurse's aide. Rather helplessly, but with intense curiosity, I watched the difference in the suffering between two patients in pain: the first, a withdrawn, lonely man, 30 years old, with multiple fractures from an automobile accident, the second, a friendly 11-year-old boy, in sickle cell anemia crisis. As the man told his story, his God was inflicting pain, punishing him for his reckless driving, forcing him live on to pay with his own pain for those who had died in the crash. He accepted God's harsh sentence by refusing visitors, pain medication, skin care, and even most of the food I brought. His wounds were ulcerating and he was starving. In contrast, the boy's God was a great comfort. His extended family was ever present and pulled him through the frightening crises with laying on of hands and passionate prayer. He believed God wanted to heal him, and that we, the nursing staff, were God's helpers.

I was worried about the man and talked to the head nurse. She told me it wasn't my business to talk with patients about those matters. It was for the chaplain. "But he refuses to see the chaplain, and he talks to me," I persisted. "Nonetheless, it's not our place to talk about it. We don't know why any of these patients are suffering," she explained. "Anyway, maybe that man is right." It was the end of the spoken conversation, but my mind kept on. What if the boy were to believe as did the man, that his pain was God's punishment? What if the nurses were to believe that?

I don't recall that I ever did talk to that poor man, but his suffering stayed with me, as did the question, Was it my business to talk with him? I agree with the head nurse that a chaplain consultation might have been ideal. Often clergypersons, spiritual companions, and pastoral counselors can speak with an understanding, a knowledge, and occasionally an authority that is unique to their expertise and helpful beyond measure. But this man would not speak to the chaplain. He was speaking to me. As nurses, social workers, family therapists, physicians, psychologists, compassionate friends, even as a young nurse's aide, if a story of spirituality is inflicting or alleviating suffering, if the other wants to talk with us, shouldn't it become the business of our conversation? When it does become the business of our conversation, when we are invited in, how can we creatively and usefully respond, knowing we do not have expertise in spirituality and religion? These are the questions that prod us.

Each of our stories gives reasons for our interest in opening therapy to spiritual stories, but we find these questions to be important to others as well, not necessarily because spirituality and religion are central to their own lives or cultures, but because they want to honor what is important to those who entrust their stories to them. Several of our close therapist colleagues were either not raised in religious contexts or have a spiritual or religious framework quite different from most of the people who come to them for therapy, yet they desire to respond respectfully, carefully, and creatively when people speak about their spiritual lives. These colleagues tell us that they do not know how to talk about these things, even as we imagine that their not-knowing could be an asset that we can only approximate. Surely our personal stories open doors, but they close doors, too.

RELIGION AND SPIRITUALITY: A CLOUD OF CONFUSION

So far, we have been coupling the words *religion* and *spirituality* as though they were interchangeable. These words are commingled by many people, with religion providing a safe and open structure within which a vital spirituality can flourish. For others, however, the two words stand against one another. Some who value such spiritual practices as meditation or ritual deny that religious practices are legitimate, at least in organized forms as they exist among mosques, synagogues, temples, and churches. They consider religion to be irrelevant, rigidly oppressive, destructive, or just boring. Likewise, some religious persons consider spirituality that is practiced outside a religious context to be self-indulgent and not accountable to the larger community. Few domains of human life are more covered by a cloud of confusion, ambiguity, and mystification than those of religion and spirituality. Books intended to make understandable their universal truths are often written using abstract words that are meaningful only to a limited circle of believers. Persons who have had powerful personal experiences often seem to feel certain that their idiosyncratic experiences ought to be the model for every other person. Others who see the divisive, destructive power of religion determine that atheism is the most ethical stance they can take, that allegiance to no sect is the way to peace. One can feel the pull of this conclusion reading George Klein's (1990) monograph *The Atheist and the Holy City*. As Klein despairingly looks over Jerusalem:

> The three great religions and their hundreds of often bitterly antagonistic sects, branches, and factions exist within a few yards of one another, but

yet they have no channels of communication. Most of them exist as if in watertight compartments, separating like oil from water.

Only a few yards above the crowd in the bazaar, the swarthy Coptic monks sit like hermits in their garret atop the Church of the Holy Sepulchre. Their isolation is reminiscent of the caves in the desert. The ultra-orthodox Jewish *haradim* are also locked in, but in a very different inner world of their own, so dominated by their eternal dispute with their God. They reject and despise the godless state, the secularized world of sin.

The houses of the Moslems are fenced in and shut, turning their backs on the unfaithful. The Armenian quarter is closed to all strangers. Even those who belong are locked in or locked out after 6 o'clock every evening, and no one can enter or leave without permission of the archbishop.

As soon as the first evening star appears each Friday night, the Jewish prayers begin at the Wailing Wall. At the same time one can year the recorded voices of the muezzins coming from awkward-looking loudspeakers atop the graceful minarets. "*Allah akhbar.*" The voices fly past one another. Words with identical meanings, wanting nothing to do with one another— they are light-years apart. (p. 200)

The spiritual domain is like a parliament with dozens of political parties represented, none of which uses a shared language in its debates while advocating with passion its own worldview. Spirituality and religion are so afflicted with such a confusion of tongues that clarity about the language used is necessary before work can be accomplished.

CLARIFYING OUR LANGUAGE

We have sought to develop methods for conducting psychotherapy to allow therapists to tap into whatever spiritual resources a person might bring, even when they do not understand or embrace that spiritual tradition. We have tried to develop a clinical approach broad enough that it could be used by those coming from traditions very different from our own. The perspectives on spirituality and religion that we have adopted are ones that facilitate this objective, so we want to be clear how we are defining the terms we use.

We offer a simple, practical definition of spirituality: *Spirituality* is a commitment to choose, as the primary context for understanding and acting, one's relatedness with all that is. With this commitment, one attempts to stay focused on relationships between oneself and other people, the physical environment, one's heritage and traditions, one's body, one's ancestors, saints, Higher Power, or God. It places relationships at the center of awareness, whether they be interpersonal relationships with the world or other people, or intrapersonal relationships with God or other nonmaterial beings. In this sense, the spiritual domain can then be contrasted with the psychological domain (organized by choosing personhood—a whole self with intentions, choices, plans, desires, and behaviors—as the context for understanding and acting) and the physiological domain (organized by choosing relationships among elements of the body—muscles, bones, hormones, neurons, and neurotransmitters—as the context for understanding and acting).

We value this perspective for the possibilities it opens in our therapies. An emphasis on relatedness is a prominent feature of nearly every spirituality we have examined. A definition of spirituality centered on relatedness thus has wide applicability in clinical settings. It provides a position from which a therapist can start addressing particularities of a spirituality as it has taken form in the life of a specific individual or within the breadth of a culture.

A definition of spirituality in terms of relationship also anticipates the clinical methods of our therapies. It fits collaborative therapies that focus on language and culture, which we illustrate in subsequent chapters. Although we acknowledge that this definition does not capture unique aspects of many spiritual or religious traditions, we use it because it positions us well to listen and to act effectively when people tell us about their lives, regardless what tradition they represent.

This perspective on spirituality is organized around a core metaphor of *attunement*. Just as a flying bird constantly attunes its wings to the air currents, responding to up- and downdrafts and changes in wind direction or velocity, so a person continuously responds to the flux in important relationships. By maintaining a posture of active, continuous responsivity and movement, the fundamental relationship can remain constant. A commitment to living within a spiritual domain means vigilance for lapses in any of these relationships and reattuning them through processes of reconciliation.

Our working definition of spirituality is closely aligned with one used by our New Zealand colleagues at The Family Centre in Lower Hutte. Working at the confluence of Maori, Samoan, and European cultures, The Family Centre organizes both its therapies for clients and families and its work in community development around an understanding of spirituality: "Spirituality for us is not centered around organised religion, but on the essential quality of relationships, and refers to the relationship between people and their environment, people and other people,people and their heritage, and people and the numinous" (*Dulwich Centre Newsletter*, 1990, No. 1, p. 7).

DISTINGUISHING SPIRITUALITY FROM RELIGION

This perspective on spirituality emphasizes what is generalizable across different cultures. When spirituality is enacted within a particular culture, however, the language, practices, and customs that evolve take on unique forms. Traditions then develop as religions that sustain these forms of language, practices, and customs from one generation to the next.

Religion represents a cultural codification of important spiritual metaphors, narratives, beliefs, rituals, social practices, and forms of community among a particular people that provides methods for attaining spirituality, most often expressed in terms of a relationship with the God of that religion. In this sense, God personifies and objectifies the relatedness of spirituality. By working out a relationship with his or her God, a religious person can bring into proper focus other relationships.

In case illustrations in the following chapters, we have tried to remain consistent with these definitions, referring to spirituality when talking about a person living within a context of relationships, and to religion when talking about specific cultural forms. Some persons embrace New Age spirituality and its selflessness, while decrying traditional religious ideas. Others live daily lives of passionate engagement between a quite solid self and the God of Christianity, Judaism, or Islam. Our mission is not to debate truths about either selves or Gods, but to establish a therapeutic conversation wherein a person can bring into the therapy whatever for that person is real.

RELIGION AND SPIRITUALITY:
ENABLER OR CONSTRAINT?

As William James (1994, p. 363) once pointed out: "The gods we stand by are the gods we need and can use." It ought to be the case that one's religion would be a reliable path to a spiritual life; this is no doubt what nearly all believers intend when they enter into religious practices. In the real world, this is sometimes the case and sometimes not. Under anomalous circumstances, religious practices can become actively antispiritual. Some clinical problems arise when religious stories, communities, and practices violate connectedness, hindering instead of helping a person to attain spirituality. Examples range from religious arguments advocating racism, abuse of women and children justified by scriptures from the Bible or the Qur'an, or Pol Pot's claiming Buddhist compassion by hurrying his victims in the killing fields through the cycle of reincarnation into a better life.

Spirituality loosed from a container of religious tradition also can do harm. Comparative religions scholar Huston Smith (2000) proposes that spirituality needs "the traction of religious tradition" to keep it accountable to a community. Otherwise, spirituality risks becoming a self-centered quest for personal growth. Smith has noted that practitioners of the eclectic new spiritualities often pick and choose beliefs and practices among Buddhism, Christianity, Judaism, Hinduism, Islam, and other traditions. However, he fears that this avoidance of commitment to any single tradition means that the person simply chooses what is easy and avoids what is hard, to the detriment of disciplined spiritual maturity.

How does a clinician respond when a person claims that a direct communication from his God warrants placing self or others at risk for harm? How does one work with a person in psychotherapy whose religious convictions advocate hatred or violence toward others? How does one converse with a person about religious practices that are coercive and controlling? How does one respond in psychotherapy to a person when it is apparent that her religious zeal is alienating important people in her life, contrary to her expectations? In Chapter 9, "When Spirituality Turns Destructive," we discuss dealing with these dilemmas in therapy.

THE INSIDE AND OUTSIDE PERSPECTIVES

As psychotherapists, we consider our value to the persons who consult us to lie in our asking questions from the outside, from the position of the stranger. The role of the curious stranger who can conduct a dialogue from a not-knowing position can be a unique and valuable one. This is a role that any therapist can fill, whether or not he or she belongs to a religious tradition or is knowledgeable about the various forms of spirituality and religion. Indeed, we specifically intend this book to serve as an aid for those who conduct their clinical work outside the domain of a particular religion.

Other professionals—pastors, priests, rabbis, chaplains, pastoral counselors, and spiritual companions or directors—make unique contributions by addressing these issues, but do so from a different vantage point. These counselors often share with their clients a joint accountability to a particular spiritual tradition. Some clergypersons can speak as authorities on sacred scriptures or as a representative of God. Counselors who identify themselves as representing a particular spiritual tradition may be sought out because they can speak from within the wisdom of that tradition in addressing problems. The pastoral counseling literature doubtless addresses the issues we grapple with in this book, but from a vantage point inside the theological world. We come to these issues from the position of strangers, no more theologically or spiritually equipped than anyone else who strives to be aware of his or her own stories and to listen carefully to others. We come with apologies if insiders feel insulted by our restating the obvious, but with hope of offering newness to other outsider therapists who yearn to be respectful, curious, and inclusive of the experiences of those persons who seek their aid.

Both the inside-spiritual tradition and outside-spiritual tradition perspectives can potentially help individuals as they respond to life's dilemmas. The two of us have often referred people to a pastoral counselor, spiritual director, or cleric when that expertise seemed a better fit with a person's needs than what we could offer. Some have accepted and profited from these referrals and others have declined, electing to do psychotherapy with an outsider. Both perspectives have their places.

This distinction is reflected to some extent in the ways people select professional assistance with their problems. Although we strive to open psychotherapy to the spiritual resources persons bring, neither of us has ever had someone present requesting help with a spiritual crisis as the stated problem. Rather, spirituality enters the therapeutic dialogue as one perspective among others that have utility in resolving relationship problems, treating psychiatric symptoms, and coping with medical illnesses. In perhaps half of our therapies, discussion about "spiritual issues" does not enter the dialogue of therapy, not because the people who consult us lack this dimension in their lives but because they do not initiate or respond to our openings by indicating that this is how they wish to spend our time together. Counselors representing different spiritual traditions work with a wide range of clinical problems, but may be specifically sought out by those who view their problems as spiritual crises. Pastoral counselors we know personally are exquisitely sensitive psychotherapists, especially in relation to the oppression of religion and how it can constrain therapy conversations as well as lives.

HOW THE CHAPTERS
OF THIS BOOK ARE ORGANIZED

We turned to cultural anthropology in our search for a conceptual framework that could embrace different religions and forms of spiritual experience. Years ago, anthropologist Victor Turner (1982) became fascinated with the uses that different cultures made of various forms of symbolic expression, terming this fascination "comparative symbology." Similarly, we have organized this text by discussing idiom, trope (metaphor), story (narrative), belief, dialogue, ritual and ceremony, spiritual practice, and community as different genres of symbolic expression in Chapters 3 through 8. Through these genres, spiritual experience enters language and is enacted in personal relationships and the organization of society. The genres that we have selected are those we believed would be most commonly employed in individual and family therapies.

We chose this organizational scheme for three reasons. First, it provides a systematic method for listening that counters cultural bias. For example, beliefs are viewed by many in the United States as the most important aspect of religious life, perhaps due to the widespread influence of Protestant Christianity in the culture. There often is less inquiry about the role that ritual or community may play. Presumably, the opposite bias might occur in another culture where the dominant forms of religion or spirituality are organized around rituals, to the neglect of beliefs. Making an effort to listen even-handedly for a half dozen different expressive forms—an activity we discuss in Chapters 3 and 10 as *multichannel listening*—can correct a prejudice toward the genres to which a therapist has been most accustomed.

Second, therapists' clinical skills are organized by expressive genres. A therapist works with a metaphor differently than with a story in therapy, and with a story differently than with a belief or ritual or community. Ericksonian hypnotists emphasize work with metaphors, narrative therapists with stories, and cognitive-behavioral therapists with beliefs, although each therapeutic approach usually utilizes several different expressive genres at some point in a therapy. Thinking about spirituality in terms of the symbolic forms through which it is expressed can help psychotherapists better appreciate what they may have to offer a person struggling with a dilemma of spirituality.

Finally, focusing upon the symbolic form of expression provides a method for avoiding too rigid a dichotomy between religion and spirituality. Although spirituality and religion are not synonymous, the division between them is not nearly so clean as the prospirituality/antireligion position in recent cultural politics often presents it. Focusing upon their expressive forms offers a common vocabulary for both spirituality and religion as they are present in daily life.

The following examples illustrate different expressive genres:

• *Metaphor that mediates a relationship with God or the numinous.* A 40-year-old psychologist described his recovery from alcoholism and his personal journey from farmer to addiction counselor. From childhood through early adulthood, he felt God was "the scorekeeper" who scrutinized his every move. After a transformative religious experience, his dominant metaphor for God had become that of a kind grandfather saying, "It's going to be okay." He described vividly how he experienced God's presence as "the scorekeeper" as different from God's presence as "the kind grandfather."

• *Religious rituals.* A 30-year-old diabetic woman was in panic from dread of being placed in an enclosed hyperbaric oxygen chamber to treat an infection in her leg. She told how she had received these treatments before, but the members of her church always would come to the hospital, lay their hands upon her, and pray over her. On this hospital admission, she had been admitted hurriedly from the emergency room, and there had been no time to gather the church members.

• *Spiritual practices as methods for attuning one's embodied being to open to spiritual experience.* A young woman practiced yoga and meditation daily in order to sustain a sense of hope and wonder during the moments of her daily life. Any sense of separateness from the universe around her would disappear during meditation. Later, while experiencing the fragmenting loss of her love relationship, these meditative practices provided as much coherence in her life as did her psychotherapy.

• *Community, constituted by the relationships among those adhering to particular religious beliefs or practices.* A 60-year-old man became severely depressed after suffering a mild stroke. He told how he continued to read his Bible, to pray, and to experience God's presence as close at hand, but he was no longer able to go to church on Sunday. As a church elder, he had for decades greeted visitors and passed the offering plate each Sunday. The members of his church were in a real sense his family, but his stroke had cut him off from their presence.

• *Religious beliefs.* To a remarkable extent, a 50-year-old man with advanced cardiovascular disease was ignoring his cardiologist's recommendations for diet, smoking, and exercise. "What I believe is that God is so powerful and we are so weak, that if God wants to save me, nothing I am doing is going to get in his way. If he doesn't want to save me, nothing I do is going to make a difference." His conviction about God's control over his destiny dominated his interactions with his doctors and the health care system.

In daily life, these different genres can each contribute to a coherent sense of religious and spiritual experience, some more than others, depending on the person, the culture, and what circumstances hold sway. For a particular clinical problem, one genre more than the others may hold crucial possibilities for resolution of the problem. Each one offers a different set of healing possibilities that can be accessed in therapy. Chapters 3–8 discuss in turn the specific therapeutic options that each expressive genre provides.

FOUR PERSPECTIVES THAT EXPAND OUR UNDERSTANDING OF SPIRITUALITY

The reader primarily interested in clinical work may wish to begin Chapter 2 at this point. Others interested in its concepts may want to examine further how this work has been influenced by ideas elaborated in related fields of study. These perspectives expand an understanding of spirituality and its contributions to clinical work. Here we provide an introductory discussion for each of these perspectives to anchor understanding of them, as they reappear regularly in subsequent chapters.

I–Thou Relationships

Martin Buber's (1958) distinction of I–Thou relations remains perhaps the best articulated understanding of the quality of relationship that fills the life of a person committed to spirituality. Buber distinguished I–Thou and I–It relationships as the "primary words" of human experience. As he noted, "Primary words do not signify things, but they intimate relations" (p. 3). Relationships between self and God, self and others, self and the environment, self and one's heritage, and self and body are in each case I–Thou relationships for a person living a life of spiritual commitment. Psychotherapy, when working within a spiritual domain, becomes a task of mapping which regions of one's relationship ecology are marked by decay from I–Thou into I–It relations. This map sets the direction for the therapy.

This perspective suggests that we think about the knowledge and skills needed to detect this decay and to restore I–Thou relationships. These are skills necessary for discerning, attuning, and acting in response to relationship events. The social poetics of John Shotter and Arlene Katz (1996, p. 216) describe them as a "practical grasp of the changing, moment-by-moment links and relations between such events and their surroundings as they unfold." Dostoyevsky (1990, p. 27) describes Father Zossima in *Brothers Karamazov*: "Many said of the elder Zossima that, having for so many years received all those who came to him to open their hearts, thirsting for advice and for a healing word, having taken into his soul so many confessions, sorrows, confidences, he acquired in the end such fine discernment that he could tell, from the first glance at a visiting stranger's face, what was in his mind, what he needed, and even what kind of suffering tormented his conscience."

Communitas and Spirituality

The relational focus of our definition of spirituality is closely akin to a social process described as *communitas* by Turner (1969, 1974, 1982). Communitas is the spirit of unity that pervades those who participate together in the performance of a ritual, the journeying together on a pilgrimage, or the solidarity of a political movement. Each participant regards the other as whole person relating to whole person. There is a strong sense of interconnectedness, not only among members of that group but often among all humankind. The dominant emotion is that of love and acceptance of the other: "When even two people believe that they experience unity, all people are felt by those two, even if only for a flash, to be one" (Turner, 1982, p. 47). The notion that there is a generic bond between men, and its related sentiment of 'humankindness,' are not epiphenomena of some kind of herd instinct but are products of 'men in their wholeness wholly attending' " (Turner, 1969, p. 128).

When communitas is strong, social structure in terms of boundaries and hierarchy disappears. Among members of the group, social distinctions regarding power, wealth, and social position are dropped. There is a powerful awareness of the bonds that connect rather than differences that separate. As Turner (1974, p. 151) noted: "These individuals are not segmentalized into roles and statuses but confront one another rather in the manner of Martin Buber's 'I and Thou.' Along with this direct, immediate, and total confrontation of human identities, there tends to go a model of society as a homogenous, unstructured communitas, whose boundaries are ideally coterminous with those of the human species."

This anthropological perspective on communitas extends our definition of spirituality by associating it solidly with the creative processes of a society. Communitas exists in the subjunctive mood of possibilities for the future. In secular settings it appears in such examples as the enthusiasm and frenzy of a political convention, the interplay of ideas among a team of research scientists, or the cross-fertilization of themes among a school of artists. In religious settings, it appears in such examples as the "oneness of spirit" among those participating in a ritual, the prophesying and listening to testimonies during a religious revival, the sharing of stories among pilgrims journeying to a shrine, or the solidarity of a moral crusade against child labor, abuse of women, or some other cause. In each, there is a free exchange and rapid turnover of ideas and images as serious questions are considered—what is real or important or useful to pursue. Old assumptions are challenged and new ones freely examined. In every culture, communitas in its different manifestations supplies a potent force for creative change, generating fresh metaphors and symbols that later are formalized within the structure of society as its cultural values.

Liminality

Liminality is a region of human experience located between subjective and objective descriptions of reality and outside the purview of routinized daily life (Turner, 1969, 1982). Liminal experience—like that found in art, play, and religion—is creative, fluid, and cannot be grasped by the logic and categories of everyday life. It can be understood only through evocative symbols. Psychoanalyst D. W. Winnicott (1975), focusing more on the individual's experience than the social processes involved, talked about liminality in terms of "transitional space," as a domain of experience that bridges the internal, subjective world of an individual with reality as it is experienced by the external, objective community.

The sacred is a form of liminal experience (Turner, 1969). The sacred refers to that which evokes reverence and awe due to its associations to spiritual or religious experience. A place, such as Mt. Sinai, can be sacred, as can totems, icons, or passages of music. Commonly, the authoritative writings of a religion, such as the Bible, Torah, or Qur'an, are regarded as sacred by believers. Events considered sacred always contain elements that the person experiences as real but that cannot be witnessed by others. In the 1963 movie *The Cardinal*, for example, Catholic believers bowed and worshipped before stains appearing on a wet wall. The believers saw the miraculous appearance of Jesus' blood where a watching nonbeliever could only see rust stains from the water. Encounters with the sacred are an important component of spiritual life, but spirituality usually covers a broader territory, including, for many people, not just the sacred but all of life, even its most profane parts.

Emotional Postures

In the 1980s, our encounters with Chilean neurobiologist Humberto Maturana presented a fresh perspective that became central in our clinical work. Maturana spoke about human emotion as a biologist, in that he did not emphasize the feelings accompanying emotions but highlighted instead the role of emotion in readying a person's physiological state to do or to express something. For Maturana, emotion was a bodily disposition for action. This understanding was strikingly different from the perspective that had dominated American psychiatry, in which emotions and feelings were regarded more or less as the same thing, with both referring primarily to subjective mental states.

Using Maturana's perspective, the two of us began interviewing clients and patients about their physical experience of their bodies— instead of asking about their feelings—when inquiring about states of emotion. This inquiry opened conversations that linked bodily symptoms to present and past relationship problems with family members, friends, coworkers and bosses, and others in the broader culture. From this vantage point it became easier to understand how the process of utilizing feelings to monitor emotional states can lose calibration, leaving a person unable to detect connections between relationships and the symptoms affecting their bodies.

Such conversations about *emotional postures* became a key element in therapies for somatoform symptoms, which we described in our previous book, *The Body Speaks* (Griffith & Griffith, 1994). An emotional posture refers to the readying of the body's physiological systems for a particular path of action. That is, an emotional posture of anger is a readiness to attack; an emotional posture of fear is a readiness to flee; an emotional posture of shame is a readiness to hide. Emotions are about doing. Feelings are a secondary process about monitoring and following one's emotion.

Thinking in terms of emotional postures has provided a useful way to understand how spiritual experience is related to the body's physiology, so often a concern for medically ill individuals seeking healing through spiritual practices. At the bedside of a patient with cancer, I (Griff) may ask: "What are you experiencing in your body? What are the sensations? Where? If you were to think about this state of your body as getting ready to do something or to express something, what would that be? When you pray or meditate, how does this state of your body change? If you experience God's presence as near, rather than far away, how does this state of your body change?" We describe in Chapter 10 a set of emotional postures, termed *existential crisis states*, that exacerbate or speed the progression of some medical and psychiatric disorders. Our work with spiritual experience in the lives of medically ill patients is in large part an effort to counter these states of vulnerability (Griffith, 2000, 2001).

THE GENERATIVE POWER OF WONDER

How can a clinician open therapy to spiritual and religious resources that a person might bring if the therapist shares no common tradition of religious beliefs or practices with the person? Our best clinical outcomes have occurred when we have been able to stay in the position of an anthropologist meeting another person from an unknown culture. We have been least successful when we felt that a prior understanding, whether from religious studies or personal experience, had given us a head start in comprehending the person with whom we were speaking because we could anticipate what to expect. The skills most helpful for opening therapy to the spiritual and religious domains have been those for preparing our own selves to meet someone not yet known—the fostering within ourselves of curiosity, wonder, and openness to the being of the other.

The good news that this brings is its dispensing with notions that special "religious expertise" is needed in order to be of help. We discuss in Chapter 2 specific methods that have aided our efforts to remain within a posture of not-knowing and noncertainty when encountering the spiritual experiences of others.

Chapter Two

Opening the Door

I (Melissa) had not seen Susan for about a month. She had been out of town on a long-needed vacation, visiting in the southern coastal town in which she had spent the happiest times in her childhood. Her other, earlier family home had been in an apartment in a midwestern city with her mother. Their life together had been beset by her mother's severe mental illness, sporadic disappearances, and male visitors who were sometimes abusive to Susan and to her mother.

In our first session Susan told me about the night she changed homes. She was 10 years old:

"Mother had been gone for days and I couldn't find her anywhere. I was later to learn that she was in the hospital, but in no state of mind to be thinking of me. I had cooked up all the food in the house and I waited and waited for her to come home. Finally I went down to the landlady's apartment. She called my brother, John. I told him how scared I was. I can remember his voice on the phone. He said, 'Stay there with the landlady, I'm coming to get you right now.' He took the train from Chicago and arrived that night. Mother still wasn't home. We packed up my stuff and he took me back to Chicago to the seminary student apartment he shared with his wife, Bethany. I stayed with them till my dad and stepmother could come get me and take me to the coast to live with them. I knew my father had always wanted me to be with him, but I had to be with my mother because of the custody arrangements. That night though, when I called John, he said he didn't give a flip about the rules. He said he was coming and that I would never be left alone again. In the end, John took care not only of me, but of our mother, too."

The home of Susan's father and stepmother was safe, strict, and sober. The structure was a haven to Susan, and the restrictions were made more tolerable through her connection with her brother, who, though miles away, kept contact through comforting telephone calls. Susan came to love the church that was the center of their family life. John became a minister in this denomination, one who was known throughout the diocese for his tolerance, openness, and defense of the outcast. He pastored several churches and settled in a church on the coast. He and Susan continued to have a close relationship that sustained both through the deaths of their father and stepmother. In recent years posttraumatic symptoms had brought Susan to terms with the sexual abuse she had suffered years before at the hands of the men who had come to her mother's apartment. She turned again to John and Bethany and found validation and support. "John felt so guilty for not having come for me earlier, but he was so young. How could he have known? I told him I always thought he was my savior. What in the world would have happened to me if he hadn't helped me? We spoke often during that last year and I believe he knew how grateful I was to him."

That last year had ended abruptly one Sunday morning as John was standing in front of his congregation. He reached for his chest and fell forwards. His heart attack was so severe that he died before the ambulance reached the church. Within 2 years of John's death, Susan's mother died. Now Susan was the only remaining living member of her original family.

She had traveled to the coast to spend time with Bethany and to visit John's old church, but instead of feeling comforted in the church she was even more aware of her aloneness. The intensity of her sadness took her aback. She could barely maintain her composure during the service when the speaker introduced her to the congregation as John's sister. The minute the service concluded, Susan rushed out to the courtyard, to the small memorial garden dedicated to her brother, but she found no peace there.

"Then," she said, "I knew clearly where I needed to go. I got in my car and drove to the beach where John and I used to walk and talk. It was just what I needed. When I knew I had done what I needed to do, I went home."

"What was it that was there that you so clearly knew you needed to do?" I inquired.

"That stretch of beach had been our place. . . . " Susan waited.

"Did you sense your brother's presence there?" I asked her.

"Yes, I had hoped to and I did. I was walking along the beach and all of a sudden I glanced down and saw this white shell. The inner part of it was gleaming in the sun—I know this sounds weird. . . . " She paused and looked at me. I was quiet. "You see, John had always worn only white robes since he had come to the church on the coast and, when I saw that shell, I immediately felt he was there with me."

"Did he have any words for you, or was he with you quietly?" I wondered.

"Not exactly words but there was a clear message. It came through in the way he was with me. The message was 'You can do this, Susan.' "

"You can do this," I repeated.

"Yes, that's all, but that was enough." Her voice was low and clear. "He knows how sad I have been and how hard all this loss has been for me. I guess he knows that sometimes I wonder if I can do this. But I am stronger now. It was good, calming, to know that he believes I can do it."

I wrote down the words as I checked with her, "Shall I write this? It sounds important to remember."

She nodded. "Yes, I want to always remember it. I think that's why I went there."

OPENING THE CONVERSATION

Conversations like this one with Susan are what I recollect when I try to respond to the set of questions that workshop participants pose to us the most often: "How do you bring up spirituality?" "Why doesn't this come up more in my therapies?" "What are the questions you ask?" While there are questions we can (and will) offer later in this chapter that convey a readiness to discuss spirituality, more often it seems to arise naturally in the story a person is telling, as with Susan. Still, a conversation can take many paths. What seems to "arise naturally" as an inviting path to me may not be noticed by another therapist or, to yet a third, it may seem a distracting detour to be avoided.

From behind the one-way mirror, we have observed superb and helpful interviews by experienced, thoughtful therapists who did not choose to follow, as we might have, clients' statements that seemed to us to be invitations to discuss the role of spirituality in their lives. "Only God can help me now" or "I know I could be well if could get back to meditating," the client would say, but the therapist would ask a question to go in another, possibly even more useful, but definitely different direction. What determines which therapists find these paths inviting and which do not? Peter Kahle's (1997) research might provide some answers. He surveyed 151 therapists about their willingness to integrate spiritual issues in psychotherapy. He wanted to learn who would be comfortable talking about spirituality, what words they would use, what circumstances would be necessary, and what factors would influence the willingness to discuss this matter. He reported that the overwhelming majority of therapists (98%) said they would be willing to talk about spirituality and God if the client introduced the topic; this number shrunk when he asked if the therapist would be willing to introduce the topic of spirituality (60%) or of God (42%) (p. 100). The question remains: Who hears clients' comments as introductions to the topic and who does not? This is a complex question to research because one cannot report not hearing. However, if we assume that the influences that guide our willingness to respond have some commonality with those that guide our readiness to hear, Kahle's study may yet provide some clues. When he asked where respondents had received messages that discouraged discussion of God in therapy, over half cited professional education, training, and worksites (p. 147), but when asked where messages came from that encouraged this discussion, clients and patients were most frequently cited. Notions that dissuaded therapists from discussing spirituality included concerns about imposing their belief systems on their clients, convictions that reliance on God was disempowering of people, and a fear that religious differences between client and therapist could put a barrier between them. We would want to respect all these concerns, but we hold that there are good guards against them: careful curiosity as to the clients' experience and its meaning for them, inquiry as to their preferences, and belief that there are always multiple, alternative stories.

Therapists, too, can be dominated by a single story of what a conversation about spirituality could mean. One of Kahle's (1997, p. 166) respondents described why one should not speak of spirituality in therapy with these words: "My task is to comfort the wounded, not to convert them." This leads us back to the conversation with Susan, for it seemed that to comfort her meant precisely to talk about her spiritual experiences. So how was it that this comforting pathway was the one taken?

I have tried to examine my own participation in this specific conversation with Susan. Three aspects stand out:

- Noticing and inquiring about the specific words she spoke.
- Noticing shifts in emotion as she told the story and inquiring about memories and experiences associated with these shifts.
- Asking questions guided by commonly told stories from the religious culture to which I assumed Susan belonged.

In attending to Susan's words, I heard her say that she knew exactly where she needed to go. These two words "knew" and "needed" were spoken with conviction. "Needed" was repeated three times, culminating in her "knowing" she had received what she "needed," so I asked more about this knowledge.

As for shifts in emotion, I heard her speak her longing for her brother, her disappointment about the loneliness at church and even in the memorial garden, where she had hoped to find solace. Then the tale shifted from desperate searching to clear direction. The question, "Did you sense your brother's presence on the beach?" opened the door to Susan's telling of her healing spiritual experience.

Finally, familiarity with cultural stories may have led me to ask about her finding her brother's presence and receiving a message from him. I guessed that Susan held a belief that though her brother had died, he lived not only in her heart, but in eternity, and that she yearned to have assurance, a word, a sign from this one who had promised her so many years ago that she would never be alone. Fortunately, in this conversation my assumptions about our shared cultural and spiritual stories fit well and extended Susan's speaking. However, my reliance on this familiarity was more unintentional than planned. In contrast to the reliability of attending to language and shifts in emotion, presumed familiarity with cultural stories can actually mislead. One can be off the mark. She might have said to me, as another person once did, "It is blas-

phemous and nonscriptural to consider that the spirits of the dead communicate with this world," jolting the focus from personal experience to
theological doctrines. Even if assumptions about a person's background
are accurate, the person may feel ashamed if his or her actual experience
does not meet the expectations of a certain religious group. Therefore,
knowing that these slips will occur, the best we can do is to listen, to remain tentative, to attempt to ask more often than to suggest, and to
show appreciation and interest when corrected.

These are some of the ways to remain hospitable to spiritual stories.
Beyond my attending to her language, noticing shifts, and suspending familiarity of cultural stories, beyond even the well-timed question to open
the door to her spiritual experience, Susan had to know that she was
bringing this experience to a space in which it would be welcome in order to enter fully the conversation. For several years this question has
held our interest: How can we cultivate the kind of hospitality that will
welcome all stories, whether illogical and contradictory, unspeakable, in
opposition to the dominant culture, or in that self-conscious category
Susan named through her pause and her phrase—"I know this sounds
weird."

Her pause, tentative checking glance, and warning of weirdness echoed another warning, an ancient admonition. "Do not throw your pearls
before swine, lest they trample them underfoot and turn to attack you"
(Matthew 7:6, Revised Standard Version [RSV]). These words I learned
as a child. But offered to me now are the stories of others, pearls born of
irritants and, through arduous labor, made smooth and beautiful. These
pearls are deserving of wonder. What are the professional habits of
thought and action that treasure and honor others' pearls, and what are
the habits that trample?

Many of the ideas and practices that guide us are drawn from our
collaborations in the late 1980s and early 1990s with Tom Andersen,
Magnus Hald, and Anna Margrete Flam at the University of Tromso
(Andersen, 1987, 1991) in northern Norway and with Harry Goolishian, Harlene Anderson, and colleagues at the Houston–Galveston
Family Therapy Institute in Texas (Anderson, 1997; Anderson & Goolishian, 1986). This collaboration examined how postmodern philosophy
could inform psychotherapy in ways that invited participation by clients
and patients by honoring the language, ideas, and traditions that they
brought to therapy, particularly when their familiar discourses were
marginal ones in our society. From this work, the following ideas have

been helpful in shaping our therapeutic dialogues to include conversation about spiritual experience:

1. *An attitude of wonder in the therapist can be cultivated only if cynicism and certainty are attenuated.* It was in Mississippi that we began to realize the immense variety and unpredictability in individuals' experiences of God. People from strict, conservative religious backgrounds would surprise us with deeply personal experiences of a soft, accepting, nurturing God. No less stunning were the harsh and rigid descriptions of God that came from people in religious communities reputed to be inclusive and liberal. Obviously, the degree of our surprise had been a measure of the entrenchment of our stereotypes.

In our therapies, we tried to notice and record those beliefs that obscured our sense of wonder and curiosity. We listened for and recorded stories that surprised us, that released us from such assumptions. The surprising moments sometimes came first, and we worked backwards to figure out what it was that we had been assuming. We called our beliefs "certainties" to emphasize that this was a word sounding an alarm for us (Griffith, 1995a).

On a recent trip to Massachusetts, one of us picked up a copy of one of the Amherst College campus newspapers. It reported that the number of students attending groups like Christian Fellowship, Hillel, Interfaith, and Koinonia is on the upswing. It told of an essay published in another campus paper by a Koinonia member titled "Converting Jews is a Christian Responsibility." Also featured was the group AAARGH (Amherst Atheists, Agnostics, Rationalists, and Godless Humans), who were making vociferous responses to the religious organizations. This may make for healthy debate for a college campus and even for society, but what happens when Koinonia and AAARGH, known to one another only by their identities of client and therapist, meet a few years later in the therapy room? Or Hillel meets Koinonia? Or AAARGH meets Christian Fellowship?

Many of us as clinicians have AAARGH responses or conversion urges. We just don't publish them in a paper or wear them on a T-shirt, and even if we do, we usually check those displays at the office door. Because we do not check our opinions at the door, how do we then maintain integrity and openness to the individuals who consult with us? In our workshops, we always invite participants to gather in groups and grapple with these dilemmas.[1] The questions we pose and the ideas we ask participants to consider are the following:

- What cues—appearances, accents, words or phrases—cause your gut to knot up, your eyes to roll, or your back to bow up?
- When this occurs, just what is it you think you already know about this person? Have you ever been surprised? Would you like to be surprised?
- Ask your fellow group members to experiment with you, finding ways to reawaken your curiosity. For instance, what questions might you pose to yourself or to the person to whom you have become closed that would hold the possibility of surprising you?
- It is possible that you honestly wonder whether you can be the therapist a particular individual needs. If this is your question, we suggest enlisting your fellow group members to role play the individual, sharing both spoken and unspoken thoughts of the individual with you. This may aid both in deciding whether you should be the therapist and in respectfully conveying your decision to the individual.

Workshop participants have given us feedback that would hearten all camps. Therapists who describe themselves as conservative and others who identify themselves as liberal are concerned about resolving these dilemmas with integrity, as can be seen by the following illustrations. A marriage and family therapy graduate student from a conservative Christian university program described a crisis of conscience in his work with a woman coming to therapy who was planning to have an abortion and who said that she was at peace with God regarding her decision. This student who asked for consultation was sincerely troubled. "She doesn't know my convictions, but I can't stop thinking about this. Should I tell her what I believe is right?" That course, he felt, would risk losing her as a client and would only increase the chance of the abortion. Or, he said, he could continue to listen to her story (she needed a compassionate listener and had made a connection with him, and he did not want to abandon her) and hope to persuade her indirectly to continue the pregnancy. I (Melissa) imagined, as I listened to his dilemma, that it might be overlaid with his sense that God may have sent this woman to him. I also imagined what a caring and attentive therapist he must be for her, and thought how courageous he was to open his concern in this workshop to more senior family therapists, most of whom, he must have guessed, did not agree with his position. In a way, this man, lower in power in the workshop because of his student status, youth, and minority religious position, was opening himself to me much as the woman he described was opening herself to him. However, he understood a bit more than did the woman about the risks he was taking.

"How is it a dilemma for you? Where do you feel the most torn?" I asked him.

He explained that he felt torn because he was not being completely honest. This lady trusted him and believed him to be an honest person, which he did indeed strive to be. I inquired about what steps he might take to be honest with her and what he might wish if he were in her position. In the end he decided to follow the admonition "Do unto others as you would have them do unto you," rather than any other dictum. He decided to open his dilemma to the woman, so that she could decide for herself whether she wanted to continue to work with him, and whether she wanted his thoughts about the abortion.

In a community workshop organized by the Salesmanship Club Youth and Family Center[2] in Dallas (Griffith & Griffith, 1997), we asked participants to consider cues that might close down their curiosity, and how they might open it again. A memorable response came from a group of gay and lesbian colleagues, who worked with people ill with HIV. The spokesperson for the group said something like this:

> "We decided we wanted to be challenged, so we tried to come up with a real live person, one with whom we were all familiar, who would get us in the gut just by walking into our office. Some of us could imagine rolling our eyes at some people, but others said they would have no trouble with that person. It turns out that we are a more diverse group than we thought—it was hard to find an individual who evoked that gut response in all of us! Finally, somebody said, 'What if Jerry Falwell walked in?' and, Bingo! We all had a visceral reaction. So we have been asking ourselves, seriously, how we could be respectful and curious if faced with Jerry Falwell. We didn't come up with any questions for Jerry, but we did come up with something that made a difference for us. We decided to each think about times we had been judgmental, dismissive, and oppressive to others. We took turns telling one another about these times, and by the time we were finished, we could no longer judge Jerry Falwell."

2. *A climate of openness and respect can be facilitated by "democratizing" the structure of therapy.* Thus far we have spoken only about the role of a clinician's knowledge and understanding in enabling per-

sons to speak about spiritual and religious experiences. There are other factors that influence what happens in therapy that go beyond the person of the clinician.

The physical setting of therapy can also be an obstacle. Several years ago when our family therapist colleague, Jerry Gross, was a church pastor, he became sensitized to the silent suffering of divorced persons who continued to come to their church even though this particular denomination with its strong antidivorce stance offered them minimal support. Jerry decided to invite them to meet with one another and with him, to support each other and to become a visible presence in the church. By establishing a meeting room and time and, to the dismay of a few church members, publicizing the meeting on the church signboard, he and the group helped to transform the space of the church to a more hospitable one for them and their stories, even when, sometimes, their stories were ones of felt betrayal by God and the religious community. The groups continued there until one night Jerry met a woman at the door of the church. Waiting and shaking, she said, "I need to come, but I cannot set foot in this church. It frightens me." Jerry responded, "Okay. Maybe we need to hold this group in another spot." He found an alternative location away from the church grounds. Sometimes the warmest of clinicians cannot overcome the chill of a space. Clearly, Jerry's commitment was first to provide a welcoming space for people to tell their stories. He privileged the inclinations of the woman over his own convenience or preferences to determine where that space needed to be.

By contrast, the very presence of a church setting or a gathering of spiritual leaders sometimes creates an environment in which people can speak openly. Recently we conducted a seminar with a group of physicians on dilemmas that arise when patients' spiritual convictions collide with treatment goals. In the back of the room was a visitor who was not a physician or a member of the group. She seemed intensely interested in the discussion as the participants posed ways they might try to make respectful inquiries in such situations. Finally, she bravely raised her hand, "I don't know much about this, but from listening to you all today, I just have one question. I come from a religious group who has strong standards about some of these things. When you talk to your patients, is it your goal to understand their beliefs or to change them?" I asked her which impression she had. "It sort of sounds like trying to change them to me." I wondered whether this might keep people in her religious group away from healthcare providers. "It happens all the time," she said. Given this, if a clinician really wanted to provide the best grouping in which to consult with a member of her group, would it be wise to offer to let the person invite another group member, or one of the religious leaders to the meeting? "Oh, yes. If the minister came, that would help a lot. It would make it much, much better. But they don't ever ask us for that." We chatted after the lecture. She told me that she was a Jehovah's Witness. I know the struggles between this group and nurses and physicians are long-standing, especially regarding blood transfusions, which are against the church doctrine. Her experience has taught her that entering the healthcare system means to be marginalized and to have her beliefs be the object of an attempted conversion, a lesson that her overhearing of our discussion did not dispel.

In the preceding situation, even with religious leaders present, this woman and the members of her church will always be visitors in the world of our medical center. A more radical approach to democratizing the structure of a therapy is for the clinicians to become the visitors in the world of the marginalized group. Colleagues with whom we collaborate at the Center for Multicultural Human Services in Falls Church, Virginia, meet Islamic clients in a counseling clinic located within a mosque. These Muslim clients present their distress to their Imam. Because he participates and mediates, they then can also open their lives to the secular therapists.

Our colleagues at The Family Centre in Lower Hutte, New Zealand, insist that a "cultural consultant" from the local community be present in each session when a European New Zealander conducts therapy with a Samoan or Maori client. More important than qualifications as a mental health professional is that this consultant is trusted, respected, and chosen by his or her community. There may be much we can learn in the United States from our international colleagues about countering in mindful ways the negative influence of cultural practices and institutions when they exclude expression of spiritual and religious experiences.

3. *Conversational participants can speak freely of spiritual or religious experience when first they feel that their personhood is respected by the clinician.* Courtesy and etiquette are necessary, but the best of intentions may be unable to provide it unless there is some local knowledge of the beliefs and spiritual practices that are valued by those involved in the conversation. For example, an Israeli colleague recently

pointed out to us that a question we ask in therapy that is entirely appropriate with most Protestant Christians—What is your image of
God?—would be difficult for someone who was an Orthodox Jew, because it is sinful to place any image on God.

It can help to study the prominent traditions of a religious group
from the published literature (Lovinger, 1984; Matlins & Magida,
1999a, 1999b; Noss, 1963) and, better, from personal acquaintances.
However, such knowledge can never be sufficient when encountering the
unique life of another person from an unfamiliar culture. After learning
what one can about custom, ceremony, and etiquette for a particular
group, the best clinical guideline is *to meet a person in a manner that is
easy to forgive.* As human beings we fortunately seem to share enough
experiences in common that humility, openness, and caring can be discerned across cultures. In the end it is usually these emotional postures,
more than correct knowledge about beliefs and practices, that enable
gulfs of misunderstanding about spiritual and religious experiences to be
bridged. These emotional postures must be authentic, not feigned.

Sonya began her 10th psychotherapy session by telling me (Griff)
how "so much has happened" since the previous session. She had been
seeing a new man, Eric, every day. Ambivalent, she was afraid he would
hurt her as had other men in her life. I expressed surprise because only a
few weeks earlier she had vowed a 2-year moratorium on any new relationships with men. Nevertheless, she had been at Eric's house every day
for the past week, talking late into the night. Sonya contrasted this new
relationship with the landscape of her present daily life—her disgust
with male coworkers at her office and frustration with her conflicted
family—by commenting that "Eric and I have a spiritual relationship."

Noting her language, "spiritual relationship," I wondered what she
meant. Uncertain whether a direct inquiry about it would be experienced
as intrusive or off-putting, I asked instead about its mirror. Like any
metaphor, "spirituality" makes a distinction between two domains of
experience, thereby implying its counterpart, the "nonspiritual": "Your
statement sounds like the flip side of something else," I commented. "If
your relationship with Eric is a spiritual one, then what is a relationship
like when it is not spiritual?"

Sonya began talking about this difference, then opened the conversation more broadly into a domain of her life about which we had never
spoken. "My spirituality at this point—I'm not into religious expression—it takes me to a deeper understanding of myself. Things happen

for a reason." She told how she had been raised Catholic, but now drew meaning from many different religious faiths. She told how, in addition to her psychotherapy with me, she was also praying for God's guidance in learning how to relate to men differently. She talked about having "an ongoing conversation with God," explaining that "I want to block out all the other voices, so that I can hear God's voice clearly."

I asked about times when she could hear God's voice clearly and let it fill her being: At such moments, what did she then notice differently about men and her relationships with them?

Sonya said she had been praying to meet a soulmate. "I do believe people come into your life to teach you something. That helps me to bear my pain."

It sounded as though this evidenced a trust in her God that I had not heard her describe with human beings, so I asked her to contrast her experience of God and her experience of people. She acknowledged that she encountered ambiguity and uncertainty with God, yet she could trust God completely. "God has not disappointed me. It's like chaos theory— there really isn't any chaos, but order and meaning."

I wondered why we were only talking about this just now. After all, the paramount issues in her therapy, now in its 10th session, were those of trust and of suffering pain in relationships. Her relationship with her God had been such a striking exception. How did she understand that we had not spoken about it earlier?

She told how she had considered therapy to be "a clinical, detached, scientific enterprise" where this would have no place. She was afraid I might make fun of her. I wondered whether it was then a measure of her trust in the therapy that she was now able to talk about these things. Visibly tensing, she nodded.

A week later, Sonya returned to tell me how she had thought about the session afterward and was surprised that she had never talked about her spirituality with me, because it was such a large part of her life. "You didn't laugh at me when I told you about my spirituality. I can tell you about other things." She then described how she had started "remembering things" since beginning therapy, but had not spoken about them. As a small child, she had been beaten and tortured by a babysitter who kept her while her parents worked. Once he stuffed toilet paper in her mouth to stop her from crying out and threatened to kill her parents if she told anyone. She now recounted episodes that had occurred periodically since then when she would lose her voice and become unable to speak. It was as though there were fingers around her throat saying, "Shut up! Don't say anything!"

Sonya's story has many aspects, but it was her omission of any talk about her spiritual life during our early sessions that most intrigued me. No one is surprised when people in therapy struggle to find ways to speak openly about sex, death, or those whom they hate. These were the kinds of things that Sonya had been able to talk about. Yet it had been harder for her to reveal a trusting relationship with her God. Why?

Our explanation is that Sonya's story is about marginalized experience that often has been excluded from the dialogue of therapy. What distinguishes a psychotherapy that is open to stories of spiritual or religious experience is not its subject matter, but its similarities to other therapies for those who are misunderstood or silenced by a dominant culture. In this sense, a psychotherapy that is welcoming for a religious person will share kinship with the kind of psychotherapy that a gay person, a person of color, or a homeless person might find welcoming. Many ideas that the two of us have found useful in opening therapy to the sacred were learned by conducting therapy with persons suffering symptoms of somatization, among the most stigmatized and marginalized persons within our healthcare system. Courtesy, etiquette, and respect for the personhood of the other necessarily characterize these therapies.

4. *Spiritual or religious experience can be available for reflective dialogue only if those present sustain embodied states that permit this experience to be recognized, understood, and expressed.* The state of the body governs access to spiritual or religious experience. This may seem an odd proposal to emphasize in a discussion on spirituality, as religious life for so many—whether Hindu, Muslim, or Christian—stresses a distancing of self from bodily desires. However, we noticed in our research interviews how seldom people discerned their God's presence through any of the five senses. Rather, they were actively using a visceral sensibility of their bodies to guide the discernment (Shotter, 1993a, 1993b). Often their words were reminiscent of Norman Maclean's (1976, p. 37) description of the mystical relationship between a fisherman and the river: "I don't know what it is or where, because sometimes it is in my arms and sometimes in my throat and sometimes nowhere in particular except somewhere deep."

Nearly every person with whom we talked described sensing God's presence through vague feelings located somewhere within their bodies. Even when a person said, "I feel God's presence everywhere," close questioning found "everywhere" was not distributed equally. Often God's presence was felt deep within the torso, literally, "in my heart." Rather than seeing, hearing, or touching, these persons were maintaining their attunement through a sensibility of the body (Griffith et al., 1992, 1995; Polles et al., 1994; Tingle et al., 1993).

Even religions that discourage gratification of bodily passions strive to access states of the body that are associated with reverence, awe, and communion with God or Spirit. This access is sought through spiritual practices—fasting, ritual dieting, ascetic practices, or other activities that place a check on physiological arousal from fear, anger, or shame. All this suggests that the sensations of the body play a larger role in the perception of spiritual experience than many of us in Western culture had supposed.

Focusing upon the body as a door to the sacred makes sense if we grasp the relationship that exists between physiology and epistemology. Maturana and Varela (1992) pointed out that cognitive processes can occur only as they are permitted by biological structure, meaning that what is knowable is limited by the state of the body. Certain states facilitate spiritual experience; others hinder such experience. In Chapter 1, we discussed this dependency of knowing on bodily state in terms of emotional postures that facilitate or hinder them (Griffith & Griffith, 1990, 1992a, 1994). What is important about this perspective is its emphasis on emotion not as something one feels but as something one does (Weingarten, 1999, 2000).

The relationship between the body, its emotion, and knowing holds two additional significances for a therapy that involves spiritual experience. First, spiritual experiences often exist only partly in language, but are felt fully within the body. When this is the case, a conversation that engages only that which is easily articulated in words can bypass that which makes a spiritual experience central in a person's life. An important sequence of questions to ask can be the following: "Can you distinguish moments when you feel intensely the presence of God [or, "when you deeply experience your spirituality"] from those moments when you don't?" . . . "How is it that you sense the difference? What do you experience in your body? What are the sensations telling you that you have entered that state of being?" . . . "When your body is in this state of being, what are you able to know and understand that you cannot so easily know when your body is not in this state?" One useful outcome of such a dialogue is that a person can become more mindful in using his or her body's sensibility as a guide in responding to spiritual concerns. The following excerpt from a research interview is one person's response to these questions (Griffith et al., 1995):

DREW: I think it is here in the chest (*pointing to the center of his chest*)— a lightness.

GRIFF: Is it present elsewhere in your body, or is it mostly in your chest?

DREW: I think it's mostly in my chest. I mean, sometimes I feel that all over, but first I notice it here.

GRIFF: Can you recall a particular time when you felt this sense of lightness in your chest and felt it intensely?

DREW: Lots of times. One I remember specifically was going to a retreat in the mountains. There was an amphitheater overlooking one of the mountains. I remember sitting in the amphitheater with the leaves were changing colors and the sun coming in from behind me . . . the air was cool and the sunlight was warm . . . I could feel God's presence. I was being caught up in what He created, just being caught up in the warmth that I felt.

GRIFF: Could we go a bit into that memory?

DREW: Okay.

GRIFF: Were you alone?

DREW: I was alone at the time, yes.

GRIFF: So this was really a private experience?

DREW: Right. I was on a retreat with other people, but I had walked out there early in the morning.

GRIFF: When at that moment you sensed God's presence, were there any words spoken? I mean, did you speak to God, or was it a communication that really was not in language?

DREW: It was all nonverbal.

GRIFF: Okay. Did it seem that God was off in the distance or very close? When you imagine the scene, where was God in it? This is more of a feeling question, not a theological one—what you immediately felt, not what you may analyze intellectually.

DREW: One of the things I felt then . . . and I feel now as I think back on it . . . is the feeling that God is behind me, with his warmth and all, encouraging me. God's there and he's behind me, supporting me and encouraging me.

GRIFF: So did it feel in this scene that God found you, or that you found God? Who spoke first?

DREW: It was more like God always was there, and he encouraged me to slow down long enough to see that. It was more a gesture than words.

GRIFF: Can you show me the gesture?

DREW: It was like God walking up behind me and placing his hands on my shoulders.

GRIFF: And if those hands could have spoken, what might they have said?

DREW: I'm here. I love you. I accept you just as you are. I'm your great-est fan. All I want is to love and support you. I don't want you to have to chase after me and find me; I've already found you. I'm right here.

As with Drew, most persons we have interviewed quickly identify a specific sense that signals contact with God or marks a spiritual experi-ence. However, they often have struggled to find language adequate for expressing what was felt nonverbally in the body and was also private, often unshared with any other person. For Drew it was only after 11 turns in the conversation that he spoke in words what he had felt so pro-foundly within his body. Once identified, such states of the body serve as gateways into important life narratives that sometimes anchor not only the person's spiritual life but also his or her identity as a person. In a therapy session (instead of a research interview), the next question asked of Drew might have been: "As you sense this lightness in your chest . . . this sense that God has approached from behind, touching your shoul-ders . . . what are some of the important stories of your life that are con-nected to these sensations?"

Spiritual experience often cannot be accessed for the work of ther-apy when individuals reside in emotional postures of alarm, particularly those of shame or blame. We became accustomed to research partici-pants commenting on the intimacy of our conversations: "I have never told anyone about this, not even my wife." Openness required for such intimacy disappears unless there is an assurance of safety. Any suspicion of prejudice against spirituality by the therapist can be enough to close the door. Inquiring about the person's state of body can serve as a reliable indicator of whether or not there is sufficient tranquillity for a meaningful conversation to ensue.

There is a cascade of threat that dissipates any possibility for therapeutic dialogue when it progresses unchecked: a lapse in empathy → a personal affront → emotional recoil → visceral disgust or alarm. Bodily signs of alarm, such as shallow breathing, averted or tense gaze, folded arms, or tight face and fists may indicate that a therapy interchange is already in the "recoil" to "visceral alarm" section of this continuum. We can heed this warning and slow down, for conversation then is more likely to be debate than dialogue, and there will be little disclosure of such important but sensitive domains as spiritual experience. The relations between body and spirituality will be further discussed in Chapter 6 on beliefs, Chapter 7 on rituals, ceremonies, and spiritual practices, and Chapter 10 on medical and psychiatric illnesses.

5. *Opening conversation to talk about spirituality or religion depends less on knowing what questions to ask and more on careful listening to what people spontaneously speak about when they feel safe and respected.* One can ask about specific words, phrases, or idioms that point to the spiritual or religious domain—"The Lord be with you," "I prayed that wouldn't happen," "Someone must have been looking out for me," "I felt so at peace," "I deserve this punishment," "Everything happens for a reason." Although the person may have been using an idiom, such as "It's in God's hands now," only as a figure of speech, one may open a serious conversation by asking, "Is that a safe place for it to be? When you think of it as all in God's hands, do you see this matter as receiving great attention or as being forgotten?" Alternatively, one may query, "All in God's hands, what is that like? Is it relief—that you have turned it over to God, and God has taken it? Or is it more like it has been taken away from you? Do you sense you still have a part to play, but you have God's help with this? Or something different than any of those?"

When no references to spirituality stand out in the conversation, one can ask more directly: "Is spirituality or religion an important part of your life?" or "Are there important beliefs that I should know about for our work together?" The two of us usually prefer, however, not to ask such questions unless we already have a sense that these questions make sense within the language and culture of the person. Rather, we start by asking how the person has responded to a current or past personal crisis in terms of universal dimensions of human experience, questions to which we refer as *existential questions*:

- What has sustained you?
- From what sources do you draw strength in order to cope?
- Where do you find peace?
- Who truly understands your situation?
- When you are afraid or in pain, how do you find comfort?
- For what are you deeply grateful?
- What is your clearest sense of the meaning of your life at this time?
- Why is it important that you are alive?
- To what or whom are you most devoted?
- To whom, or what, do you most freely express love?

Although not every one of these questions would be relevant, *if* spirituality is important to a person, then one of these simple questions may lead directly into a discussion of how it is important.

WHEN NOT TO PURSUE

Examining one's certainties, democratizing the therapy context, respecting the personhood of others, and using bodily expressions of emotion to guide the dialogue are therapeutic practices that usually facilitate open conversation about spirituality. At other times, however, these same practices argue for caution in asking about spiritual matters. Sometimes a person has good reasons not to speak about spiritual or religious life, even if it is important and valued, and even if the therapist is respectful, open, and trustworthy. Under these circumstance a therapist's questions about spirituality may digress from a more necessary conversation, or, worse, be intrusive or threatening.

As in other social groups, it is important, therapeutically and ethically, to negotiate which conversations about which topics are appropriate for which groupings of people. In addition, it must be remembered that God and other spiritual beings at all times are also part of the conversation for many religious persons. Failure to attend appropriately to needed boundaries can bring inadvertent harm.

In one instance, I (Griff) failed to attend appropriately to such boundaries when they were needed. Several years ago a priest from an Orthodox church sought couples therapy with his wife. The complaint she raised, his discomfort with intimacy, appeared to be too humiliating for him to address directly. Suspecting that he must encounter the same struggles in seeking intimacy with his God, but on terrain where he might feel more comfortable, I asked, "How do you face this question in your relationship with God?" I then asked him to role play, by his assuming God's persona, some interactions around questions of trust and intimacy with God. The priest went through the role play compliantly but tensely, with beads of sweat forming on his forehead. The role play seemed empty of authentic emotion, and the couple discontinued the therapy after four sessions. He stated his belief that they should be able to work out their problems without professional assistance, even though she disagreed and wanted to continue. My errors were multiple. Too late I realized that I had placed the priest in a double bind. It was his sense that he was not only his wife's husband, but her priest and spiritual leader as well. From his perspective, I had asked him in front of his wife to bare the same shortcomings in his relationship with his God that she complained about in their marriage, yet he did not feel comfortable declining the exercise because he had initiated the therapy. Furthermore, I had introduced a manner of interacting with God, through role play, that would have been comfortable within many American Protestant Christian traditions but may have held very different meanings for an Orthodox Christian church, about whose beliefs and practices I had only a superficial knowledge at that time. Finally, I noticed the tenseness of his body and sweating forehead yet pressed ahead, instead of letting his physical expressions of alarm pace my words and actions.

Sometimes a conscientious effort to include a spiritual or religious dimension in therapy, while not antitherapeutic, still constitutes a digression from a person's agenda. I (Griff) once met an Orthodox Jewish couple in therapy. For each, their religious observances were central in organizing their daily lives. I spent much of a session seeking to understand how their religious beliefs and practices informed their relationship and the hopes they held for our therapy. At the next session, however, they each said that my questions had been thought provoking, but that they

were more concerned about the fights that were threatening their relationship. They wanted immediate help with practical strategies to stop
the fighting. Was it a better idea, despite this, to have taken time to learn
how their relationship and its problems were contextualized by their
religious beliefs and culture? Or was I imposing upon them a spirituality-
in-therapy perspective that held my interest at the time? Or both? Spirituality and religion are probably no different than other perspectives—
sexuality, power, intergenerational family patterns, gender roles—that
can capture a clinician's fascination at the expense of the client's or
patient's concerns. Any perspective for understanding other human
beings, whatever its merits, can become an imposition.

In recent years, much of our clinical work and teaching in workshops has focused on learning how to ask questions that are carefully
tailored to open dialogue, to foster reflection, or to prompt therapeutic
change. Good questions can make wonderful openings, but they can also
close off the conversation. Too many times I (Melissa) have had empathic disconnection in therapy sessions—the kind that confuse the client
and myself—when my attention was captured by preoccupation with
asking the "right" questions. However, preparing my mind and spirit to
hear others' stories and clearing the assumptions that obstructed my
curiosity about their experiences have always fostered the connection
and the conversation. As Susan's later comments will subsequently show,
sometimes, even when I think a good and timely question has sparked
the telling of a story, the truth is that the story was waiting only for me
to be quiet and ready to listen.

THE UTILITY OF NONCERTAINTY

As these vignettes suggest, the two of us seek a posture of noncertainty
when conducting therapy. This does not mean that we each do not have
beliefs, convictions, opinions, or prejudices, but that we have adopted an
intentional plan to foster curiosity, openness, and wonder as our dominant emotions in the therapy room.

Most religions and spiritualities seek both to build community and to
define what truths are of ultimate concern. Sometimes the building of community is limited to those who adhere to the tradition; sometimes the aim
is to foster connection among all people. The search for truth appears in
many different forms—seeking enlightenment, discovering hidden mean-

ings with sacred scriptures, or gaining direct revelations from one's God. In organizing psychotherapy, each of these aims tends to recruit different and contradictory emotional processes in the treatment relationship. A focus on "What is truth?" evokes emotional postures of certainty and judging, whereas a focus on "How can relationship come into being?" evokes emotional postures of curiosity, openness, and wonder.

Some therapists' work is modeled on convictions gained through powerful spiritual experiences during which compelling lessons were learned. Others conduct therapy guided by the belief system of a religious or spiritual tradition. Our proposal differs from both approaches in the extent to which we adopt an intentional noncertainty about "what ought to be" in order to stay as open as possible to what the person desires and "what can be" in relationships with others, self, and God or other spiritual beings.

WORKING WITHIN A PERSON'S FAMILIAR DISCOURSES

When we talk with people in therapy, we attempt to meet, understand, and get to know their accustomed discourses, to the extent possible. This is the position of an anthropologist who wishes to learn about and to contribute usefully to a not yet known culture, but not to disturb or harm it by intruding.

Discourse describes the ways a system of language and relationships has become institutionalized among a particular group of people (Davies & Harre, 1990; Weingarten, 1995a). It provides a way of being for those who belong to that group. A discourse is embedded in the customs, manners of speaking and relating, institutions, and written documents of a culture. As Kaethe Weingarten (1995b, pp. 10–11) has put it, "Discourse works through language and through language it shapes what we can know. In fact, a radical view of discourse holds that our conscious and unconscious thoughts and emotions, our sense of ourselves in the world, and our ways of understanding our relation to the world are constituted through language and discourse." Overlearned and well practiced, the influence of a discourse in structuring conversation and relationship typically lies outside the awareness of those who use it. It is too close to be easily seen and too much at hand to be easily discovered.

It is important to note that each person lives within multiple discourses. There are discourses that define the culture of the workplace, one's national or ethnic identity, one's gendered identity as a man or woman, and other coexisting or competing identities. There are discourses through which the spiritual domain of life is experienced and expressed in daily life.

The different expressive forms with which we articulate our work in this book—metaphors, stories, dialogues, beliefs, practices, rituals, ceremonies, and communities—can be considered as different genres for the discourses within which live those who come for therapy. In addition to these expressive forms, each discourse is characterized by its idioms. Religious idioms are shorthand expressions that point to a spiritual or religious domain organized within a specific culture.

Our task is learning to enter competently into a particular discourse in ways that enable conversation to occur on ground familiar to a person. When one does not already possess such competence, it is critically important to stay in the position of a learner, open to new ideas, asking questions of curiosity. Awareness of the different genres and idioms of symbolic expression helps us both to listen for spiritual experience and to ask questions that can generate a therapeutic dialogue.

A discourse is highly politicized. Certain ways of talking and relating appear because they have been afforded special status while alternative ways have been forbidden. Class, gender, ethnicity, and socioeconomic status have much to do with what discourses have been selected through history as acceptable ways for expressing spiritual experience (Foucault, 1980; White, 1995a). This means that one always risks inadvertently offending, attacking, or silencing another person, depending upon how the talk is handled when discussing spiritual issues. We hope to listen and to speak sensitively with heightened awareness for the power issues that are unavoidable when conversing with another person about spiritual experience. In Chapters 6, 8, and 9, respectively, we will discuss therapeutic work with religious beliefs, community, and ways in which a spiritual or religious discourse can foster harm and destruction. In these chapters we discuss situations in which it becomes important that power relations implicit in a person's discourse of spirituality or religion be made explicit so that they can be incorporated into the therapeutic work.

This chapter began with Susan's story, and she has offered her reflections to close it. It is my (Melissa's) practice to offer my writing to

persons who have been generous enough to allow me to write my ver-
sions of our conversations so that they may read and revise in any way.
At these times I explain that, unlike a therapy session, this is a meeting
to help me to write in a way that best honors their experience. Months
after the conversation described in the chapter's beginning, Susan agreed
to meet with me for this purpose. Her reflections taught me more about
the significance of her dialogue with John, explained how it fit with and
expanded the story of her spiritual, relational, and work life, and, quite
unexpectedly, gave me a glimpse at the tangible symbol she kept of what
had become a sacred metaphor for her.

After Susan had read the opening vignette, I asked if she remembered the moments I described, how she might describe them differently,
and whether she felt they were a part of our exchange that mattered.
"Yes," she told me, "That did matter. . . . I knew when it happened on
the beach that I wanted to tell you about it. It's funny, I thought I would
find John in church, but it didn't happen there. I think God led me to the
beach. As soon as the thought came, I knew it was right."

"So when you came that day, you already knew you wanted to tell
about this?" I asked her, a bit chagrined that I had thought I needed to
work so hard to facilitate her telling.

Susan then began explaining to me the significance of that dialogue,
and in so doing, led me into her story. "The talking with John on the
beach . . . it was like a stepping stone. . . . I could stand on it and see
from whence I had come. I could see all I had been through and how far
I had come. I could see how much stronger I had become."

"And from that stepping stone, do you also see the future differently?" I asked her.

"Not that I know how it will turn out," she said, "but I am confident in my strength to handle whatever comes. I have never before been
sure of that."

"So John's words, '*You can do this,*' are your words for yourself,
and they go into the future, too," I reflected.

"I have not felt his presence this much since he died. It's a big
change. And it feels like a change that will last."

"What all is it changing for you?" I queried.

Susan laughed. "See, I could sit here today and read what you've
written and talk about it and feel sad, but not traumatized or upset. I am
calm. Now, you know me and you know that's different. I've been getting there, but this is a new plateau. . . . And I think it has upset the ap-

ple cart with people connected to me. My boss isn't used to me being this strong. She knows I'm different. What she doesn't know is that I'm actually putting out feelers for another job and getting some encouraging responses. I just thought I was trapped there for life, and that I had to endure whatever they handed down to me. Now I can imagine other possibilities. My family isn't used to me being this strong either. I've stopped doing some things with them that aren't good for me. I should have stopped them long ago."

Susan dug down into her deep bag and found the shell. "Remember the white shell, the one that reminded me of John in his white robes? I brought it home. I keep it here and pull it out sometimes." She held it in her hand, turning it over and rubbing it with her thumb as we talked.

"What is it like for you to hold the shell?" I asked her.

"Look, it's not perfect," she mused. "It's quite ordinary. It even has an edge chipped off, or maybe it's worn away. That's good. It's more realistic."

"More like life?" I asked.

"More like John." She talked a while about some of the struggles her brother had suffered. Continuing to rub the shell, she commented, "It is calming though, to hold it. I hadn't thought about it before, but it's hard and strong. I believe I could throw this shell down on the floor and it wouldn't break."

Susan's rich metaphor informed and undergirded her story, and recollected for her the dialogue with John. I was grateful for the depth of explanation she gave me, and hope that the act of bearing witness will help to ensure that though the shell may someday be lost, the metaphor, story, and dialogue with John will endure.

NOTES

1. If or you wish to do this, we suggest doing it with at least one other person and preferably more. Working to loosen strong biases is a dialogical process.
2. The Salesmanship Club Youth and Family Centers, Inc., is a nonprofit agency (sponsored by the Salesmanship Club of Dallas) serving children and their families through outpatient counseling, a therapeutic camp program, and an early intervention neighborhood school.

Chapter Three

Metaphor and Spirituality

"My friends call me to tell me that I should divorce Frank. They say, 'It's all right, Mary. Just look in the Bible. Divorce is permitted in cases of adultery.' They don't understand. My covenant was with Frank and with God for this marriage. It would be different if Frank were continuing to betray me, but he has repented and he is doing all he can to change, to be honest, and to be a better husband. He's still got a long way to go—but I see him changing. . . . I'm still angry. . . . I'm not completely open to Frank yet. I'm not ready. He can't devastate me now because I'm not open. But if I do open myself and he hurts me again, well, I know the marriage would be over. That's no decision. What I fear in that case is that *I* would be over, that I could never recover from that hurt."

Mary and I (Melissa) had met for several weeks. I could see why her friends wanted to direct her out of her marriage. She had recently discovered that for many of the 30 years of her marriage she had been deceived. Frank had been involved in a long, lingering affair. Mary's suffering was now compounded. Not only was her trust in Frank broken, but this revelation had made her doubt her own ability to perceive and make judgments. I was tempted to encourage her to leave the marriage, as had her friends, except that she was clearly not requesting my direction. Mary had sought God's direction and felt that God had bid her to stay in the marriage. This decision was further buttressed by her witnessing Frank's recent efforts to change. Still, this was a hard decision for her. Some of her friends had admonished her for choosing the "easy way"—staying with Frank—rather than making the hard decision to divorce him. She did not see it this way.

"But divorce would be the easy way," she protested. "To protect myself and to give up on him and leave. . . . No, this way is the hard way. . . . Taking this way, I've learned a lot about faith."

"What have you learned?" I wondered.

"It's like things are falling down all around me, crumbling and cracking," she explained. "But I will be okay."

"The picture that I get is one of a storm, with things swirling around you. Is it like that?" I asked her.

Mary nodded.

I wanted to understand how it was that she could "be okay" in the midst of this. "Is there a buffer protecting you from the falling objects, or is it like objects could fall on top of you, like a board might fly by and slice off your arm or a nail might puncture your shoulder?"

"There's no buffer, really, but it's funny you mention the storm," Mary reflected, recalling a story. "When I was in nursing school a terrible tornado struck. We called it the Palm Sunday Storm. I remember I was at my grandmother's house after church services, the Sunday before Easter, when a neighbor ran in with the news. We were all gathered round the table for dinner. I got right up from the table and left to go help out. Being a nursing student, I knew I could be useful and that my skills were needed."

"I will never forget what I saw. The devastation. There were bodies, dead and wounded out in the open, homes demolished. We worked for days afterward, cleaning up the debris. . . . In fact, that's more like where I feel I am now, rather than in the middle of the storm. I'm cleaning up the debris."

"As you are cleaning up debris, where is God?" I asked.

"Just beside me," she said softly. "Right next to me. As I pick up a board, he's picking up the heavy end, making the board somehow supernaturally lighter."

I sat in silence with Mary. Her eyes were wide and mirthful, and her smile was quiet and thoughtful. I mused, "Surely this is a person who routinely and graciously picks up heavy ends for others." I did not voice this thought. It seemed more important to have the silence, which seemed to be one of peace. However, my thoughts were not peaceful.

They were fretful: What would befall Mary if her husband betrayed her again?

"I guess you learned as a young nursing student that in the middle of a peaceful day, storms can come quickly, without warning, bringing great devastation," I offered.

"Yes," Mary said. "That is a lesson one never forgets."

"If you were out there steadily cleaning up the debris, with God alongside you, lifting heavy ends of the boards, and, suddenly, another storm hit, then where would God be?" I asked.

Mary answered without hesitation. "Where would he be? I'm not sure. But I do know that he would know what to do. If there were a ditch he would grab me and run there. He would put me down in the ditch and lay on top of me."

It seemed she anticipated my next question as she continued. "Or, if there was no ditch nearby, or if we couldn't get to the ditch in time, he would get my body on the ground and cover my body with his own till the storm passed. . . . I guess I don't really know exactly what he would do. Maybe I don't have to know, but I do know that he would know what to do."

During the moments of this meeting a rich and unforgettable metaphor had been developed that gave structure and meaning to Mary's suffering and to her spiritual sustenance. It informed much of the therapeutic work that would follow. In that conversation, Mary and I developed this metaphor together. When Mary said, "It's like things are falling down all around me, crumbling and cracking, but I will be okay," her rich sensory words formed a picture in my own mind. I then proposed a candidate metaphor, one of a storm. She nodded, then began to expand her story, enlivening the metaphor more.

This process was a close-working, back-and-forth collaboration. The image of a storm came to my mind because of connections in my own life, growing up in the South, heeding tornado warnings, and fearing the big storm. Had I been from California, I might have reflected differently: "It sounds like you're in the middle of an earthquake!" Perhaps that image would have been too cataclysmic for Mary. Another experience might have led me to say, "Is it as though the house around you is rotten and decaying, but that somehow you have found some firm piece of the foundation?" I cannot know now if those words would have opened or closed a door. I do know that when I contribute to the co-creation of a metaphor, I must hold my offerings loosely and assume that if they are tossed out, a richer one may be in store.

SPIRITUALITY IS EXPRESSED THROUGH
LANGUAGE AND RELATIONSHIP

Mary's commitment to Frank is mediated by her relationship to her God. This relationship is one whose physical presence she can feel. It is described in vivid, sensory language: "He would get my body on the ground and cover my body with his own till the storm passed." Her sense of this relationship with God is expressed through her metaphor of a storm, her story of dealing with the aftermath of a tornado, and her belief that God would know what to do. When a person describes his or her spiritual experience, it is in terms of particular relationships and specific language that shape the form of those relationships. For most religious persons, a relationship with God is at the center of spiritual experience. For those who follow spiritualities that are not God-centered, spiritual experience may be located within relationships with other people, within nature, or with one's ancestors. In therapy, the relationships and language of spiritual experience can provide means for resolving the problem that has brought a person or family to therapy.

Language and relationship, while akin, are not the same. Although language and relationship are both called upon to express a connection with religion or spirituality, they do so in different ways. A person who experiences the presence of God does so with an immediacy that extends beyond the limits of what language can express. Such a person may describe the felt presence of a personal God as "warmth," "light," or "peace," as though it were sensed within one's physical body, yet clearly more is denoted than can be captured by these words. Martin Buber (1958, p. 104) observed that "We speak with Him only when speech dies within us."

Our research with people about their religious experiences has impressed upon us how much a person often must grope to find words for spiritual and religious experiences that cannot be adequately expressed in language (Griffith et al., 1992). Therefore, it is a challenge that encounters with the sacred can be made understandable to others, and reflectively to oneself, only when they are expressed in language. As Buber (1958, p. 101) also noted, the relationship between humans and spiritual beings is one where "the relation, being without speech, yet begets it." People often seem driven to speak of important encounters with the sacred even as their words fail them.

It is because language both expresses and constitutes spiritual experience, however, that the tools of psychotherapy can open healing possibilities out of spiritual experience. Because language *expresses* religious experience, religious experience can enter meaningfully into psychotherapy via its metaphors, stories, and beliefs. Because language also *constitutes* religious experience, new meaning that arises out of the dialogue of therapy can transform reflexively the experience itself. Therapists have long noted that changes in a person's relationship to a personal God and religious community often occur spontaneously during a psychotherapy, even when religion had not been a focus of the therapy (Meissner, 1984, pp. 5–6).

That expression of religious experience in words and sentences secondarily reshapes the experience, leaving it different than it had been, creates a dilemma for many. What once had been formless and primordial is now stamped by the cookie-cutter distinctions of daily life—God is a "father," the spirit is like "a river" or "the wind," heaven is "above." William James (1994, pp. 224–225) recorded the words of Mr. Hadley, "a homeless, friendless, dying drunkard" who had a religious conversion so life-changing that he never again touched alcohol: "I said, 'Dear Jesus, can you help me?' *Never with mortal tongue can I describe that moment.* Although up to that moment my soul had been filled with indescribable gloom, I felt the glorious brightness of the noonday sun shine into my heart. I felt I was a free man" (emphasis added). The incomprehensibility in language of the experience to which Mr. Hadley alludes has been echoed by countless believers across a range of religions who try to report their experiences with their God.

Similar issues hold when an experience is spiritual but not God-centered, as in a moment of enlightenment, when sense of self disappears and all is unity. Mystics over the ages often have been loathe to speak of their powerful spiritual experiences, lest the effort to speak prose change the poetic. A desire to protect the passionate intimacy of such moments is set against desire for community, for sharing them with others, and for hearing others' experiences.

RELATIONSHIP EXTENDS BEYOND LANGUAGE

Spiritual experience is expressed not only through language but in the immediacy of bodily experience. It exists not just in words and sentences but in the sensations and movements of our bodies. This is how all relationships are experienced, with both material and nonmaterial beings. For example, a 45-year-old woman preparing for a heart transplant told how she had coped with the stress of the medical treatments and diagnostic tests. When undergoing lengthy, painful tests such as coronary arteriography, she sensed the constant, hovering presence of God: "My body can feel his presence. I know I am not alone." She showed little fear in approaching the diagnostic procedures and little stress from the trauma afterward.

Relationships between individuals and spiritual beings—ancestors, saints, spirits, angels—bear many of the characteristics of human relationships. However, they also possess some unique aspects that can enable them to serve as resources in ways that human relationships cannot, as many of the vignettes of this text will illustrate. Some of these unique features are the following:

• *The personal relationship between self and one's God or other spiritual being may be the only relationship in which there are no secrets.* A religious person commonly assumes that God knows all. The same may be true of relationships with other spiritual beings who are not considered limited by their materiality. Consequently, it can be asked in a therapy interview: "What does God understand about this situation that other people involved in the it do not understand?" "Are there concerns that you can take to Saint Theresa that seem too difficult to talk about anywhere else, even here? Is this sufficient, or would you like to be able to have another person in the conversation?" Particularly when there is an impasse in a therapy, such questions can open new layers of dialogue.

• *A personal relationship with one's God, or other spiritual beings, may provide the only relationship that can be counted upon to be always present and available.* A religious person usually assumes that God or other spiritual beings have no geographical limitations, so one is never alone anywhere in universe. Despite their best human efforts, family members and friends cannot meet this standard. It also means that God or other invisible beings, as a spiritual community, can provide a felt network of support when human beings are unavailable. When this is the case, a focus in therapy on experiencing fully the felt presence the spiritual can be critical for coping when isolation, anomie, or alienation are major elements in a person's problem. Perhaps after eliciting and listening to a richly detailed story of this felt presence, one could ask, "What words (or images, songs, or reminder objects) will help you remember this story and to know that you are not alone?"

• *A relationship between a person and God or another spiritual being can provide a continuous source of meaning.* Dostoyevsky defined a human being as a creature capable of bearing infinite suffering. Based on what we have experienced in our own lives and witnessed in the lives of the people and families we have known, we concur with this definition—but only with these provisos: Human beings can bear infinite suffering provided that they do not do so alone and that the suffering has meaning. Amidst the chaos of disease, loss, and random violence, a relationship with a spiritual being, beyond the capacity of human relationships, can provide a well from which new meaning can be endlessly drawn.

• *A relationship with a spiritual being can stand as witness to what is just and unjust.* For persons who have experienced hidden abuse or injustice, the query "What in this situation do God's eyes see that no human eyes can see?" constitutes a question of justice. When no person can know and understand, God is available as witness to the truth. When all potential observers are excluded or deceived, the awareness of an omniscient witness may make the unbearable situation bearable (Griffith & Griffith, 1994).

GENRES FOR EXPRESSING SPIRITUAL EXPERIENCE

Whatever the immediate felt presence of spiritual experience, it is given form—shaped, constrained, transformed—by symbolic language and actions. Some common forms in which spiritual experience is expressed include:

• Metaphors and other tropes
• Stories, or narratives
• Beliefs
• Dialogue
• Rituals
• Ceremonies
• Practices
• Community

Within different spiritual and religious traditions, these various expressive forms are elaborated into different genres of spiritual experience.

What is important about our selections for this list is that these are expressive forms that are familiar *both* to psychotherapists of every ilk *and* to those who consult with them who value spiritual experience. Nearly every therapist has specific therapeutic practices for working with metaphors, stories, dialogue, or the other listed forms. As we will illustrate, most religious and spiritual traditions utilize more than one of these expressive forms, although different traditions rely more on some than others.

There are other expressive forms important for particular religious traditions but not usually found within the repertoires of psychotherapists. Interpretation of oracles, divination, communication with spiritual beings, prophecy, scriptural exegesis, and preaching are religious genres unfamiliar to many psychotherapists in Western cultures, excepting those who have personal histories or current affiliations with religions valuing these practices. Most communities in the United States have counselors or psychotherapists who identify themselves publicly and professionally by an association with Christian, Islamic, Jewish, Buddhist, or other religious tradition. Sometimes these clinicians can utilize these less common genres to aid people, using healing practices that are inaccessible to secular therapists. Those outside that religion lack this competence and, more importantly, the confidence of the believer that comes from trusting that the therapist endorses the practice in his or her own life.

In our work, however, we do not identify ourselves with any specific approach to spirituality or religion (McGoldrick, 1999). Instead we have aimed to develop clinical practices that permit a psychotherapist working with a person who does *not* hold beliefs or spiritual practices in common nevertheless to conduct psychotherapy in a manner that makes use of healing possibilities inherent in that person's spiritual experience.

For practical purposes, these listed genres are ones most psychotherapists call on in conducting therapy. Each of them presents unique therapeutic options. Just as we might discuss meter, imagery, and rhyme as important but different devices a poet might utilize in composing a poem, we can distinguish different uses of metaphor, story, belief, or dialogue in conducting psychotherapy.

SOCIOBIOLOGICAL DIFFERENCES AMONG THE GENRES OF SPIRITUAL EXPERIENCE

Various forms of symbolic expression play distinct roles in human life. Of particular relevance for psychotherapy, different forms work differently in coordinating a person's language and relationships with his or her physiological state. Metaphors and other tropes, for example, play a key role in coordinating mental and physiological processes of perception. Stories are particularly important in the organization of a sense of self and other processes of identity formation. Both ritual and conversation help choreograph the experience of community. Spiritual practices and ritual can engage bodily experience in ways that genres relying more on language cannot. Life in community orchestrates all the other expressive forms in a grand movement that enables culture to come into being.

THE DIFFERENT GENRES ARE INSEPARABLE

Although we at times will focus on their distinctiveness, the expressive forms are also inseparable. Most of them appear within any given therapy interview. One could argue that many of the vignettes told in these pages might, with a change in emphasis, have been used to illustrate yet a different genre—belief rather than story, or community instead of dialogue—making our distinctions among them seem artificial.

In real life the conduct of therapy is a sequence of aesthetic compositions. Questions weave back and forth among these expressive forms as a dialogue is composed during a session. One does not necessarily take priority over another, although each opens a different avenue for therapeutic change.

MULTICHANNEL LISTENING

Multichannel listening is a systematic effort to hear each of these expressive forms as they appear spontaneously during an interview. Multichannel listening responds to expressions of spiritual experience in whatever forms are familiar and comfortable to the speaker. The interview becomes organized around the consultee's preferred, sometimes tradition-directed, modes of expression. For one person, a powerful metaphor—a mental image—organizes spiritual experience. For others a pivotal story, of blessing or betrayal, positions them in the world. For yet another, it is participation in rituals and a sense of belonging to a community. For others, it is commitment to specific beliefs and doctrines.

Forms favored for expressing spirituality or religion may be selected in large part by the tradition. A Southern Baptist Christian may focus on beliefs about Jesus Christ and conversational prayers with his or her personal God. An observant Jew may focus mainly on participation in ritual and commitment to the community of Jewish people. Multichannel listening seeks to elaborate the therapy within whichever genres are familiar, well-practiced, and chosen by the person.

For our purposes here, we feel it is helpful to separate the strands of the process by examining how a therapist works differently in each of these genres. An examination of all the ways in which each of these genres can be employed would yield a cumbersome book. However, a few illustrations can show how each contributes uniquely to a psychotherapy that includes spiritual or religious experience as we survey the language of those who consult with us.

The next five chapters are organized according to these different genres. In each chapter there is a dialectic between language and relationship, with relationships to God (or other spiritual beings) bringing forth language, and the questions, reflections, and responses in the dialogue of therapy then reconfiguring these relationships in reflexive fashion. Chapters 3–8 each detail how a therapist can work with spiritual expression as it is mediated within one of these genres. We begin with a discussion of metaphors and other tropes.

THE "PLAY OF TROPES" IN HUMAN LIFE

The tropes—metaphor, metonymy, synecdoche, irony—are figures of speech used to express meaning poetically. For many psychotherapists, the different tropes exist only as vague memory traces from a high school English class. However, anthropologists utilize tropes as a coherent conceptual framework to describe how people express meaning through activities and events of daily life (Fernandez, 1986, 1991).

In literature, the different tropes convey to the reader the writer's personal experience. By using a particularly evocative metaphor, the reader can more vividly enter into the writer's experience than if the writer tried to state only the facts of the matter—"I feel lonely" versus "My life has become a sepulcher." What anthropologists have noted, however, goes beyond this: People not only use tropes when writing and speaking words to others, they also *perform* tropes, that is, enact them in behavior as well as in spoken words. The performance of a trope weds unseen meaning with behavior that is visible to others, thereby providing a vocabulary for the unspoken communication of meaning.

Through the performance of tropes meaning becomes incarnate. When a trope is performed, a particular cultural world opens. Some examples of the performance of tropes include the handshake as a social greeting (demonstrating that there is no hidden weapon), purchasing a new sports car (communicating to others that one has personal wealth), celebrating a wedding anniversary (publicly recommitting to marriage by honoring its past), and a myriad of ways that worship is expressed in churches, temples, and synagogues (kneeling and bowing before God to symbolize a relation between a vassal and a king; removing shoes before entering the temple to symbolize leaving behind the contamination of the world; offering gifts and alms to the poor to symbolize the relationship between God and human beings). Understanding this "play of tropes" in human life has been a central preoccupation for anthropologists attempting to understand particular cultures (Turner, 1991).

Tropes differ from referential uses of language, that is, when words—like "car," "dog," "brown"—denote specific objects or qualities of an object. Particular words or expressions can, of course, be used in either manner. Consider "There are a lot of cars on the freeway" versus "Public transportation has lost its battle with the car," or "The leaves are already brown this autumn" versus "With winter's approach, my world turned brown."

Tropes serve a key role in human life as points of junction where physiology and language meet. Tropes engage the body as much as the mind. When one lover says to another, "You are my sunshine!" the beloved feels in her body the warmth of the sun's rays. When one whispers to a friend, "This loss is too heavy to bear," the metaphorical weight of the burden usually shows in the speaker's posture, tone of voice, and facial expression. Tropes can shift attention, posture, voice, heart rate, and blood pressure in ways that ready the body for specific action or expression—to love, to fight, to flee, or to reflect quietly (Csordas, 1994).

The performance of tropes is instrumental for constructing a society

(Durham & Fernandez, 1991). They put together a world that holds meaning and orients people in their relationships with one another. For one friend to say to another "You have my stamp of approval" makes a statement about meaning and hierarchy in that relationship, which would differ from the words "We are of one heart and one mind."

Tropes help create possibilities for spiritual experience by enabling a person to perceive every thing in the world as connected in some way to every other thing, which is a key aspect of spirituality across most cultures (Friedrich, 1991). As with the canon of steps and poses in classical ballet, tropes flow together in compositions that express spiritual experience. Rituals, prayer and meditation, beliefs, and other uses of symbolic language utilize different tropes to sustain their emotive power.

METAPHOR

Metaphors play a critical role in most forms of spirituality by posing abstract concepts in terms of images and events drawn from daily life. A metaphor is a way of conceiving one thing in terms of another. Lakoff and Johnson (1980) describe this as mapping from a source domain to a target domain. Source domains are familiar life experiences, mostly taken from the physical world, that are well understood and easy to think about, such as traveling on a journey, watching a tree extend branches into the sky, or feeling oneself to be trapped in a closed space. Target domains are abstract conceptual domains, like love, happiness, or spiritual experience: "My life with God is a long journey," "I am planted by still waters," "Life is a jail cell." A metaphor maps from experience that is well understood to experience that is not. As such, a metaphor is perhaps the most useful way we have for comprehending partially what cannot be comprehended totally: our feelings, aesthetic experiences, moral practices, and spiritual awareness (Lakoff & Johnson, 1980, p. 36). Some would say we only speak in metaphors, and many have claimed that we cannot speak of the sacred except through metaphors.

Metaphors, like poems, present multiple levels of meaning, reverberating differently with different aspects of experience (Lakoff & Johnson, 1980). By modulating cognition and body experience, a particular metaphor opens possibilities for making certain aspects of spiritual life more vivid, while obscuring alternatives. Lakoff and Johnson (1980,

p. 141) noted the countless metaphors that have been applied to love—"a rose," "fire and ice," "sweet nectar," "invisible chains," "thirst," "a cup that overfloweth." As they observed: "Because a metaphor highlights important love experiences and makes them coherent while it masks other love experiences, the metaphor gives love a new meaning. Metaphors can thus be appropriate because they sanction actions, justify inferences, and help us set goals." The use of a particular metaphor for God both helps and hinders the experience of the relationship. Addressing God as either "Eternal Creator" or "Our Mother" defines a relationship that is quite different in quality, hierarchy, and intimacy, and different yet again from one brought home by soldiers in World War II: "God is my copilot." As Paul Friedrich (1991, p. 24) once put it: "A trope may mislead in exact proportion to the amount it reveals, but that is the price of any revelation" (see also Tyler, 1978). The two-sidedness of this equation—metaphors enable, metaphors constrain—lies at the heart of work conducted with metaphors in therapy involving spiritual experience, to which we will soon turn in this chapter.

LISTENING FOR METAPHORS

Listening closely for the metaphors a person employs when talking about spiritual or religious experiences helps a clinician to craft questions and make comments that bear significance for the listener. In Chapter 2 we proposed "noticing and inquiring about specific words spoken" as a step to words opening the therapeutic conversation to talk of spiritual experience. Most often this means, as with Mary, asking questions about a person's metaphors. Sometimes a word or phrase is offered directly—"Peace, for me, is flowing with the river," or "I am wrapped in a cocoon of the Spirit." As we enter such language, we enter new worlds and the possibilities they add to our everyday experience. We may wonder with the person who speaks of "a river": "When the river hits a bend, or if there are rapids, what is it like for you? Or is it a river that is always peaceful?" Or we may ask the person who speaks of "a cocoon": "What is happening to you in this cocoon? Is it a place of rest or of transformation, or both? Does it ever seem constraining? How does one know in the dark of the cocoon when one is closer to a butterfly than a caterpillar?"

HOW METAPHORS OPEN
POSSIBILITIES FOR HEALING

Whether a metaphor is useful or not depends upon whether it can fulfill the purpose for which it was intended and whether its usage carries any unsought, adverse consequences. One task of therapy is to clarify the limitations of the dominant metaphors that influence how a person perceives, thinks, and acts in daily life. This can be done by exploring the multiple dimensions of important metaphors, as a kind of "environmental impact" study for the metaphor within the life space of the person. Rarely is a person fully aware how a particular metaphor may be placing painful limitations on possibilities for his or her life. Anthropologist James Fernandez (1986) has discussed how metaphors are often organized only within primary process thinking, such that a person, like Shakespeare's Macbeth acting upon but not understanding the witches' prophecy, is usually not cognizant of the full meaning or tropic capacity of a symbol. This awareness of the meaning of the metaphor only becomes available when sudden revelatory incidents occur in the person's life that make the meaning clear. Macbeth only appreciated the full meaning of the witches' prophecy—"Macbeth shall never be vanquished until Great Birnum Wood to high Dunsinane Hill shall come against him"—when he was staring into English swords camouflaged by Birnum Wood tree branches that the hidden soldiers carried (Act IV, scene i).

Therapy can provide a setting in which such revelatory incidents can be deliberately sought. For one person, "a river" may have become a customary metaphor for talking about the life of the spirit. However, a therapeutic conversation may clarify how useful "a river" is as a metaphor as for fostering acceptance as one flows through the vicissitudes of life, yet a poor metaphor for helping one strategize how to take charge of a situation when there are active threats of harm.

Sometimes it is a priority in therapy to search for new metaphors that can make intelligible those experiences that had seemed inchoate, beyond the reach of language. At such times, the therapist can pose tentative, candidate possibilities, but must be ready for these possibilities to be altered or rejected, as well as accepted. For instance, if a person says, "I am cold and empty. I need to feel the warmth of the Spirit again," one might ask, "What is that warmth you have known it before? Is it like the warmth when the sun comes out? Or is it like the warmth of a bonfire, that you draw near to? Or maybe it's like something different from either of these." It matters, for while one has to wait for the sun to come out, one can find the bonfire, maybe even stoke it. As it often happens, the person says, "No, it's different than either of those, it's more like. . . ."

One intent in asking questions that identify dominant metaphors is to heighten a person's conscious awareness that this is a metaphor. Often this awareness itself has profound effects, in that it so often prompts a wondering: What if I were to have chosen a different metaphor? I (Griff) remember several years ago leading a discussion of uses of metaphor with a group of students when one interjected, "But I don't use metaphors!" He had never thought of his language as anything separate from the various physical objects in his daily life to which he applied his words. By the end of the academic year, he had become skilled in crafting questions based on the therapeutic use of metaphor. As he found, mindfully selecting which metaphors bring into being preferred worlds of experience can multiply one's sense of control over one's destiny and provide a sense of accountability for how one's use of language creates the world of experience.

ELICITING MULTIPLE METAPHORS

One of the most powerful therapeutic methods is the asking of questions that do no more than elicit additional metaphors for understanding a problem. Any single metaphor, no matter how compelling, is too unidimensional in perspective to illuminate fully the richness and complexity of a lived experience. Fortunately, where there is one metaphor, there are many. There are always multiple metaphors for God, spirit, and sacred experience.

Janet was a young woman still coping with the traumatic loss of her brother several years earlier. She had described how their Methodist faith had been central in the life of their family. She attended one of our workshops in which we were asking volunteers to show how they experienced God's presence. Janet offered to show her experience psychodramatically. Starting, then stopping, Janet puzzled, "It's different at different times." I (Griff) asked if she could show the different ways. On one side of the room, she stood arms outstretched and welcoming, her face relaxed; on a different spot across the room, she stood with arms folded and face taut and harsh. I asked what names she gave each portrayal. The first she called "angelic Christ" and the second, "angry God." I asked how close or far away she felt from each. The "angelic Christ" was felt to be so close that she could touch his garments; the "angry God," however, seemed distant, as though he was on a mountain top and she was peddling her bicycle up a winding path to reach him but making no meaningful progress and becoming very fatigued. Janet felt baffled that her religious experience not only held dual metaphors for God, but that they could be so disparate.

ELABORATING A METAPHOR

Because Janet was portraying her images psychodramatically, much could be seen about the details of her metaphors from observing the contrasting postures and facial expressions she portrayed. Without the tools of psychodrama, much still can be learned about a metaphor through conversation. Curiosity is contagious. When questions about the details of a metaphor are posed, they often bring forth a new metaphor in the making, and the describer becomes as curious as the therapist in wondering how it will turn out.

I (Melissa) had been consulting with Ann about some serious family problems. On this day she appeared particularly fatigued. She explained to me that a bacterial illness she had contracted overseas years ago had once again invaded her gastrointestinal system, causing abdominal pain and sapping her energy. During the hours that she was pain-free, she said, she tried to give first to her daughters and then to her ill mother, and rarely got to the last priority, her own relaxation. Relaxing for her meant being creative, throwing pots. She was actually quite a skilled potter and had hopes of someday making this into a career, but for now just to get to the community studio regularly would suffice.

When I asked how she made it through these difficult times, she replied that prayer had been a great help to her in the past. Lately, though, she had not been able to connect with God. I wondered what was in the way. She said she felt that God was letting her down—maybe worse. In a Bible study at her church they had been studying the meaning of the chastisement of God. An explanation for Ann's suffering had been proffered: Sometimes God humbles people to help them, to instruct and strengthen their spirits. Ann was working to accept that, but it just made her more despairing. "What do you want?" she said she asked God,

"Isn't this humble enough? Do you want me to fall apart completely?" She had received neither answer nor relief from God.

"Does this God who humbles people for their own good fit with the God you have known and gone to for help in the past?" I asked her.

"Well . . . no," she said, but she also didn't disbelieve that God would chastise. I asked what that God she had known before was like. Ann began to tell me about her beliefs, but I stopped her, explaining that I was actually asking more about her experience, if she would be comfortable speaking with me about that. She nodded, and I clarified. Was being with God like being with any person she had known in her life? "No," she said, "different than that . . . bigger and quieter."

"If you were sculpting God, or God and you together, what would it look like?"

"Get this right," she said, playfully correcting me, "I'm not a sculptor, I am a potter. I believe in making beautiful but practical things. So, if I were making God . . . , " she looked up and away, considering this project, "it would be a huge earthen bowl," she crooked one arm to show me. "And I would be down here, kind of curled up, resting on the bottom." She laid the other hand in the crook of her arm.

It seemed to be a peaceful image to me, like someone cradling a tiny baby, but I was not sure. "Is it a good place to be or a bad place to be, in the bottom of the bowl?"

"Oh," she assured me, "it's good, safe, restful. Like a womb, except that I can come and go."

I told her I would like to know more about this bowl. It sounded sturdy and beautiful. I was sorry that our time was nearly gone.

"It is supposed to be sturdy, though some days it feels more like a colander, with me trickling out of the holes!" she laughed. "But I like thinking about it. Beats the heck out of thinking about God wanting to humble me."

She opened our next session with a surprise. "I have designed the bowl." And she had. "It is still big, as big as I can make, and it is rimless. It doesn't have a flat bottom, but it is rounded, so that it rocks ever so slightly, yet it is heavy and wide enough to always maintain its stability. You never have to wonder if it will tip over. That was like the image I was forming last week. But I've changed the glaze. It will have a Raku glaze. Inside will be earthy swirling shades of blues, browns, purples, and greens, very warm looking. The outside will have a shiny metallic glaze, for God, and a little spot of that same glaze will be inside, me made in God's image, being gently cradled." I didn't know about Raku, so she explained to me that with this glaze the luminous patterns emerge differently in the firing depending on how much or how little oxygen the pots are exposed to. Because of that, the potter is never fully in charge of the outcome. "You can try, but you can never control it completely," she said.

Resting and being gently rocked in the bowl became a space for a different kind of knowledge in our therapy and, I hope, in Ann's life.

SEEKING ALTERNATIVE METAPHORS

New metaphors tend not to blend with older ones but to displace them, much as the Republican and Democratic parties in Congress displace each other from their committee assignments and leadership posts depending on which party led in the congressional election returns. Openings toward therapeutic change can appear when a question invites consideration of a new or alternative metaphor. Questions that can elicit alternative metaphors include the following:

- Was this always the way you experienced God, or was it quite different when you were younger?
- Are there ever times now when you experience God in a different way?
- When your mood is different—you are not depressed, you feel inspired by life, you feel joy—does a different image or sense of God then appear at such times?

For instance, Miriam was a woman suffering diffuse pains and muscle stiffness throughout much of her body. She was frightened by the difficulties her physicians were having diagnosing her illness. Afraid that her symptoms might represent a dread disease, she felt agitated through the day and unable to sleep at night due to the anxiety she experienced. "This is a time of waiting and uncertainty?" I (Griff) asked. She nodded. I wondered how she could best fend off the anxiety that uncertainty was generating. What helped most? She said she would rely on her faith: "I believe there is a purpose to everything, and that God will take care of me." I asked whether this represented a belief that existed only within her mind, or whether God was a presence that she could feel in her body? She paused quietly, then said, "I want it to be a felt presence, but it isn't right now. I don't know how." I asked what images and stories of her experience with God brought comfort. "I don't feel comforted at all when I think about God as a 'heavenly father.' " I remembered earlier conversations in which she described long-standing conflicts with her father, whom she found intrusive and controlling when she was a child. I assumed that these struggles so contaminated her associations with "father" that imagining God as a father distanced her rather than drawing her close. I asked whether there were any other images of God that she ever held. She paused, then recalled from the Bible the story of "the Good Shepherd who watches over his flock and knows each sheep by name." When she entered into this story, she felt comfort in her body. There were also times when she thought of God as "a judge." This again made her body tense and vigilant. When she dwelled upon the story of the Elect from the Book of Revelation—the 144,000 souls supposedly chosen by God to go to heaven, with everyone else going to hell—she felt most apprehensive of all. God as "heavenly father," God as "the judge," God as "Jesus, the Good Shepherd," God as the "Ruler who selects who goes to heaven and to hell"—of these four metaphors, only the story of the Good Shepherd seemed to hold potential for bringing peace to her body amidst the waiting and uncertainty. With this recognition, she mindfully adopted an image of Jesus the Good Shepherd during her daily prayer time and spoke about the palpable difference this made in the anxiety she felt within her body.

Metaphors have no intrinsic goodness or badness. However, like tools in a tool chest, the choice of which metaphor for which situation does matter, in that a specific metaphor opens some possibilities and closes others. Because metaphors help create the worlds that are possible for us to experience, they must be chosen wisely. When they work poorly, it is a task of therapy either to expand their unexplored possibilities or to find a better metaphor as an alternative.

FROM CULTURALLY PRESCRIBED
TO PERSONALLY CHOSEN

Language shaping experience is only one side of a dialectic; culture also selects what uses of language are acceptable or unacceptable. Every metaphor has its cultural history. Janet's dual images of "angelic Christ" and "angry God" can be found in the religious imagery of three centuries of American Protestant Christianity. Similarly, Miriam's four metaphors for God each had long histories of usage in her Christian tradition. Neither Janet nor Miriam considered such metaphors as "a raindrop rejoining the ocean," which might be provided by a Buddhist, or "a Golden Mean," as in the Confucian tradition.

People are handed metaphors for the spiritual by their culture, family, or religion. For some, this transmission may so endear the metaphor to them that it fits them like their skin, and there never occurs a felt need to change it. For others though, this very act of transmission may make the wearing of the metaphor like clanging manacles, which must be unshackled for the person to be free enough to connect with others, maybe even to survive. No person has given me a more profound awareness of this than Michael Dixon. Michael is a talented therapist in British Columbia who works with young people whose lives have been captured by alcohol and substance abuse. Michael and I (Melissa) became acquainted through the annual Narrative Ideas and Therapeutic Practices conferences sponsored by Yaletown Family Therapy in Vancouver. A requisite of these conferences was a commitment by all participants to make visible the unseen influences of racism and sexism in our psychotherapy theories and practices. As a person of color whose lineage includes First Nations,[1] African, and European people, Michael has been a steady and forthright friend in engaging with me, as a white person, in recognizing and countering racist influences. Through conversations together over 3 years at the narrative conferences and letter writing in between, Michael has shared with me much of his story of spirituality. We have both been well aware that we were not just coincidental conversational partners. We were embodied, "in-cultured," "in-raced," he carrying the heritage of a people oppressed, and I the heritage of the oppressors, including that of the white Christian church that "didn't seem to want [Michael] around" when, as a child, he had nowhere else to go. For this reason I was humbled when Michael offered to continue our conversation through my interviewing him at the workshop in the conference. Afterward he sent his story in written form so that it might be useful to others.

"My earliest recollection of the introduction to God was at the age of 7½ years. I had been apprehended from my mother, along with my two brothers and my sister, who was sent to another foster home. I was enrolled in a Catholic school, St. Andrew's, and expected to go to church on Sundays. After being called Mike for 7½ years, I struggled with being called Andrew, the decision of the church and school. At home I was still called Mike, home being my foster placement."

Michael was profoundly alienated—called by a name he knew himself not to be, assigned a family and a church community he could not make his own, and handed a spiritual metaphor, a Father God he knew could not be his father.

"The Jesus and Mary were white, like my foster family," he explained as we spoke in Vancouver. "I couldn't believe God could really be my father because God was white, too. And I really was a good little altar boy, but I never could be good enough for those people. They just didn't seem to want me around." He paused, shifting from his memories to the present. "You know," his tone lifted, "I didn't realize till I was an adult that all that stuff was not even about me. There were no other people of color in the congregation! It was a huge relief when I realized that what was going on there was just racism."

Then, turning back to his boyhood again, Michael continued that he wasn't sure he wanted God as a father anyway. "I had been taught that God was punishing, so punishing that he allowed his own son to be whipped, and ridiculed and nailed to the cross, and when he asked for water they mocked him and gave him vinegar to drink. As a kid, I remember thinking that must have really hurt. I remember feeling fear and sadness, fear that I would be abused and that he wouldn't help; I mean, if God didn't care for his son, then why would he care for me? And the sadness I felt was because it was true. The foster parents were abusing me and it went on for all 5 years I lived with them, and God was not there to protect me. He proved that every day of those 5 years. Soon after I left that foster placement, I quit church. I held God in contempt and did not trust him after that. This continued till I was 34 years old."

At that time, Michael relayed, lost in drug and alcohol misuse, he turned to Narcotics Anonymous and Alcoholics Anonymous. It was suggested to him there that he find a Higher Power. He resisted this, but asked them what else that could be, if not the religion and God of his childhood. They said it was okay to have a God of his own understanding, that his Higher Power did not have to be the same as anyone else's. "I remember this guy told me, 'You've just got to find a God who's little bit slicker than Michael.'"

"And who did you find?" I inquired.

"I don't think I would say it was someone," he paused, looking off and away. I asked him if there would even be a word. "I don't know. . . . It would be . . . 'Peace.' That's it. That's it. It would just be 'Peace.' And it's an encompassing. . . . It's around me."

I asked him if there was a story to go with Peace. He returned to his treatment days. "It was suggested to me that I look back on my life, for some kind of intervention that saved me from harm in one way or another. I was asked to just consider that it might have been God. It was not hard. There was this time I was on a fishing boat going from Vancouver to Campbell River across the Georgia Straight. I was 16 years old then, 4 years after I decided that God would not be there for me. Anyways, we got into some really bad weather. The seas were rough and the wind and rain were coming down hard. The boat operator told me and one of my shipmates to go out and make sure everything was tied down so we wouldn't lose anything. I went down one side of the boat to start securing the equipment, and, while walking by the wheelhouse I grabbed what I thought was a handrail. It shifted and I let go. In seconds I found that I was being tossed about in that big ocean. But I felt no panic, no fear. I was overcome by a sense of peace. I heard someone yell out, 'Man overboard!' I could see people scrambling around on the boat in a panic. We had been towing a canoe behind the boat. I reached out to the canoe. It was like a magnet drawing me to it. At the time this happened, I never thought that God was a part of that. But today I give that moment to God. The only explanation that I can come up with for why I do this is the peace that engulfed me in the midst of chaos and fear that was happening for others."

This was a very particular kind of peace. As we talked further I asked about his present experience. "Is it around you? Inside you?" I inquired.

"It's around me. And it's like I am in the middle of it. It would be like . . . it is like being in the eye of a storm." Michael thought a while. "You can be inside that tornado, or that storm, or that hurricane. And you know that if you step out of that eye, you're going to be in that turmoil, turbulence, and a whole bunch of that kind of stuff!"

"Are you all alone there in the eye?" I wondered.

"I sense God is with me, too," Michael explained. "I'm calling it 'God' because it seems people easily relate to that word."

"But that is not your word," I added.

"It's really—it's not my word," he responded.

" 'Peace' is your word?" I checked.

Michael confirmed, "Yes, 'Peace' is what it is. It's when I'm actually . . . even in heavy feelings, if I'm feeling really sad, when I don't allow that out and I keep it in, I'm in that storm. When I allow it out, then I'm in that place of 'Peace.' And it's that process of coming out of my pain. Back to the eye."

"And it sounds like such a life-sustaining experience to be in the eye of the storm," I said. With an easy flow, we talked on for a while, and I wondered if the old stories of a punishing God ever intruded on this Peace. Michael said he had fears about that, was aware of his vulnerable places, of what would throw him back out into the storm. He also had some strategies to deal with that, some ways to find his way back to the eye. These were not just solo strategies, but community strategies.

"Because you have to get through the storm first before you can get to the peace and tranquillity," Michael explained. "I have some really close friends who have survived through the storm and still hang with me. And they . . . I don't want to sound egotistical about this . . . have reaped the benefit of the peace I have, that I am able to share with them."

The culture that Michael was thrown into as a child prescribed a metaphor of a punitive God, a father who could not be his father, promoted by a church and family that produced isolation. The metaphor he found in the community of healing, the metaphor of Peace, could be felt in his body, as he recalled the story, and in the moment he was speaking. It has just the opposite effect of the metaphor handed to him. It connects, sustaining not only Michael but others, reaching out to calm them in the chaos of the storm.

At our last correspondence, Michael used both words at different times, God and Peace. I think that still, if we ever get to speak of this together again, unless he urges me to do otherwise, I will not speak in the metaphor of the Father God. I will speak in the metaphor of Peace.

A therapist thus can inquire not only how a particular metaphor is shaping a person's experience, but also how the person's culture is influencing which metaphors can be easily chosen for the discourse of daily life. Here culture means "the shared understandings people hold, that are sometimes, but not always, realized, stored, and transmitted in their language," that characterize a family, a workplace, a region, or a people of a particular ethnicity (Quinn, 1991, p. 57). Each culture encourages use of certain metaphors while discouraging use of others. Cultural values, institutional rules, poetic traditions, and social situations all play their roles in this selection. Which metaphors can be experienced as real is largely governed by constraints from family, ethnic, and religious traditions. For this reason, a particular person typically has multiple metaphors, but only a limited number of them can be applied to God and spirit in a manner that feels real.

In public conversation, the officially sanctioned metaphors of the culture predominate, and the unique metaphors of each person's private experiences might never be guessed. For instance, if one were to listen in on Sunday morning services attended by most of the participants in our Mississippi research project, one would hear the congregation say the Lord's Prayer beginning with the words "Our Father who art in Heaven." Initially, this metaphor was echoed in the research setting. When we asked participants, "What is God like?" many people indeed started their responses with "like a heavenly father." However, we heard a wide range of images of God once we entered further into the conversations. As we inquired about the specific instances in which people had intensely experienced the presence of God, the answers to "What is God like?" became as varied as the lives of the participants:

"Like a warm cocoon, enclosing me as the world falls in around me."
"Like an exasperated mother whom I have disappointed and been ungrateful to too often."
"Like a nourishing, flowing river that comes to me, the parched dry river bed, and gives me life."
"Like an Olympic coach who does not model my task for me, but delights in my potential and pushes me to it."
"Like the silence in a deep, waterless cavern where I finally arrive after swimming down through a troubled lake."
"Like a nursing mama who is happy to be close to me and always has plenty of milk. As I lay my head on her breast, I feel her breathing and hear her heartbeat and I am calmed."

After eliciting people's metaphors we asked them, "What human relationship in your life most reminds you of the one you have described with God?" Some who had begun with a description of a kind father God did, indeed, recall their own kind fathers or grandfathers. But many others who initially described a kind father-God then associated to relationships with women:

"My mother, who kept calm and kept things in perspective."

"Our housekeeper, who taught me about love that lasted through hard situations."

"My grandmama, who always had a lap available."

"My women friends who are closer than family, who confront me, encourage me, and support me no matter what."

"My other mamma, my Italian Catholic neighbor lady, who always had room at her table for one more, whose house was liberatingly messy and filled with laughter, who, when she gave of herself, became more, not less, of herself."

Though the publicly spoken metaphors, constrained and influenced by culture, were masculine, a wealth of varied, layered, deeply felt feminine metaphors could be heard in these personal associations. These and other experiences have taught us to look past the public and more general metaphor to the private and particular experience.

Tracey helped teach me (Melissa) this, for her private meaning was so joltingly different from the understanding I assumed from her public metaphor. I met with her the day after she had been to church. Though she was a diligent worker, she could never make enough as a nurse's aide to meet the necessities for the three children for whom she was the sole support. This meant she did without for herself. Some friends at her church had collected money and had surprised her with bags of groceries. Her head was down, and she said she was still feeling the pain and embarrassment of receiving their gifts.

"I know these gifts came from God. I guess I should be thanking God, instead of complaining," she said. "Those people didn't have to give me anything." But in her eyes was only humiliation, not gratitude. "I'll just have to pray about this some more."

"Could you tell me about when you pray? What is your experience of God? Not what you believe, but what you experience," I requested.

"I'm a Christian. I really do believe in God, but it's so hard. I don't hear him or see him or feel him. I know other people do. I have a hard time with God."

"So when you pray, you can't see or hear or feel God, but what do you feel like?"

"Like I am a tiny speck calling out, 'God, I need to see you.'"

"You are tiny. So how far away is this one to whom you are calling?"

"Far, far away."

"Can we get up, I'll play your role, and you show me how far and what you can make out of this one far, far away?"

(I assumed the role of Tracey, scrunched down like a speck, and called out "God, I need to see you!")

Then I walked over to consult with Tracey, at the edge of the room. "So what is here? What can you see of God?" I asked.

"God is like a light, very bright, too bright to look at. I can't look at him."

"What kind of light? What color? Yellow or white? And glaring, but is it warm?"

"It's a cold light," she said, "like the one in a doctor's office. You don't want to be there, but you have to be there."

"Is there a voice that goes with the light? Words?"

"No, all the words have to come from me. You know, like having a spotlight shined on you on a stage."

"So you can be seen well, in detail, but you can't see anything out there but the glare?"

She nodded.

"And is it like there's someone operating the spotlight? Can you imagine what the operator is like behind the spotlight?"

"He's just waiting to see what I'm going to do wrong next. Like my dad, I know," she said in a bored voice. "People think God is like their dad. I've heard that before. But it doesn't help me."

"Well I don't know about that theory," I responded tentatively, "but in whose presence do you feel this way—like they can see you but you can't see them? Like you don't know if they hear you? Like they are waiting to see what you will do wrong next?"

"Actually, that is like I feel with my dad. I mean, I love him," Tracey explained, "but he just doesn't let me know him. And that's how I feel when I pray."

"No wonder you don't want to pray. But still you pray. Have you ever had any other experience of God?" I inquired.

"No, never," she said.

"But still you pray. And you think it was God who answered your prayers this week, who got money to you?" I was trying to understand.

"I know it was God because it was so unexpected. It was out of the blue," Tracey explained.

"Did it seem to come from the light?"

"No, it came out of left field. I really wasn't expecting it."

"Left field"—I thought of a baseball game. I imagined God coming in with a surprise from left field. A much more welcoming metaphor than a cold, glaring, silent light.

"Gee, I'm guessing that in that baseball game you might have thought God would be the pitcher or the coach, but not some surprise coming in from left field."

"What? You're losing me." She reined me in from my metaphorical wanderings.

"Well, tell me what this is like—something coming in from left field. That would be coming at you from . . . ?"

She gestured to her left and behind her.

"Oh, out of your line of vision?"

"Yeah, just someone approaching me to help."

"What is this God like, the one who comes over from left field?"

Tracey sat shaking her head back and forth, looking puzzled, thinking. "Attainable, close in. Maybe approachable." She sat pensively and silently, looking first to her left, then in the direction of the cold light. "I'm just thinking of the difference in the two. This is so different. I don't know. I've never seen this one."

"Perhaps you were blinded by the light. Maybe this is a good place to leave it tonight," I said. "It looks like there's lots more to think about, like I'm dying to ask you what that one from the left field sees when he approaches you, but for now just 'attainable' and 'close in,' that's a lot."

"I'll be looking to my left all the time now," she said.

"And I can't wait to hear what you'll see when you look to your left."

I sat alone to complete my notes after Tracey left our meeting, astonished and grateful for the conversation. I knew that it had been a near miss. "Light" is a word for God that I hold dear and have held so long that, for me, light *is* warmth in the cold, comfort, a guide and a safety in the darkness. "God is like a light," Tracey said. "Yes," I thought. "I understand. I know." But I knew nothing of her light, the light in a doctor's examining room, a light that brings the expectation of pain, a light like a spotlight, one that brings isolating scrutiny. In this realization, I was grateful to all my colleagues (especially Combs & Freedman, 1990) who have urged me to inquire about words and metaphors, to value the not-knowing more than the knowing, and grateful to Tracey for releasing me from the confines of my experience.

And what, I wondered, will be the story that will develop of God who comes out of left field, a story that is just beginning to come into language? If Tracey develops that story in her relationship with God, who will join and support her—perhaps the church friends who bought the groceries for her? Could it even be that her inscrutable father would be happy for her to meet the One who comes in from left field? What difference will that One make in how she relates to herself, her financial struggles, her church, and even to that harsh and scrutinizing light?

NOTE

1. The term "First Nations" originates and is most widely used in Canada. This designation draws attention to a particular geographical positioning of people and reveals a lack of otherwise assumed (by members of the dominant culture) homogenization. It underscores the diversity of tribes via the acknowledgment and various affiliations and separations between each sovereign nation. As such, "First Nations" represents a more inclusive and accurate term for identifying indigenous peoples of Canada (M. Roguski & S. Motch, personal communication, August 2001).

Chapter Four

Stories of Spiritual Experience

Several weeks after Mary had told the story of the Palm Sunday storm (see Chapter 2), she opened a therapy session by stating that she was "stalled" in her marriage. She could not go any further in opening her own heart until she knew more of what Frank was thinking. He talked with her about lots of things, she said, "but not about his innermost feelings." I offered, as I often had before, to include Frank in our conversations. This time she accepted.

When I (Melissa) met Frank, I could see why Mary wanted to try to stay in this marriage. Frank was genuinely sorry for his past actions, acutely aware of the pain he had caused Mary and that her trust would take a long time to rebuild. When I inquired about his own concerns, he replied that his greatest fear was that he was not worthy.

"Not worthy?" I inquired.

"Yes, not worthy," he said. "That I'll get there and she will see me and she'll discover that I'm not the one. That I just don't have what it takes." Mary began to seethe. She was worn out, she said, with Frank's low self-esteem. She couldn't fix it. She wanted him to take care of it. When he said things like this it made her think he would burn out before he got there. I wondered what "getting there" meant. Frank said it meant changing into the man God wanted him to be. "I'm working at it

81

every day, but not enough hours. I get so tired. Either I'm not changing fast enough or it doesn't show enough, or both, probably both."

Mary had already acknowledged the positive changes she had seen. They mattered, but she needed to see more. Frank said he knew he was changing, but the biggest changes were on the inside, and became obvious only slowly to others. I wondered if he imagined that God could see these changes. "Yes," he said, "for better or for worse, God sees all of me. I can't choose to slowly reveal myself to him. Yes, he knows I'm changing." I asked Frank how he experienced God responding when he saw these changes. "I don't anthropomorphize God that way. God is more like a force to me, more like nature. But I'm afraid he's disappointed in me."

Frank had used the pronoun "he," but had said he didn't experience God in human form. I could not come up with a more imaginative, nonanthropomorphic question, so I asked Frank, "If there were words from God for this disappointment that you fear, what would they be?"

Looking back now on our conversation, I believe it was in response to this question that Frank spiraled down into a story that had *lived him* in the past. "Oh," his voice dropped to an almost inaudible level, "D+, C–, I guess." I thought I had misheard and asked him to repeat his reply. Frank's volume increased a bit, but his head lowered. "D+, C–," he repeated.

"A grade?" I was puzzled. "God would give you a grade?"

Mary turned to him and sympathetically sighed. "That's never stopped tormenting you, has it?" Then she turned to me—"It's an old, old story," she explained, "a job evaluation, years ago."

I could imagine how devastating the evaluation must have been 20 years ago. But why, I wondered aloud, had it lasted so long and become so strong? How had this particular event become a key story? Frank then told me about his legacy of unworthiness. His father, a smart, charming traveling salesman, was a womanizer who left Frank and his mother when Frank was 5. Although he didn't see his father often, Frank knew he was disappointed to have a son who pursued music and literature instead of following him, competing in the business world. Frank said that he knew the D+, C– wasn't really God's voice, but still he heard it. "It's like God might say to me, even today, like my dad, 'You just don't have what it takes, Frank. You have become the product of your fears. I can't really help you. Maybe you can help yourself, but I can't help you.' "

The three of us talked together a while about the power those old stories sometimes held over Frank, and over his relationships with Mary and with God. When I asked Frank if he ever heard anything different from God, he said no. Even so, he said, he didn't believe that the critical voices he heard were true. At the end of our session, he was bent over, as if bearing a burden. We all felt sad. Frank seemed to want to reassure me and Mary. "I'll be all right. That was just emotion, only emotion talking," he said. "It's not what I believe."

The weight of the discouragement that Frank and Mary bore seemed to hang in my office after they left our meeting. I felt called to re-examine the conversation and my participation in it and used the lens of narrative therapy to do so.

NARRATIVE APPROACHES TO THERAPY

In all of the work we each do, but most centrally in working with stories, we are influenced by narrative theory. Our book *The Body Speaks* (Griffith & Griffith, 1994) is informed by these ideas. Because a full discussion of narrative approaches is beyond the scope of this book, we refer the reader to an extensive literature that has become available in recent years (Epston, 1989; Epston & White, 1992; Freedman & Combs, 1996; Freeman et al., 1997; Friedman, 1993, 1995; Gilligan & Price, 1993; Hoyt, 1996; Madigan & Law, 1998; Madsen, 1999; McNamee & Gergen, 1992; Monk et. al., 1997; Parry & Doan, 1994; Smith & Nylund, 1997; Tomm, 1989; Weingarten, 1995a, 1995b; White, 1989a, 1989b, 1995a, 1995b, 1997, 2000a; White & Epston, 1990; Zimmerman & Dickerson, 1996).

Here we will consider five ways in which the narrative metaphor guides our work with spiritual stories:

1. To a great extent we are *lived by* our stories. While we are always shaping and creating our life stories, we are also shaped by the stories we tell ourselves and are told by others about who we are and can be (Epston et al., 1992; Gergen & Gergen, 1985; Mair, 1988). Our stories influence to whom we are bound and from whom we are separate.

2. These stories are not just independent creations by us or our families, but are made within the forces of society, beginning before our birth in the ways our ancestors treated others and were treated. Indeed,

our stories precede us not only through our bloodlines, but through the forerunners of our racial groups, social class, nationality, gender, and religious group. Previous and present distribution of power among these groups determines "who gets a say about what." In this way the discourses, values, politics, and standards of the society in which we live continually open space for or constrain the self-narratives we can entertain (Madigan & Law, 1998; Shotter, 1993a; White, 1989a).

3. There is always more lived experience than has yet been put into our stories of ourselves. There are always multiple—and sometimes contradictory—stories of our identity and relationships, our limits and possibilities (Bruner, 1986; Geertz, 1986).

4. Some narratives about our lives are already known, readily articulated to others, and easily received by them. Some are known to us, but difficult to speak to others. Still others are not yet formed, existing only as sketchy outlines at the edge of awareness. Therapy is a forum to entertain both stories made and stories in the making, and to reflect on which stories one desires to be guided by and which stories one desires to resist (Freedman & Combs, 1996).

5. Therapists have a particular privilege and responsibility to the people who consult with them as both witness and co-creator of stories of their lives (Epston & White, 1990; White, 1990). Due to power imbalances both within the therapy relationship and within the larger culture in which the therapy occurs, the therapist is called to "radical listening" (Weingarten, 1995b) that listens first and foremost to what the storyteller thinks about the story he or she is telling. The teller's expertise about its meaning and primacy are privileged above the therapist's impressions.

Considering this responsibility in relation to the session with Frank and Mary raises several questions. How is it that the story of a critical, harsh God, and not a story of the God in whom Frank really believed had been told in our session? Did the way we conversed loosen or tighten the D+, C– story's grip on Frank? What discourses in our culture were at work in sinking Frank into this story?

I regard it as a mistake to have asked Frank a second time to describe his experience of God in human-like form. He had said the first time that this was not his way of experiencing God, but I retained this characterization in the question. Frank still heard the "D+, C–" from God, even though he realized that his hearing was affected by voices of other authority figures—his boss and his father. Perhaps he made good use of my mistake. Perhaps Frank's putting those mundane terms on the lips of God made for an unbelievable incongruity, loosening the power of that story over Frank's life. Narrative approaches would further influence me not to stop at this immediate circle of Frank's father and boss, but to consider that they, like Frank, were affected by standards and specifications for manhood that value men for success in commerce and competition, and give short shrift to men whose passion is for the arts. If I had given Frank the opportunity to speak to this, he might have explicitly rejected these specifications, and might have had much to say about their widespread impoverishing effects. After all, he seemed to reject them with his life, tutoring young men in music, rigorously studying Dante, serving as an encouraging, nurturing leader of a men's Bible study. However, even though Frank and I did not converse about this perspective, it had therapeutic utility for me, informing me of what Frank was up against. A narrative perspective intensifies the question: When surrounded by a culture that reinforces the image of this critical, specifying, disappointed God, how did Frank hold fast to the knowledge that it was, as he said, "not what I really believe"?

His statement suggested an alternative story, but to make this alternative full and rich, I would need to know more of the God in whom he did believe and to hear the stories—landscapes, plots, and characters—that had made this God alive and real for Frank. After that session I made a note to remember that Frank had said he did not relate to God as a greater, wiser human. When he tried, his human-like God was shaped and scripted by the story of his father, his boss, and his culture. I needed to respect that and try to enter his experience, rather than fitting his experience into easy metaphors. The couple's therapy went along, gradually building trust and hope, for several months before the subject of God came up again.

Then some events outside their marriage triggered Mary's pain and fears once more. It was hard for her to feel safe or close with Frank and hard for her to tell him why. Again, she said, she first needed to hear more of his innermost thoughts. Frank responded, "I know she wants me to tell her more, but what can I say? Talk is cheap. Only my actions will convince her and that just takes time." Mary wanted to be included in some of Frank's spiritual developments. She needed a window into them to continue to nourish her hope for their marriage. When Frank said, "Talk is cheap," we all knew it was code for his commitment not to be slick like his father. However, that left us in a bind. Words were needed to build trust, yet words were inherently untrustworthy.

I admitted to realizing how much they were suffering and to being uncertain of how to help them in that moment. Because they prayed and turned to God with their daily concerns, it seemed quite natural to somewhat playfully ask them, "If you were to have God for a therapist this morning, instead of being stuck with just me, do you have any ideas about how the conversation might go?"

Frank said he couldn't know. His explanation recalled the previous session to my mind. "I can't imagine that because God is not like a person for me. I just can't anthropomorphize God. I don't have the words to speak about my experience, though I know it's real. But maybe God will speak through you," he said encouragingly.

"I don't think so," I laughed. "I don't sense any inspirations coming on, but would it be okay today for me to ask you a bit more about your experience of God?"

He nodded, and said he learned about God "through the Word," but the place he most experienced God, most knew God's quiet surrounding presence, was in nature.

I could see nature as he spoke. Outside my big office window, in my line of vision but not in theirs, was a path leading into spring green trees. I spoke my wish that we could be out there now, in nature, on this cool misty morning. If we could be, I wondered aloud—and if Frank could sense God's quiet surrounding presence—how might that influence his thoughts about this conversation? Frank replied that it probably would influence his thoughts, but he didn't know just how. It was lovely out there, though, he noted.

I proposed that, though we could not go out, we might just be quiet for a while and look into the trees, and if thoughts happened to come, they could be spoken. Frank and Mary, familiar with contemplation and comfortable with silence, readily agreed and turned to face the trees.

We all looked into the forest for such a long time that I thought we would end the session in silence, which might have been a fine conclusion, but then Frank turned back into the room, calling the conversational circle into being. His eyes were brimming as he began to speak. "Do you know the part in the novel, *Les Misérables*, the part where Jean Valjean has stolen the priest's silver candlestick? The priest was kind enough to take him in, give him bread and a place to sleep, then Jean

Valjean leaves, repaying the priest for his hospitality by stealing from him—do you remember? . . . And the police catch Jean Valjean, recognize the candlestick, and bring him back to the priest. The priest, who could and should condemn him, tells the police, 'No, this was once my candlestick, but it is his now. He didn't steal it. It was a gift. I gave it to him.' " Frank paused. He wept quietly. "And Jean Valjean goes from that moment and is a changed man. He spends his life doing wonderful things for people, all only possible because of the grace of the priest, the priest he stole from. It's grace, that kind of grace. That's the best I can tell you about my experience . . . just grace."

How different the story of God Frank told on that day was from the one he told months ago. The first was a story of despair, the second of hope. Each involved a recognition of a failure, but one led to an old, stagnant evaluation, and one to grace and a changed man. What made for the difference in these tellings? Time, perhaps. Frank had come to know his God in a deeper way during those months, and had more steady, faithful hours logged in the marriage, but perhaps the way the stories were called forth made a difference. When my earlier questions forced Frank to respond in a form that he had said was not his own—a human-like God with face and voice—Frank was swayed by the recollected voices of men. However, when invited to go to his own source—nature—and when the imperative to speak at all was genuinely lifted, Frank was able to passionately articulate his experience. Now the window to his inner life was opened a bit wider for Mary.

STORIES AND TIME

Stories differ from metaphors. Through stories, people give meaning to their experience of temporality and personal actions (Polkinghorne, 1988, p. 11). Stories describe sequences of particular events; they have a beginning, a middle, and an end.

The organizing metaphor for Frank's story in the first session was "unworthiness." This metaphor served as an anchor for multiple stories about the worthiness or unworthiness he felt in relationships with Mary, his father, and his former boss. "Unworthiness" as an isolated metaphor would do no more than establish a vantage point from which Frank might view his life. Its associated stories are needed in order for the past,

present, and future of Frank's life to unfold. A story, or narrative, organizes human experiences into episodes that make sense over a stretch of
time.

Stories connect multiple metaphors and different kinds of metaphors, with each metaphor bringing forth its unique world of possibilities and constraints. A single sentence from the account of Frank's conversation with Mary—"Yes, not worthy," he said. "That I'll get there
and she will see me and she'll discover that I'm not the one. That I just
don't have what it takes."—holds five different metaphors: "worthy" (a
metaphor of commerce), "get there" (a journey metaphor), "not the
one" (a metaphor of idyllic love), "don't have what it takes" (a metaphor of measurement against a standard). Each of these metaphors
repositions the listener a bit differently, flowing together as do the notes
that make a musical theme.

Although a story relies upon its embedded metaphors, it transcends
the limits of each metaphor's world. A metaphor opens a monological
perspective, a unitary world in which all the parts fit and are consistent
with one another (Lakoff & Johnson, 1980). Alternative realities cannot
be imagined within the limits of the unitary reality of any particular metaphor. A story, however, can link multiple metaphors to its story line,
even some that are inconsistent with one another. The plot of a story comes to resemble an electrical cord with its metaphors attached along the
way like spotlights, each pointed in a different direction and each illumi-
nating a different patch of the darkness. As the multiple perspectives of
its different metaphors are brought into relation with one another, the
story introduces a new, encompassing version of reality.

Stories make individual events comprehensible by locating them
within the whole to which they contribute (Polkinghorne, 1988, p. 18).
Ordinarily, both the conversation 20 years past with his boss and the
Hugo novel read years ago would have faded to blurs in Frank's memory. Instead each persisted, standing in sharp detail. For different reasons, each story became imbued with meaning, promising reproach or
redemption for Frank's life.

Like metaphors, stories are intrinsically neither good nor evil. By
our individual and cultural values, we determine them to be "good" or
healthy or healing when we believe they point to solutions for life's
problems, when they provide meaning, when they engender communion
with others, and when their real effects on self and others move toward
justice. We consider them "bad," unhealthy, or pathogenic when they

obscure solutions, when they foster despair, or when they isolate people or generate animosity among them. Hence a story that is "good" to one person's ears may be "bad" to another's. Both Mary's and Frank's stories illustrate this. Through the dual filters of my own life experiences and my understanding of Frank and Mary, I heard inspiring stories that provided a sense of connection and hope. Other therapists may have heard Mary's story of protection in the storm as one that endorsed an oppressive religion, hiding the problem and forestalling the solution by fostering the illusion in Mary that she had protection and help when she was vulnerable and alone. They may have heard Frank's story of transformative grace as an unrealistic romantic identification with Jean Valjean, ignoring the messy realities of his life. The "radical listening" to which Weingarten (1995b) refers respects how Mary and Frank heard their own stories, how *they* each desired these stories to inform their lives. A narrative perspective would also inform me, as their therapist, to be authentic with them as to whether I could honor their stories and desires, possibly even to tell them the influences that fostered or hindered me. When we offer to others the context of our own responses, it is to give them the benefit of informed options, so that they can determine whether or not our thoughts are relevant for their situation.

CO-CREATING STORIES

We participate in the co-creation of stories by our way of listening, our questions, and our reflections. As stories are told, the response of silence, raised eyebrows, leaning forward, or distractedly doodling becomes an edit, a punctuation, influencing the teller to shift topics, say more, soften a point, or cease speaking. Appreciative intense attention may be the most powerful way of all to co-create stories. Other ways to participate in story making, commonly termed reauthoring in the narrative literature (Epston, 1989; Freedman & Combs, 1995; White, 1989a, 1989b), involve questions that are crafted to assist a person in choosing which stories to live within, and how these stories can best be told, disseminated, and honored. We prefer to speak of co-creating because it represents the wide spectrum of this activity and reminds us of its constancy, not only in therapy but in life. Hence, even as we engage in therapy, we are aware that other co-creating influences are at work, both helpful and harmful ones, inside and outside of our therapeutic relationship.

Narrative approaches have highlighted the influences that constrain or liberate the stories people speak and are lived by. The power holders in any culture favor particular stories as the guides for the living of life, whether that culture is a family, a community, or a nation. These favored, or dominant, stories, are the ones that would be expected to appear in a conversation. Marginalized, or nondominant, stories are those that may also exist but typically are ignored or, in some cases, may be literally prohibited from being told. As with the secular stories in a culture, there are certain stories of spiritual experience that are expectable ones, easy to elicit, tell, and hear because they are undisturbing. They fit the social context within which the teller and listener are interacting. There are other stories that for the same reasons usually go unnoticed and unspoken.

Jane was telling me (Griff) about her new experience of spirituality. She had volunteered to participate with us in our research project (Griffith et al., 1995). In the interview, Jane had already described the image of God that had constrained her past spiritual life, one of an elusive "Rescue God," to whom she was always calling out but who never really delivered her from the stresses of her life. She was contrasting this with her current experience. "Now, when I think of God, I think of abundance," she said, opening her arms wide, "abundance of love, abundance of presence, abundance of beauty." She added that she was a babe to this abundance, and had only known it for the last few years.

"When do you experience this abundance?" I asked her.

"All the time! When do I not? I experienced it last night when my friend brought over a great suit that she had bought for me in the thrift shop. I experience it right now in having this interesting conversation with you."

I asked her further about when the shift occurred. She began to tell a story, one that she said she had kept to herself for quite a while, but had recently begun to entrust to others in her Baptist church and friendship circles.

> "Well, I had what I guess people would call a mystical event. It was with my friend, my next door neighbor, who was dying of AIDS. At that time, we had not become good friends, and I was trying to judge how much he wanted my friendship. . . . He was a professional seamstress, and I was making some drapes, so I asked him if I could borrow his tables to cut out some panels. He said, 'Why don't you come over and I'll show you how to do it right?' Like I told you

earlier, I was in a lot of emotional distress at that time. Things in my life just were not working out, and I didn't know what I was going to do. I needed God. I was in almost constant turmoil, so going over to sew with my neighbor seemed like, if nothing else, a good distraction. In the course of that evening, this person that I did not really know very well at all, unsolicited, just began to tell me his story while he was sewing. As he sewed I noticed how beautifully, how gracefully, he moved. It was like an art form. Really, the entire evening was like being in a work of art, something holy. We went on and on and we weren't even tired. Around midnight, he was showing me how to use a particular machine. I was standing next to him watching. I was not in any particular state of mind. I was just watching him. That's when the experience came over me. I was standing, behind him, looking over his shoulder. This sensation, this warm feeling, came over me. I looked at my friend and he appeared to be glowing! I believe it was an inner sensation, like I was seeing with my eyes what I was feeling inside me. I said to myself, 'Wow, this is amazing! Finally, God has come to me. Come in this gay, AIDS-stricken man. Sewing!' "

Jane added that she wouldn't say that everything in her life fell into place after that. Far from it. But as the friendship with her neighbor deepened, and as she stayed close to him through his last days, her perspective shifted from one of looking to be rescued from difficulties, to one of expecting abundant grace and a gift in the midst of difficulties.

We think about Jane's story as a marginalized, nondominant narrative of spirituality for several reasons: the mystical elements of seeing a glow, the physical experience of warmth, and the appearance of God through a man who, in that particular culture, was considered dubiously credentialed to serve that purpose. Dominance of stories is a culture-specific phenomenon, so it is risky to speculate what may be a dominant or marginal narrative for another person. The two of us venture to make a judgment about this story because we and Jane had much commonality in our cultural backgrounds. But better is to listen to Jane's words. She gave a clue that could inform a therapist from any culture of the story's dominance status when she said that she "kept this" to herself for a while, that only later she "entrusted" it to a few friends. When I (Melissa) called Jane to ask her about publishing her story, I explained this idea of marginalized stories and asked if that had anything to do with her keeping the story to herself for a while.

"Heck, yeah," she said. "I was afraid it was too New Age-y, too wacky."

I inquired, "You were questioning it yourself, or . . . ?"

"No, no, I knew it was real," she clarified. "I didn't want people to think I was wacky. Also, it was pretty intimate. I felt protective of it. I think I didn't want it to be held up to the eyes of a skeptic. I didn't want to have to prove it to anyone."

"Was it mostly the mystical part that you thought folks might be skeptical about, or was it also about God coming to you through a gay man?" I asked her.

"Oh, it was both. But what a great vehicle for God! To lots of people, he was doubly untouchable, both gay and with AIDS, and I wanted to protect him, not to put him in a position of being before skeptics."

Jane's words elucidate what people encounter in speaking marginalized stories, the fear of being written off, the possible intrusion on intimate experiences, the risk of being called on to prove themselves, and, most tenderly, the peril of participating in hurting others they love.

I thanked her for letting us write about her story, and she said, "Thank my friend."

COMPOSITION AND CHOICE

One aspect of co-creating stories focuses on the process of composing stories out of one's experience. A second aspect focuses on the relationship between the person and stories that are told. Jane's composition involved actions and commentary. She reported events that happened—her neighbor's invitation, their cutting fabric together, and her observation of his graceful movements—while her interpretation ("The whole evening was like being in a work of art, something holy") spoke to the pattern she began to witness that connected all these events. Jane implied how she related to the contrasting stories she told. She wanted distance from the disappointing stories of a God who was supposed to, but never did, help her escape difficulties. Her nicknaming him the "Rescuer God" seemed to be a way of gently poking fun and reminding herself of this pitfall. On the other hand, she was making clear decisions to let the story of abundance live through her, by opening to a full friendship with her neighbor and even by her enthusiastic participation in the research interview. Determining to tell the story to listeners who are likely to believe, appreciate, and encourage her—friends, church members, us—and her choice to let us tell it here becomes yet another way to meld her identity with her story.

Co-creating stories in therapy focuses on the back-and-forth of quiet appreciation of the teller's composition and on asking questions out of curiosity that introduce new distinctions, elicit stories yet unnoticed, and prompt reflection. The therapist serves as a consultant who assists a person in articulating his or her experience in ways that establish meaning, facilitate relatedness with others, and maximize personal agency (White, 1988). By asking questions that externalize and objectify stories whose influence has been to isolate, disempower, or demoralize, a therapist aids a person in choosing how he or she can live differently in relation to such stories. The following illustrations show some directions that can be taken with stories of spiritual experience.

Eliciting Alternative Stories

One can always assume that, noticed or unnoticed, multiple stories are available for the work of the therapy. Bringing forward to center stage a story that has gone unnoticed can become the most important step in the therapy.

A college professor spoke bitterly about the family from which he came. "We were a dysfunctional family." In rapid succession, he told me (Griff) different accounts from his childhood: His father drank too heavily and beat him and his mother; his mother was intrusive; his siblings fought and argued. Moreover, he had suffered from severe asthma, missing long periods of school.

As the professor told his story, I puzzled that it did not seem to fit the distinguished man before me. I finally asked, "How did your story come to have the ending it has had? The story you have been telling might as well have ended with your being jailed as a juvenile delinquent, or with your committing suicide as a depressed young adult, or with your becoming an alcoholic. . . . How is it that you came to be a scholar, to have a wonderful family, to have a rich life in which you have given much to others and they to you?"

He paused thoughtfully for a few moments. Then he responded, "I'm not religious now. But I think what made the difference during those years was that God was very real for me. God was dependable. God was present in a way my family members would never be. At a cer-

tain point, it was like I realized that if my life would amount to anything, I had to make it without my family, so I exercised even though I
had asthma; I studied; I learned how to dress appropriately and how to
act in social situations. I believed God was with me."

As a young adult, he became disillusioned with the reluctance of his
church to confront basic issues of social justice. His passion gradually
shifted from participation in an organized church with its worship of
God to political activism. At this time, 25 years later, he had almost forgotten the early origins of his moral commitment.

The professor had started by telling me a story that fit well within a
common metanarrative in the culture of Western psychotherapy. In the
discourse of psychotherapy, an account of parental failure, abandonment, and neglect ordinarily brings an empathic response from a therapist and a request for more details about loss, abuse, and deprivation. It
is an underlying assumption that the problem of the therapy can be explained in part by these losses. Perhaps he was surprised that I did not
respond in that vein. When asked instead about the gap in his story, he
searched for and located yet another narrative that could better encompass both his childhood of deprivation and his adulthood of accomplishments. This alternative story introduced a new character—his God—
whom he drew from forgotten shadows of his past.

Which was more valid—the story of the professor as a neglected
son in a dysfunctional family, or his story of being sustained by an
ever-present God? I supposed that they both were valid accounts, in
the sense that both were real for him and consistent with accepted
facts of his life. As a therapist, however, I wanted to know the effects
of highlighting one version or the other in his canon of "Who I am as
a person" stories. How does each story influence what he subsequently
can witness in his life and the lives of others? Which grants him a
sense of self-appreciation? Which helps him to act effectively in his
world? Which opens more possibilities for him to solve the marital
conflict that brought him into therapy?

Anchoring Chosen Stories

Jean, in 1 year, had experienced loss at almost every level. Her mother
had died, her father had developed Alzheimer's disease, dramatic workplace shifts had severely diminished support for her, and her marriage, a
secure source of joy for many years, now felt threatened. For several

months she had spoken with me (Melissa) about having a hard time "coming back" to herself. She wanted to respect both her anger and sadness, but instead she felt controlled by them. "I used to be a person who gets excited about a beautiful sunshiny day," she said. "Now I may not even notice it."

I had not spoken much with Jean her about spirituality. Early on in the therapy, she had told about being raised in a very religious family, and said that was not for her. For her, spirituality was different—very personal, very private. It brought her tranquillity and a sense of connectedness, she said, but it was not always easy to find these days. She did not want to talk about it, but said she would let me know if the time came when she did.

Accustomed to herself as a competent, steady, secure, fun woman, Jean felt racked by the heaviness she felt and the inconstancy of her emotions. She had suffered for several months, and we both were worried that nothing she or we together were doing seemed to bring significant, sustained relief. So when she came in one evening, her face, body, and voice relaxed, reporting peaceful sleep, I wanted to know what had happened. She explained, backing up in time to set the context, "I think I finally know what did happen to me: I lost my faith."

"Your faith in . . . " I floundered.

"In life," she explained. "I lost my faith in life. Trusting life. For a long time now, I have trusted life. I lost that. And now, I have regained it."

Recalling her earlier wishes, the private nature of her spirituality, I asked if this was a time to talk about it, or if it would be best kept private. She said it would be fine to talk, so I asked about her regaining faith, trusting life. She described it with words like "letting go of control," trusting that she should just "do this day" and the next thing would be clear to her. She said that it was about being able to just "go with the flow." In fact, she recalled that we had spoken months earlier about spirituality and that when she was in touch spiritually she could go with the flow.

"So this a familiar feeling, a familiar ability, to go with the flow?" I asked her.

"Oh, yeah, *it is me*, it is the way I have been in so much of my life. Other people have been amazed at how I could do it, you know," she laughed. "I've had some pretty wild things to go with the flow with, and sometimes, I have been amazed myself." She looked up and away.

"Are you thinking of one of those times now?" I wondered.

"Yes, I was, I was remembering when my son was 16, and—this was years before lots of kids were doing this—he dyed his hair green and spiked it. I didn't know he was doing this, and I walked by the bathroom and there he was, looking in the mirror, preening and adjusting the last spikes. I was horrified! But I knew that would be no good, so I took a few steps away before I expressed my horror and instead I asked myself, 'Now if I were going with the flow what would I do?' I went back down to the bathroom and said to him, 'I'm just amazed at how you do that. Would you teach me how to do my hair like that?' And he did! The gel, the spikes, he got all my hair standing up like his. We laughed and laughed and we decided to take a picture."

Jean and I laughed and laughed, too, until both of us had tears in our eyes. It was a story to celebrate, a heroic, wise, and outstanding illustration of Jean's spirituality at work. I had to thank her, too, for the unforgettable lesson she had taught me for my own mothering life. I wondered if she still had the photo, if it would serve to remind her of her history of faith in life, of letting go, and going with the flow. She was not sure about that, but sharing the story and the laughter had made the memory more vivid.

I still do not know how to understand what created the change whereby Jean regained the faith she had lost. Neither of us expected smooth sailing from that point on, but for the moment in that session, the calm in Jean's body created unique possibilities for reflection and recollection. Her recalling, and my witnessing, a story that spoke of her going with the flow anchored her chosen way of being—attuned with her spirituality, a sturdy truster of life. For our ongoing conversation, we began to collect a canon of calming stories to steady her in the midst of the present chaos.

Externalizing and Countering the Influence of Destructive Stories

Jack was a man who began therapy deriding himself as one who "couldn't even make a decision about what pants to wear each morning." He hated his job but could not make a decision to leave it. He had promised family and friends that he would stop using drugs but once again was wasting money on marijuana and alcohol. He had been reared as a

Southern Baptist and still stated his commitment to those beliefs, although he felt he had broken so many promises to God that he no longer prayed. He saw himself as a "weak" person who could not make commitments—to himself or to others or to his God—and keep them.

I (Griff) wondered with Jack what we might notice differently about his life if the influence of these stories of weakness were to be less pervasive. He had in fact sustained many commitments in his life. He had been more consistently attentive to his widowed mother than his other siblings. He could name relationships in which he had been a loyal friend. He worked conscientiously even when not closely monitored by a boss. Prior to our first meeting, he had made decisions to start psychotherapy and to return to Alcoholics Anonymous (AA) meetings, commitments that he had kept.

Jack and I began meeting weekly in psychotherapy with a focus on protecting his renewed sobriety. One looming risk factor was the role played by certain stories of past failures that he would think about, dwell upon, and become demoralized by. He had saved $25,000 but lost it all while abusing alcohol and cocaine. He felt that his family had once viewed him as their most talented and promising child, the one who would bring pride to the family. Although he completed college and worked successfully, he felt he had never fulfilled this promise. When despair and self-hatred from dwelling upon these stories of weakness grew stronger, his commitment to his recovery program would dissipate. He would begin lapsing in his commitment to daily AA meetings, talks with his sponsor, and avoidance of bars and substance-using friends. Relapse would eventually follow.

From my personal familiarity with Baptist doctrines and worship, I offered a Bible verse to Jack from the Book of Philippians for framing the work of our therapy, a verse with which I was confident he would be familiar: "Finally, brethren, whatsoever things are true, whatsoever things are honest, whatsoever things are just, whatsoever things are pure, whatsoever things are lovely, whatsoever things are of good report; if there be any virtue, and if there be any praise, *think on these things*" (Philippians 4:8, King James Version [KJV]). The last phrase—"think on these things"—would mean dwelling mindfully upon stories that facilitated his recovery, not on ones that undermined it. To "think on these things" resonated with his Baptist background, with his Twelve Step approach, and with his own sense of his situation. He agreed to spend out-of-session time selecting carefully the stories on which he would permit his mind to dwell. My questions during therapy sessions sought to bolster his efforts.

Eight weeks later he was continuing to adhere to his recovery program. In an interchange with me, he expressed poignantly the difference it had made that he could push stories of past failures—"stories of weakness"—to the periphery of his awareness. I had read aloud to him some notes I had jotted down from the first session: "Tells story how he can't even make a decision 'about what pants to wear.' Hates job but can't make a decision to leave it. Sees self as 'weak.' Can't keep promise to God so stopped praying. Now he can't even keep promises to self."

"If I were to be a devil's advocate," I asked him, "What would be my best strategy if I were to try to tempt you into living within stories of weakness?"

"By pointing to the past. You would remind me of my past failures," he responded.

"Pointing to the past?" I wondered.

"Yes. The past may haunt me, but it won't control me."

*   *   *

Dan and Cynthia had begun couple therapy a month earlier. On this day they both looked dejected. I (Griff) asked what had happened since our last session. Cynthia told about the argument they had had during their long-weekend vacation. After what had seemed to her to be years of futile requests that they have more fun in their lives, Dan had spontaneously planned a wonderful trip to New York City for the family. To Cynthia, this seemed like a redemptive moment for their marriage. They began the trip buoyant with enthusiasm, but then an argument began over money, ruining what had seemed so wonderful. From what had seemed like a fresh start, they were back in the same old rut, Cynthia arguing the necessity of their "getting a life"; Dan arguing the necessity of "not spending tomorrow's money today."

As I listened for the expected ending to this story, I was caught off guard when it took an unexpected turn. Cynthia told how in the middle of the argument she had said a prayer, then stood her ground with Dan, not backing down. This was in sharp distinction to her usual modes of responding, either to withdraw passively or to explode in angry tears. I asked what she had prayed. She explained that she had asked God to help her to be strong and to speak the truth. Dan then listened quietly to her.

"You were different then, in the car, than you were when you came in the room with Dan and me this morning. Help me understand the difference," I requested. Cynthia said there were times when she could sense "protective armor" that would appear around her like a shield. When she felt its presence, she knew she would be safe, and she could feel her strength. "How is it that you sense its presence at some times but not other times?" I asked. She said she did not know a sure answer, but did believe that the power of the shield was from God. "In your relationship with Dan, how are you a different person when you sense the presence of the shield versus when you do not?" I asked, followed by "Are you closer and more intimate with Dan when the shield is present, or when it is not?" Cynthia described how she stood up strong and could take care of herself when she sensed the presence of the shield. She then could feel closer to Dan because she was not afraid.

I then asked Dan whether he had been aware of this "protective shield" in Cynthia's life or its importance for their relationship. He shook his head. I asked whether there might be anything analogous in his life. He told how Cynthia's anger would often hit on an old sensitivity—"the destructive power of an angry woman"—which he believed to be a legacy of his childhood. When Cynthia would raise her voice, he would emotionally "go to the ground" and retreat from her to an isolated place. At home he would lock himself in his study. There he would pray and meditate. I asked Dan what happened when he prayed and meditated in his study. He said that he repeated the Twenty-third Psalm over and over. Then, at a certain moment, he would feel "serenity" building within him. When the serenity grew strong, he could then face Cynthia again.

I asked whether there were any moments when Dan, as a serene person, and Cynthia, with a clear sense of her protective armor, were simultaneously present with each other in relationship? They each thought not. I told them I was intrigued by that possibility and asked whether they would be willing to work on it at home, as an out-of-session assignment—that they carefully notice whether there were in fact even occasional moments, however rare, when they were together as serene and protected partners. What if we were to work toward identifying such moments and finding ways to help them to occur more frequently and to

last longer? Learning to meet each other from within a sense of "protective armor" and "serenity," each anchored in their spiritual beliefs and
practices, became a frame for therapy to which we regularly returned
during a lengthy couple therapy that addressed many additional issues.

Collecting a Wide World of Stories

I (Melissa) was connected with Mr. Mahmed through a project that links
professionals and refugees who have survived political torture. In his Middle Eastern homeland, he had been a member of the opposition to the
dictatorship. For this reason he had been detained and tortured. The tor-
turer's goal was to extract the names of his comrades, although he gave no
names and the torturers eventually gave up. Later he escaped and came to
the United States. We were discussing the progress he had made, his determination and strong will, and the life he had made for himself here. He was
fluent in four languages, but I only in English, so he, with the help of Gabrielle, an interpreter colleague, has accommodated me.

"When the torturers tried to get names of other people from you,
you gave them no names. You said they failed, that you remained strong,
that it was a victory, yes?" I asked him.

"Yes, it was a victory," he nodded.

"And they wanted you to give up on life. Now you are taking your
life back, going to school, regaining your health. Do you see this as evidence that they failed again? Is making a life for yourself again another
victory over the torturers?"

"No. It is good to take my life back, but is not a victory. Victory is if
I help other people, people in my country who do not have a good life.
But for now to help my country. . . . " He lowered his gaze.

"Is not possible?" I offered.

"Yes, is not possible, for now. So I can help people here in America." He went on to detail his plans for bringing local refugees and people born in the United States together in a group, to take away stereotypes, he said, and to make friends, to help one another, so that our
children and grandchildren could be friends, not enemies. He paused
and held his head high, "The purpose of a human being is to make the
world a better place for all humans."

He spoke this sentence as if it were an important saying. He had told me about other proverbs as we had worked together, so I asked him, "Are those words from the Qu'ran?"

"Sure, sure, this teaching is in the Qu'ran, but it is in the Bible, too, the Torah, too. The holy books, they are all written. . . . " He had an exchange with Gabrielle.

"Same author," she supplied.

"Yes, same author," Mr. Mahmed said. "He does not change the message when he writes a new book," he laughed. He returned to the topic of his plans for the citizens and refugees group, wanting to tack down some specifics, get it going. Gabrielle and I joined in, appreciating his enthusiasm, but also concerned, wary of the difficulties, the time it might take, to get such a project off the ground.

"Of course we can do this!" Mr. Mahmed said, not the least dissuaded. He was absolutely certain that there were many Americans eager to meet with refugees to engage in a mutually beneficial exchange. I marveled at his optimism after suffering such cruel treatment, but I kept these thoughts to myself because I knew he did not want my marveling and my reflective questions. He wanted to make some concrete plans. I thought of his remarks in an earlier session, when I had asked about the source of his strength. "My strength—not so exceptional," he said. "But I have hope. Other things are not exceptional. I have very big hope. Life is hope. My father and mother told me, 'All things, they change. Don't worry.' "

I mostly listened as he and Gabrielle worked on sketching out the various details, how and with whom to set up the meetings. Mr. Mahmed was exuberant, and I mentioned, "Big hope. You do have a great amount of hope."

"Look!" he said. "Look what happens in the world. In this decade, what has happened. The Wall has fallen down in Germany. Gone. Look what happened in Russia. In America, too, the parties both agree that they must care for the people. The world changes."

It seemed he was an encyclopedia of signs of positive change. "I see now how you keep your hope so big. You pay attention to the stories of hope. Is that how you do it?" I asked him.

"Yes! And do you know about the meeting of women in New York? Women from many countries. Together. Women from the United States bring what they know, but they say, 'We have only a part.' Women from Africa bring what they know; they have a part that the women from the

United States need. Women from other countries bring other parts. It will change. The world will change."

Mr. Mahmed is not naive, nor is he in denial. The pains in his body remind him often of the torture. His life is full of struggle, learning a new language, mastering the daily nuances of a new culture, but he says, "Life is hope." He practices hope (Weingarten, 1999) by collecting and telling stories from all over the world. He knows that it is impossible to bring about changes in his country, *for now,* but he keeps possibilities alive for the future by noting changes toward tolerance and cooperation elsewhere. His spiritual foundations, to which he claims no exclusive rights, guide him to create new stories for others, refugees and American citizens.

Chapter Five

Conversations between Person and God

"I am still waiting to hear God's voice." Ann smiled wearily. She had a difficult decision to make and had been struggling with it for several weeks. She was not waiting for a particular sound, a tone that would register on her eardrums, or, for that matter, for any kind of unequivocal directive. She knew there were no clear answers. It was that the context of this dilemma was isolating, and she wanted not to be so alone. She and I (Melissa) had been turning it over for the last few sessions.

"I told my senior pastor that I was waiting to hear God's voice. He laughed knowingly and told me, 'Sounds like you're listening, but She's not talking. Or maybe She's giving you some clues, but you want Her to be a bit less cagey.' Actually," Ann continued, "I have been reading a book about discernment to try to gain some perspective on all this. This notion caught my attention. The author said that not hearing God's voice is also a part of discernment. Hearing the silence is just as significant as hearing the voice. So I've been trying to listen for the silence."

"Listen for the silence as opposed to hearing nothing . . . I don't think I understand," I told her.

Ann helped me, "It's like . . . I remember when my sons were very small. And how I came to know and feel their sounds and their silence and be okay with that in a way that only I could because I was their mother. Even lying in my bed, which was next to their room I could hear their sounds turning in their cribs, or breathing, or not even hear them but hear their silence and feel their presence. And I could know that all was well and that I could be next to them or be apart from them and that, though there were no sounds, they were okay."

"Oh, it is an alive silence, a present silence," I ventured.

"Yes," Ann said, "quite alive, but quite quiet. So I am standing at the intersection of this crossroads, holding my breath."

"Holding your breath?" I asked. "Maybe I still don't understand." I could not fit it together. That sounded like something one did when afraid, not like the all-is-well maternal sense I had just understood.

"Yes. Waiting and holding my breath. Being very still on the outside, but lots happening on the inside. I remember when I was a little girl, being with my grandfather. He used to take me and my brothers out fishing. He knew what to do with the boys, but I could tell he didn't know quite what to do with me. He was glad for me to come along, though. Sometimes he would put his hand on my head and I remember liking that feeling. I remember wanting to be very still, to not move or talk, because I didn't want to do anything that would scare him or make it stop."

"Knowing the presence and being very still with it. Is it like that?" I wondered.

"Yes. It's like I finally learned to be about making love. At first I just focused on thinking, 'This is not going to be bad. It is not going to hurt,' and I could do it and it was okay, but not good. Then I worked too hard at trying to feel great and that was too much, but I remember when I learned just to be. That the touch was subtle and pleasurable and that I could just be available to it and not worry about bad or great and that is when sex got good."

"Just to be available to it?" I commented that this sounded like the way she had been learning to be with people.

"Yes," she responded. "I seem to have two options to elicit closeness—to please people or to be sad. This is neither, this is just to be me, to be available."

"So," I glanced at my notes, scribbled phrases from all of her lovely metaphors, and spoke quietly and slowly, "with God, your part is to be available? To be still? To know the touch is subtle, to know the presence even when unseen? To hold your breath so you can hear the voice?"

"Yes," Ann spoke quietly also. "And maybe it won't be through a voice, maybe God speaks through a touch or in other ways, but I don't need to feel alone, just because I don't hear an answer."

CONVERSATIONS WITH GOD

Could Ann's experience be described as a conversation? We are choosing to answer yes, because in the therapy community we have a way to speak about conversation, just as Ann could describe her way of being with her sons, her grandfather, and her husband, so that she and Melissa could speak about her way of being with her God.

Throughout the world, spiritually minded people communicate regularly, sometimes many times each day, with invisible presences. Jungian therapist Mary Watkins (1988) draws on the wisdom of Jewish tradition to harken us to these "imaginal dialogues":

> In the Hebraic tradition human beings were distinguished from all other living creatures not by virtue of their capacity for reason but by virtue of their engagement in three kinds of dialogues: dialogues with neighbors, with themselves, and with God. At first glance, in our own time and culture, dialogues with ourselves and with the gods seem dim and almost silent next to our dialogues with our neighbors. These dialogues seem to flee from listening ears, hiding out in the most private parts of our solitude and fantasy. They abandon speaking aloud, or otherwise manifesting themselves, as though shrinking from the pejorative labels "pathological," "immature," or "superstitious." But if we approach without such critical predilections, we can begin again to hear the voices of these other dialogues—these, let us say, "imaginal dialogues." (p. 1)

While we understand that there are many descriptions of beings—spirits, saints, ancestors, angels—with whom people engage in rich imaginal dialogues, we will focus this chapter primarily on conversations with a personal God. This is simply because we can only write of what we know. Both in our own spiritual experiences and, with rare exceptions, when people in therapy have told us about dialogue with a spiritual other, they have spoken of dialogue with God. Undoubtedly this reflects our own cultural heritage as well as the heritage and traditions of the people who consult us, and probably also reflects what experiences people expect we will be open to hearing.

Such conversations can be the only fully open conversations in a person's life, the only ones that hold no secrets. Sometimes there are words, but often, as with Ann, the nature of these conversations goes beyond the expressive capacity of language and is so intimate that no words are used to communicate.

DIALOGUE, A PARTICULAR FORM OF CONVERSATION

If conversation is a general, colloquial term for the back -and-forth talking and listening between persons, dialogue is more specifically the kind of conversation that ensues when (1) each participant senses that he or she will be heard, understood, and taken seriously, and (2) multiple perspectives can coexist simultaneously within the conversation (Anderson, 1997; Braten, 1987; Buber, 1958; Shotter, 1993a, 1993b). Dialogue represents a shared inquiry in which participants puzzle, muse, and reflect together (Anderson, 1997). There is a sense of commitment and belonging to the conversation as a joint enterprise (Shotter, 1993a).

Some conversations, such as debates, are not dialogues but monologues (Anderson & Goolishian, 1986). Monological conversations are organized around certainty and closed opinions, rather than wonder and openness to novel ideas (Anderson, 1997). Voices compete to dominate or to convert. In their politics, monological conversations are unsafe for the weak and the quiet—only the powerful or the loud get to speak or to have points of view seriously considered. Biologically, engagement in a monological conversation tends to bring forth emotional postures that hinder a transition to dialogue. Such conversations usually carry a subtext about attacking or defending, dominating or submitting, rather than listening and reflecting (Griffith & Griffith, 1994).

Conversations between a person and his or her God, like other kinds of conversations, can be either monologues or dialogues. This distinction is a critical one. Norwegian sociologist–philosopher Stein Braten (1987) has argued that dialogue, with its "criss-crossing of perspectives," is necessary for the kind of problem solving that must be sustained over time, whereas monological conversations, even those among brilliant intellects, progressively dissipate in their creative potential. Although a singular point of view may be compelling, it quickly becomes impoverished in creativity if it is the only perspective represented in the conversation. Person–God conversations, like human conversations, need to become dialogical rather than monological if they are to provide the creativity needed to solve life problems.

Consider the following transcript from a research interview (Griffith et al., 1995): Priscilla, a colleague who participated in the study, relates her encounter with the "I am."

GRIFF: Does your God have a name?

PRISCILLA: Not really. I think of him[1] as having every name that has ever been used for God. . . . You know, whether that is "Allah" or "Spirit" . . . or "God" . . . sometimes, I guess the "I am" comes closest. I don't really much like the word "God," but it's pretty handy shorthand. So I can use that word for now and incorporate it in the way I have redefined it, different from the way I understood it earlier in my life. . . .

GRIFF: Can you tell me about this "I am" God? How do you sense the presence? What sensations tell you that the presence is there?

PRISCILLA: Well, it's really light and warm and big.

GRIFF: How do you sense the lightness or the warmth? Is it anything that you see, or anything you hear, or anything you feel?

PRISCILLA: Yeah. I guess it is a feeling of . . . visually, it's almost a light. It is like light, a radiance, and it radiates warmth and feeling . . . somewhere over in this side of my body (*pointing to her lower chest*) . . . farther down, around the middle part of my chest, real full. It radiates out and can fill my body with a feeling of nurturance and . . . this complete peace.

GRIFF: What posture does your body go to when you feel filled with that radiance? What posture of your body would most express that? Can you show it?

PRISCILLA: Yeah. (*Kneels silently with head bowed, hands moving first to her heart, then upwards in a posture of praise.*) . . . I can feel it. From here I can feel it.

GRIFF: If that is your posture, what would God's posture be?

PRISCILLA: (*Silently shows how the "I am" approaches, placing supporting arms beneath her extended arms, gently uplifting them.*)

GRIFF: Is that right?

PRISCILLA: (*Nods.*)

GRIFF: And would there be words spoken between you and God?

PRISCILLA: I don't think so.

For Priscilla this conversation is dialogical. She experiences the "I am" listening, watching, appreciating her opening, lifting up and supporting her, as her whole being responds to this response. Later in the interview she contrasts this with the relationship she had with the God she knew as a child, whom she called the "Thou-shalt-not" God— "Thou shalt not talk back, thou shalt not think, thou shalt not laugh, thou shalt not ever enjoy thyself!" She psychodramatically portrayed him as a scornful father-God, saying "I hold all the cards here, and you just need to get it. I've allowed you to play around for a while, but now it's time to get in line. You think you make the rules, but you're wrong. I make the rules here, and you've got to do what I say." Her response back then was a muttered "Well, that may be how it is. If it is, then I guess I do have to fall in. I may do it, because I have to do it, but I sure won't like it, and I won't like you." Priscilla left the church and this God behind at her first opportunity, when leaving home for college, and did not return for many years. When she did, it was to search for and find the Spirit of Light and Warmth, one who wanted her to think, speak, and laugh and who would respond with embracing, supporting, and lifting her up. Fewer words than the God of her childhood, but much more dialogue.

And what did she call this One? In listening again to the research interview from which this transcript was made, we heard Priscilla search for a word to describe the one with whom she sensed such closeness. "Spirit," "Allah," and, most of all, the "I am" were words that spoke more to her experience than "God." In review, Griff noticed that, even after her search, he slipped into using the word "God" again. We imagine that, more often than we will ever know, we both slip into using our own language for another's experience, and that the other person accommodates us. Priscilla was forgiving, but her word for this kind of accommodation, "shorthand," is a word to be highlighted. It so vividly conveys a language code that compresses, that strips away unique personal utterances and meanings, thus reminding us of the rich text we may be missing.

WHY THESE CONVERSATIONS MATTER

Compared to metaphors, stories, beliefs, and other forms of symbolic expression, what place does conversation hold in human existence? How do conversations between persons and their God matter in human life?

Conversation enables community to be built between and among individual persons. When we talk about metaphors, stories, and beliefs, we categorize some of the ways in which language often expresses and shapes an individual's experience of his or her world. But words are spoken to be heard, and with their hearing a response is expected from the other. This back-and-forth speaking, listening, and reflecting brings forth a community of people in conversation. Although we might consider the roles that metaphor, story, and belief play within a single life, the notion of conversation necessarily invokes a conversing community, at least two participants, though one of them may be unseeable by most human eyes. Conversations between a person and his or her God, and conversations among members of a spiritual community (Chapter 8), are each important and reflect different sectors of spiritual experience.

In a community, each individual operates with a dual sense of identity, as oneself and as a member of the community. For some religious people, God may be a key member of every other community in which the person participates. Person–God conversations can help sustain the integrity of human communities, as well as the integrity of a person's sense of self.

This fundamental insight was explicated early in this century by Mikhail Bakhtin (1990), an idealistic young Russian who suffered under Stalin's reign. Bakhtin was struggling to articulate the relationship between "I" and "another" in human life and how language as dialogue enables this relationship to come into being. He noted that no person as an individual is able to know even the physical aspects of his or her body without experiencing how that body is witnessed within the consciousness of another person. A superficial but common example might make the point: The clothes we put on in the morning are fully visible to every person around us but largely hidden from us, in part by our limited line of vision. We can try to bypass this physical limitation by looking in a mirror, but seeing our own reflection is never the same as hearing a friend describe us. The image in the mirror is one-dimensional; what we need is an aesthetic interpretation. Because this flat image falls short, we turn away from the mirror to ask others: "How do I look?" It is a hint of our need to know how we are experienced in the consciousness of another.

Bakhtin's recognition of one's reliance on others to know fully even the physical aspects of one's being becomes a more pressing truth when the wish is to know nonphysical aspects, such as one's personality or character. Am I strong or weak? Am I courageous or cowardly? Am I wise or foolish? Like Sartre's characters in *No Exit*, we can see ourselves only as we are witnessed through the eyes of others. Bakhtin (1990) described humans as having an "interlocutive self"—one must constantly change places with the other in order to see where one is and who one is. As he noted, we are "fated to need the other if we are to consummate our lives. . . . We must share our mutual excess in order to overcome our mutual lack" (pp. xxv, xxvi).

Bakhtin also noted the theological implications of this process. He believed that people need God as witness and author in order to experience aesthetically the drama of their lives. Selfhood is composed not only through others' eyes but also through the witnessing of God's eyes. "God is now the heavenly father who is over me. . . . What I must be for the other, God is for me" (Bakhtin, 1990, p. 56). Only God can witness all of me as a person; only God knows all the facts of my life; only God understands both the perspectives of other involved persons and my experience as I live within my dilemmas. "As God is my witness . . . " permits me, through God's eyes, to know myself.

One can think of "God" as an epistemological position to which a person moves when it is important to witness the whole of one's life. This self-reflective knowing often takes place through prayer and during meditation. In addition to having the panoramic view of a person's life, the position of God is of one whose vision has no time constraints. According to many believers, God has knowledge of the past, the present, and the future. If people are conversing with or being counseled by an Other who fully knows them, knows the hearts of people around them, and knows their past and future, then it might enrich our conversation to give ear to this Other. This practice often holds surprise for us.

The therapy with Vanessa was supported by voices of spirits that I (Melissa) could never have imagined and in ways I could never have predicted. Earlier, we mentioned that there were some rare exceptions in our experiences when people spoke of conversations with spiritual beings other than God. This was one such time. Vanessa had told me earlier how both her parents' lives had been overshadowed by addiction, her mother's by alcohol and her father's by heroin. She held the addiction responsible for killing her father when she was only 6 and then rendering her mother unable to care for her. Vanessa knew she was vulnerable to addiction. In her teen years she was nearly captured by it, but she had reclaimed her life and, with the aid of her strong extended Catholic Latino family, had completed college and was on her way to a promising career. Even more remarkable than her academic achievements, Vanessa had remained sensitive, compassionate, and optimistic. However, these very qualities seemed to endanger her as she considered spending time with an old friend. She understood the pit he was in and she thought she might be able to help him out. He was actively using and dealing illegal drugs. He wanted Vanessa's friendship, not to help, but to join in.

Should she try to aid him or to avoid him? As Vanessa struggled with this choice, she told me, she had been awakened in the middle of the night by a terrible dream. "I kept hearing, 'Come on. What are you scared of? Let's just have some fun. It'll be okay!' He was saying that, but it was like I was saying that, too. And it felt like I was going there again. It was so real. I woke up the middle of the night and I was paralyzed, terrified. So I asked my father's spirit and my grandmother's spirit to let me feel their presence in my bedroom, and they did. I mean, they are always there, but I don't always know it. They did let me know it that night, thank God. I knew that the reality was that they were there, and that the dream was just a dream. And I knew about the voice in the dream." I asked what she knew about the voice—was it her old friend's voice or hers? "Oh, it doesn't matter. It could be anybody. It's his voice, but it's been mine, too. I've said those exact words. I mean what I knew when I woke up was that those were just empty promises." She spoke the last two words emphatically.

"Empty promises," I repeated, "These are the important words." The most important, she agreed. I wondered how it was that these words came to her mind so clearly in the middle of the night. Without hesitation, she told me the words had come from her father's spirit. "So he came to protect you from the voice, the seduction, of Empty Promises?" Yes, she explained, adding that she was not surprised. Her father had often helped her before. She imagined that he was so sad that he hadn't stayed to help her in life, to do the kinds of things fathers usually do for their children, but he did all he could now. You know, she explained, he never wanted things to turn out the way they did. Stunned, I needed to slow down, to take a moment to collect my thoughts. Vanessa's father was the last one whose voice I would have invoked for discernment and guidance. Her open-hearted receptivity to his protective spirit made my close-minded attitude toward him all too apparent to me. Though I did not speak of it, I almost felt the need to apologize to him.

Vanessa, however, was not slowed down. "You said seduction, and they really are seducing, even though I know they are empty promises, they are so persuasive." I asked how she could resist them. "I don't know," she said. "That's why I came to you."

"But who really and truly knows Empty Promises? Your father named them. If he can help you identify them, maybe he can help you resist them. He knows them well, right?"

"Yes, I've only told you a little bit of what my father knows now. I've found that people, after they are dead, are so much calmer and wiser. I believe that's why God lets them come back to us." Vanessa looked straight into my eyes. She must have seen the fascination there. She cocked an eyebrow and quizzed me, "Are you thinking that all this is strange, Melissa? It may be, but it's not strange to me; my whole family is this way. It's part of our culture. You've never been visited by someone's spirit, have you? You can't fool me, I can tell," she chuckled. I told her she was a good guesser, that this was all new to me, but that I could see that her father's spirit was a great ally, and I wanted to know more about how he would help her to resist Empty Promises. "Yes, he is a good ally, and I'll tell you exactly what he would say to me, because I've heard him say it. He'd say, 'Don't believe that guy Vanessa, don't believe those empty promises. Look at what happened to me. Please, baby. Learn from my example. You stay away from that guy." And he will be watching me, my grandmother, too, because they can see me everywhere now.

Several times after that in the therapy, when difficulties arose, I would ask Vanessa to imagine how the spirits of her father and grandmother might aid. Sometimes she would know, for sometimes they had already helped her, and other times she would resolve to be more aware of their presence. They were invariably comforting and steadying, calm and wise.

HOW PERSON–GOD
CONVERSATIONS ARE UNIQUE

In many ways, conversations between a person and his or her God show all the vicissitudes of human exchanges. A person pleads, thanks, demands, offers, puzzles, and muses in conversation with God. Some conversations with God are formal and stylized, befitting a more distant, hierarchical relationship. Thus the Psalmist spoke: "As a hart longs for flowing streams, so longs my soul for thee, O God. My soul thirsts for God, for the living God. When shall I come and behold the face of God?" (Psalm 42:1–2). Other conversations are colloquial and spontaneous, an intimate relationship between friends. In the 1998 movie *The Apostle*, Sonny, a Pentecostal evangelist, paces his bedroom, demanding that God help him out of the entrapment of his dilemma. Sonny has learned that his wife is having an affair with the youth minister of their church, a church that Sonny founded and pastored. Moreover, while Sonny was away from home evangelizing, she mobilized the church to expel him from the membership. Agitated, he fled his home and his church to retreat to his old room in his mother's house. In the middle of the night, he paces the room, waving his arms, and shouts to his God:

"I always call you Jesus. You always call me Sonny!"

Sonny then exclaims: "Somebody—I say, somebody—has taken my wife and stole my church! That's the temple I built for you! I'm yelling at you because I'm mad at you! I . . . can't . . . take it! Give me a sign, or something! Blow this pain out of me! Give it to me tonight, Lord God, Jehovah! If you won't give me back my wife . . . give me peace! Give it to me! Give it to me! Give it to me! Give me peace! Give me peace! . . . I don't know who's been fooling with me, you or the Devil. I don't know. . . . And I'm not even going to bring the human [the other man in the affair] into it . . . he's just a mutt. . . . I won't even bring him into it. But I'm confused! I'm mad! I love you, Lord! But I'm mad at you! I'm mad at you! . . . Deliver me tonight, Lord. What should I do? Now tell me. Should I lay hands on myself? What should I do? I know I'm a sinner, and once in a while a womanizer, but I'm your servant! When I was a little boy, you brought me back from the dead! I'm your servant! What should I do? Tell me! I always call you, Jesus, and you always call me, Sonny! What should I do Jesus? This is Sonny talking now!"

An awakened neighbor calls Sonny's mother, who has been sleeping downstairs: "It sounds like you have a wild man over there, carrying on and hollering or whatever. Is that your son? Who is that?"

Sonny's mother responds: "That is my son. Ever since he was a little, bitty boy . . . sometimes he talks to the Lord, sometimes he yells at the Lord. . . . Tonight, he happens to be yelling at him."

The three ways in which person–God conversations differ from typical human conversations that were mentioned earlier—the potential for intimacy, the scarcity of spoken language from God, and the vantage point God holds for witnessing the whole self—all can be seen in Sonny's conversation with God. His conversation illustrates other differences as well. Not only do human interactions with God usually have few words, but the verbal aspects are usually one-sided. People sometimes speak volumes to God but rarely expect God to respond with so many words. God's response is often sought in expressions that are nonverbal—a person suddenly discovers a particular verse in the Bible, divines signs in nature, notes a serendipitous occurrence of events that seems to hold special meaning. As Sonny exclaimed to God, "Show me a sign!" Even when words from God are heard, the response by most accounts consists only of phrases or even a single word, whose meaning must be further pondered and interpreted.

These unique aspects also change the structure of interpersonal relationships and conversations in which a religious person is engaged. During a family therapy session, for example, a person can be in conversation with the therapist and other family members while also engaged in intrapersonal dialogue with God. Unlike the other conversational participants, God's voice can be heard only as revealed by individual family members, who themselves may then be hearing differing messages. Although God's perspective may powerfully influence what is and is not possible in the therapy, God does so as a hidden participant, like a family patriarch who declines to attend a family therapy session yet holds sway over what happens there.

Tom Andersen (1987, 1991) has regarded many human problems as maintained by "inner and outer conversations," with therapeutic change ensuing as shifts in these conversations occur. Andersen's perspective expanded family therapy beyond its traditional focus on the interpersonal dialogues and behavioral interactions in therapy sessions. It emphasized that there are always three concurrent conversations ongoing during a therapy session: the interpersonal conversation that includes therapist and family members; the inner, intrapersonal conversations within each person sitting in the role of client, patient, or family member; and the inner, intrapersonal conversation of the therapist. Intrapersonal dialogues with God can be among the most important of these inner conversations. In therapy with a religious person, or a religious family, the challenge is to find a way for God to enter the therapy room more overtly, and for God's voice to enter the interpersonal conversation more explicitly.

POWER INEQUALITIES LIMIT
THE CAPACITY FOR DIALOGUE

With a conversation, what matters is not so much its content, but the positions of the participants relative to one another. Who is included in the conversation and who is left out? Among the conversational participants, who can expect to be heard? Who can expect to be taken seriously? Who feels constrained as to what can be said, so that certain things must remain unspeakable? Is the conversation dominated by a single perspective, or can multiple perspectives coexist? These questions concern the act of composing—"words in their speaking" as John Shotter would say—rather than the finished composition (1993b, p. 13). Conversation is language being created in acts of speaking, listening, and reflecting. In other chapters, metaphors, stories, and beliefs are discussed as "already-spoken words" that, in boomerang-like reflexivity, return to constrain or to enable what the speaker subsequently can perceive, think, say, or do (Shotter, 1993b, p. 13).

Psychotherapy involving conversations between a person and his or her God does not focus so much on the content of what is spoken or heard as helping the person to stay positioned in relationship with God so that unconstrained speaking, listening, and reflection are possible. Does the person feel too afraid, angry, or ashamed for a reflective dialogue with God to occur? Does the person sense that his or her prayers are heard? Is God an abstract idea or a felt presence in the conversation? Is the person open to hearing what may be unexpected? Can the person sustain curiosity or does certainty about what God will say produce disinterest?

Joanna suffered from multiple sclerosis and was referred to me (Griff) to help her to cope with her medical illness. She belonged to a theologically conservative Protestant church and considered the heart of her religious practices to be her Christian faith—a commitment to her beliefs, among which were beliefs that God was constantly present, God was caring for her, and God was intervening actively in the world for the cause of good. In describing the recent exacerbation of her illness, she mentioned that she had been avoiding prayer lately. I asked what happened when she tried to pray. "I say the words and read the Scriptures, but it feels mechanical." I recalled other occasions when she had talked about prayer and meditation with the Scriptures as her solace during the darkest times as she struggled with her illness. "There is so much pain in the world. It is hard for me to understand why God doesn't do anything about it." She told about fresh doubts that had been intruding into her thoughts—Is there a God? If there is a God, does God care? If there is a reason for my suffering, why can't God reveal what that is? The fact that these thoughts presented themselves was itself a source of self-condemnation and depression: She saw them as evidence that her faith was weak. I asked whether there was any person whose presence lifted the burden she felt. She told about a close friend, Susan, with whom she shared her fears and worries. "I don't understand why I feel so uplifted after talking with Susan, but so much of nothing when I pray."

"Maybe it's because you aren't angry with Susan," I mused. I was guessing that she had realized this already.

Joanna laughed. "I think I've been more angry with God for longer than I have admitted to myself. . . . I just don't understand why things are the way they are." I shared with her the idea guiding my comments: Perhaps she was struggling so much with prayer because she was pushing faith and beliefs to do more than they can do. After all, one doesn't turn to arguments or faith to convince oneself that there is love in a human relationship when warmth and joy are spontaneously stirred by the presence of the other. Why should a relationship with God be different?

Joanna and I then discussed a friend of hers who seemed to find faith in God to be a simple and easy matter, even though he had suffered enormously from a medical illness. It was her guess that he felt so clearly the immediate presence of God that doubts simply did not arise. We agreed that the next series of therapy sessions would focus upon what stood in the way of her experiencing God as a felt presence, rather than trying harder to believe that God was present. Another way of putting this would be to say that her aim became that of entering into an open dialogue *with* God, rather than asserting what she believed *about* God.

Dialogue quickly deteriorates when participants cannot sustain certain bodily states of being—emotional postures associated with curiosity, reflection, listening, and musing. One might remember failed conversations that have been regrettable, where dialogue never again could be established once an argument or debate intruded. In such conversations, arguing and debating recruit emotional postures best fitted for attacking or defending. Anger, resentment, blame, and shame take a person out of a physiological capacity for entering into dialogue.

A therapist can influence what emotional postures characterize a conversation in therapy by guiding its pacing, turn taking, and conversational content (Griffith & Griffith, 1994). Conducting therapy in a sub-junctive mood of noncertainty and "as if," as with Joanna, helps conver-sational participants to sustain states of being within which dialogue can occur (Anderson, 1997). A commitment to "not understanding too quickly" permits the other to discover what he or she thinks and feels authentically (Weingarten, 1994, p. 179).

Dialogue is also difficult unless the power relations of a group guar-antee a participant democracy, in which each conversational participant is assured he or she will be heard respectfully and given a thoughtful re-sponse by the other participants. When dialogical encounters with God occur, they often model the story told about God and the Hebrew prophet Elijah: Bitter and furious with God, Elijah stole away into the wilderness and hid in a mountain cave. God sent first a whirlwind, then an earthquake, then a firestorm, each of which Elijah ignored. When Eli-jah responded, it was when God came as a still, small voice asking a question: "What are you doing here, Elijah?" God and Elijah then dis-cussed how angry and abandoned Elijah was feeling, and where to go in their relationship (I Kings 19:4–15). In this encounter, God, obviously the more powerful participant in the conversation, provided a space from which Elijah could speak a heartfelt response without fear of intim-idation.

This dialogical encounter can be contrasted with a monological one, in which a believer receives marching orders from his or her God that are to be simply implemented without questioning the orders or making a reflective commentary on them in prayer to God. An encounter be-tween Abraham and God was a monological one, when Abraham heard God instruct him to slay his only son, Isaac, on a mountaintop as a sacri-ficial offering. Abraham responded with obedience, rather than conver-sation about the strangeness of this request. He stopped only when God issued a second command to terminate the enactment (Genesis 22:1–14).

CREATING A SPACE FOR THE VOICE OF GOD

Family therapists have long understood that impasses in relationships sometimes can be resolved by adding a new voice to the old conversation that has evolved around the problem. In this vein, new possibilities sometimes can appear when the voice of a person's God is added to the conversation of therapy. However, many persons with religious lives do not speak in therapy about experiences and conversations with their God unless the therapist first offers an invitation. Sometimes this reticence, as for Sonya in Chapter 2, is a fear of being humiliated by a therapist who may be a religious skeptic. At other times it is a fear that therapy may undermine one's religious faith. For others, the idea of bringing up conversations with God seems never to occur, as if it there were a common understanding that talking about spiritual matters is not part of the etiquette of therapy.

In Chapter 2, we discussed ways to break the ice when opening a dialogue about religion or spirituality. Questions sometimes need to be directed specifically to the interaction between the person and his or her God, if God's voice is to enter the conversation. Any dialogue has three positions: the speaker, the listener, and the reflecting position in which one steps back and observes the interchanges between speaker and listener (Andersen, 1987, 1991). In a person–God dialogue, the person and his or her God each typically shift back and forth among these three positions during the conversational flow. When attempting to think systematically about what questions to ask, it can be fruitful to consider how questions might inquire about both person and God in each of these three dialogical positions of speaker, listener, and the reflecting position:

- When you pray, what words do you speak? [self as speaker]
- Do you sense that God hears those words? What seems to be God's response? [God as listener]
- Have you ever sensed a communication directly from God? [God as speaker]
- What sorts of responses have you had to communications from God? [self as listener]
- If you were to look down on this situation through God's eyes, what about it catches your attention? [God in the reflecting position]
- When you stand outside this situation and look on your dealing with it, and your involvement with God in dealing with it, what do you notice? [self in the reflecting position]
- What other people do you trust to help you discern if you are understanding God? [self and community in the reflecting position]

This series of questions moves back and forth among these dialogical positions, inquiring about each communication expressed—self to God, or God to self. It examines how the person and God each respond to the other and what each witnesses when standing outside the conversation looking on as an observer. After speaking aloud what previously may been addressed to or heard from God only privately, the person can ponder it in a new way. A fresh response to God, an expansion of the conversation with God, or a broadening of the conversation to include other trusted people may then ensue. Such an inquiry can gently open a therapy session to intrapersonal dialogues between a person and his or her God.

ENLIVENING A CONVERSATION
THAT HAD BECOME STAGNANT

When human problems become chronic and entrenched, conversations among those participating in the problems may become monological, stagnant, devoid of creative ideas. This often is the point at which a person decides to seek psychotherapy or family therapy. When an intrapersonal conversation with a personal God has contributed to this stagnation, reflective questions can be asked that enliven this conversation as a renewed source of therapeutic change.

Asking questions that expand the characterization of God (or the numinous) is a method for enabling such a transformation. A thinly characterized personal God is one hallmark of a stagnant person–God dialogue. As in human relationships, this can represent an inattention to aspects of the Other not fully contained within a dominant story of the relationship. Reflective questions can be asked that heighten curiosity about unexpected aspects of a personal God. It is helpful to keep questions in the subjunctive, "what if" sense. Sometimes the question "Has it ever been different from this?" can help locate a voice of God with which the person can enter into dialogue.

It can also be useful to ask questions that invite curiosity about complexities in God's perceptions, thoughts, intentions, or reflections:

- If you believe God caused this to happen, do you sense that God intended good to come from it, or do you sense that God intended harm? If you sense that God intended good, what is that good that God intended? How do you suppose God thought this through?
- What do you imagine that God felt when he witnessed this event happening?

- Do you suppose God might have had any mixed feelings, or second thoughts, about this?
- At a different time, have you ever experienced a different side of God than at present? What do you suppose accounts for the way you are experiencing God now?

Martha was a young woman who had spent her life in the bosom of the church. She had been supported and nurtured by scholarly, missionary parents who taught her about a loving and wise God. She told how her close relationship with God usually enabled her to discern truth from hypocrisy, and faith from platitudes. She believed her God held a specific purpose for her life and had given her the ability to fulfill that purpose. When she then sensed a clear calling to become a nurse, she felt certain that obstacles presented by her learning disability could be overcome. Three years earlier, I (Melissa) had worked with Martha while she was waiting and working to gain admission to a nursing program. I had heard, and she and I had relied on, the clarity of her sense of purpose to steady her through that time. During that ordeal she had educated me about living with her disability, which presented problems not with grasping the material, but with demonstrating her knowledge in timed multiple-choice test situations. Year by year, hurdle by hurdle, Martha and her advocate educated the college on adaptations needed for learning-disabled students. She made it through the nursing program by working twice as hard as most students, while coping with slurs from some that she was lazy or dumb to insist on special test situations. She did not need the assistance of therapy to get through the program, for she was well equipped with her own considerable system skills and with a foundation of clear messages from her parents that she was bright and able and that she should trust her sense of mission to be a nurse. I was delighted to receive Martha's graduation announcement in the mail, and took it as a sign of a victory won. I knew there was another step to practicing as a registered nurse, that of passing the state examinations—the registered nursing boards—but imagined this to be minor after her achievements in a challenging academic program.

Shortly after graduation Martha called, trembly and teary, "They're not letting me take the nursing boards. I have a job to start, but I can't start it without my boards, and a move to make and an apartment to pay for and I can't do anything. I sent my accommodation requests in months ago. They told me they had acted on my requests, but they had not. They lied. It's still on their desk and now all the test sites are filled. They won't give me the three kinds of accommodations I need to take the test. I settled for two out of three things I needed to expedite the process, but they did nothing! They tell me to keep waiting. I have fought for so long. I don't know why God is doing this to me. Why doesn't he help? I thought he wanted me to be a nurse, but he's making it impossible. I just feel like giving up. I can't fight anymore." Martha was in an awful dilemma: If she demanded swift justice from the Board of Nursing, she might alienate them and lose any chance of getting the accommodations she needed, but if she waited, ignoring their poor track record and hoping that they would act soon as promised, she might be forgotten.

We talked on the phone a while. She was adamant that God was betraying her and did not agree with my suggestion that maybe there were just some horribly careless people in the board office. She figured she would win this battle eventually, but the time lost would be costly—her apartment, a longer time lapse between preparation and test-taking time, maybe even her job. She had indeed, done everything right and, in her words, had only gotten "punishment" for it. She wondered, in fact, if God was punishing her for something, though she didn't know what. With God, as with the Board of Nursing, she felt helpless; at once both furious and silenced, constrained from expressing her fury because she was dependent on the good graces of both God and the board.

I wondered aloud if she felt God might also be furious with the board. "Well, then why did he let this happen to me?" she said. I understood then that her belief was that God was in control and asked her if she felt God could handle her anger. "I guess he could handle it, but I'm not supposed to think those things." However, as the dilemma wore on even that night, she did rail at God, having decided, she later said, that God could take it whether she was supposed to feel those things or not.

When we met the next day she was much calmer. She was still striving against overwhelming odds, though she had taken actions to counter the passivity that contests with large government agencies so often induce. She had begun to draft a letter to the board and had made more phone calls. I asked her about her statements on the phone concerning God's part in this, the question of punishment, and her self-doubt about her vocational calling to be a nurse. "I got over all that by the end of the night. Anyway I don't think even God is that cruel," she said. I asked how God had responded to her fury. "It was like he stood there, big, while I beat my fists on his chest. Then he hugged me. I am still not finished being mad though!" she added.

In our next meeting, the dilemma was still before her. She talked again about how tired she had grown of fighting and how God had strengthened her in the fights up to now. She had in her hands a beautiful cross-stitch she was embroidering, a gift for her parents' anniversary, of a psalm. This was the blessing spoken in her family before all leave-takings. I wondered what it was like to be stitching these words of God while things in her life were in such disarray. "It's calming," she said, "Anyway, like I told you, I got over that."

"I have wondered about that. When you said you 'got over it,' how was that, what happened that got you out of that sense that God was doing it to you?"

"It was just a feeling that changed. My heart changed," she said.

"Can you put words to the change?" I asked her.

"No, more just a feeling of peace that came, not like happy or it will all be all right. It well may not be all right, but I am at peace now."

"And when you are at peace, you don't wonder if you should be a nurse?"

"No."

This seemed quite important to me. I wanted to know more about this peace. And supposing that there would be more bureaucratic chaos ahead, I wanted to give Martha the opportunity to put words to it. "And when you are at peace, where do you sense that God is?" I asked.

"Just with me, beside me. Helping me through."

"If in the next fight, the next crisis, you could keep this peace, this knowledge that God is beside you, rather than imposing it on you. . . . "

"Well, then," she interrupted me, " it wouldn't be a crisis. The crisis is not what the board is doing. It's that I feel abandoned by God. I know it's not true, it just happens sometimes."

"I wonder what it is like for God to know that you are not only being treated unfairly, but that you feel he is directing it," I mused.

"I think he probably hates that. He can take it, but I would think he would want me to know he was beside me."

"What would it be like if you and God, with God beside you, were to step apart from the crisis and look back at it and talk together so that you could plan for next time? I wonder what might come of that conversation."

Martha wasn't sure, but she took the question with her in her mind to consider in the time between our meetings.

As long as Martha felt punished and silenced, she heard only God's silence, and the conversation had remained stagnant. For these waters to flow again, she had to meet her God in the torrent, speaking thoughts to God that she was not supposed to be even thinking. Grounded in the belief that "He can take it," she moved to another, more complex dialogue, that had space for support, peace, and safe expression of her anger. It seems not coincidental that after she spoke uncensored to God, she was able to risk composing a letter of protest to the Board of Nursing.

NOTICING MONOLOGICAL CONVERSATION IS KEY

Monological conversation signals a clinician to become active in promoting dialogue instead, to help transform the conversation. It is important to notice monological conversation when it appears in a person's account of relationship with his or her God. Such monological encounters can be identified by examining prayers and other person–God conversations using the following questions:

- Are the words spoken, or a nonverbal message exchanged, between a person and God always repetitive and unchanging?
- Does a person show a lack of interest or curiosity about what God might have to say?
- Does the person experience a lack of interest or curiosity on the part of God?
- Does God come across in the encounter as a thin character who is unidimensional and lacking in complexity?
- Can the person articulate a clear sense how God may have thought through a decision to communicate this message, or to communicate it in this form?

Therapeutic change usually requires an infusion of creativity—fresh ideas and novel behaviors. Monological conversations are typically empty of fresh ideas, and they support old habits rather than innovation. When person–God interactions are monological, it is more likely that they help sustain problems rather than contribute to solutions. As in therapies involving human participants, changing the monological character of a conversation between person and God can be a key step.

THERAPEUTIC CHANGE BY
SUSTAINING THE DIALOGUE

Other ways to facilitate dialogue between person and God seek to provide a context for dialogue when adverse conditions otherwise would hinder it, or to help someone to extend dialogue with God past the point where it customarily would have stopped. Many problems in human life, whether involving human or divine beings, will not be solved unless those involved in the problem can stay sufficiently engaged in a serious process of speaking, listening, and reflecting together. Therapeutic change therefore can be facilitated not by pressing for a particular outcome from dialogue, but by taking steps to help those involved to stay in dialogue long enough for change to occur. This strategy attempts to provide necessary preconditions for change, rather than specifying how or what change should occur.

Psychodramatic techniques, such as enrollment, role reversal, doubling, and mirror position provide powerful methods for extending a conversation in ways that are concrete and visible. We have utilized these methods in our research interviews and at times in therapy (Griffith, 1986; Griffith & Griffith, 1992b). Detailed guidelines for utilizing psychodramatic techniques are available elsewhere and are beyond the scope of this book (Blatner, 1994; Moreno, 1965). However, the following transcript from a research interview illustrates how role reversals—during which therapist and consultee each take turns playing the role of God in a simulated conversation—can be used, first to enact a conversation between person and God that previously had been private and largely nonverbal, and then to extend the conversation beyond its usual point of termination. This extension of the conversation propels expansion and elaboration of the relationship between the conversational partners. The participant who volunteered for this interview was Randy, who is a therapist and a minister.

EXTENDING THE CONVERSATION AND
EXPANDING THE CHARACTERIZATION OF GOD

According to our usual interview format, I (Griff) began by explaining to Randy that we were interested in learning, in as much detail as possible, how he experienced his God. He explained to me that his experience of God would be best understood if displayed against the backdrop of how his life had gone. Randy was struggling with thorny dilemmas that arose during the coparenting of his child after a divorce. Several years prior to the interview, he had experienced a reawakening of his religious faith. He now felt sustained by this faith and by friendships in his church. However, these were not resolving the conflicts that continued to appear when interacting with his former wife. I (Griff) suggested that he "sculpt" his struggle. Sculpture is a psychodramatic technique with which he would show by his body posture how it felt to be trapped in this struggle:

GRIFF: If you were going to embody that torn position, how would you sculpt it? . . . If you were going to show me with your body posture what is your dilemma, how would you show that?

RANDY: I could do it either of two ways . . . one, like being pulled between horses, with ropes tied to my arms and legs (*shows what it would look like to be drawn between horses*) . . . or, the other, like going into an embryonic position for protection (*curls up into a fetal position*). . . . (*pause*) I guess I can also image being humped over with the load on my back, almost like Jesus carrying the cross up the *via dolorosa* (*bends over*). It is as much as I think I can take.

Randy's psychodramatic portrayal displayed his isolation and paralysis such that I could see it concretely, an example of the poetic truth it can provide. A possible way to reopen the possibility of resolution within such an impasse is to introduce new meaning into Randy's intrapersonal dialogues. Awareness of the presence of God can be a way through which new meaning enters. I suggested that he introduce God's presence into the dilemma. I would sit in his place as Randy while asking him to show me his God by his assuming the role of God for a moment[2]:

GRIFF: Let me sit in for you. . . . Can you stand up for a moment? (*Takes Randy's position seated on the sofa.*) Now how does God come to Randy? At the moment when you begin to experience God's presence—Where does that experience begin? Is it like God is far away approaching, or already close and immediate?

RANDY: It's like this. (*Stands behind Griff, placing one hand on Griff's right shoulder.*) That is exactly how it is. And that may be all that it is.

GRIFF: Just an awareness of a touch on the shoulder?

RANDY: Yes. When you asked that question, I immediately pictured a hand on my shoulder . . . and that was all. . . . That is all that is needed.

Randy talked briefly about a deep relaxation and comfort he felt with the touch of God's hand. I then asked him to translate these bodily sensations into language:

GRIFF: If God's hand could speak, what would it say?

RANDY: (*role playing God, touching Griff's shoulder*) "I am here. . . . " That's all it says. "I am here."

GRIFF: Can we switch roles again? (*Stands again, assuming God's role. Randy again sits as himself on the sofa. Griff, as God, touches Randy's shoulder gently and repeats those words to him.*) "I am here."

GRIFF: (*Steps out of role to address Randy*) And if there were words that would speak your body's response as you hear these words and feel the relaxation within your body, what would they be?

RANDY: "I know."

GRIFF: And would there be another response in turn from God?

RANDY: I don't know if there needs to be. I don't demand one.

GRIFF: If you lean back and relax, where do you sense God's presence with you at this moment? Is the hand staying with your shoulder or has it changed?

RANDY: (*leaning back*) No. I feel kind of relaxed. It is like God is sitting in a chair beside me. I know God is present. I can sense it. The touch on the shoulder just reminded me. I don't have to have an extended conversation. The presence is plain.

These back-and-forth exchanges—"I am here," "I know"—appeared to articulate what usually occurred in a powerful, deeply felt, but mostly nonverbal encounter between Randy and his God. The next step was to see whether this simple articulation could be carried forward into a more expansive conversation. Additional questions were then asked that alternated between Randy and his role-played God, such that Randy and his God each would take turns speaking from each of the three basic conversational positions of speaker, listener, and one who reflects on what has been said:

GRIFF: Where would the relationship go from here?

RANDY: As far as the conversation goes. . . . There probably wouldn't be an active conversation, . . . although there have been times I've been in this place when I've engaged in a dialogue with God or a prayer.

GRIFF: What would be some of the things you might say?

RANDY: Things like—"God, I know you are here," or "I know that you help with whatever it is I am facing. And I need that help." "Show me what I need to do. Help me understand it when I see it." "Give me the strength to do what I know is the right thing to do. . . . " Those kinds of things.

This point in the intrapersonal dialogue between Randy and his God seemed to represent a natural stopping point in the conversation. However, it was possible to extend the conversation beyond this point by asking Randy, using role reversals, to continue moving back and forth between his position and God's position, responding to the previous utterance with each turn of the conversation.

GRIFF: (*Stands and exchanges places with Randy.*) Switch places with me. (*Assumes Randy's position.*) Be God again for a moment . . . sit as God . . . whatever you would imagine God's posture to be, assume that posture. . . . Do whatever you need to do to experience what it might be like to be God. (*as Randy, addressing God*) "God, I know you are here. Help me to understand those things I need to understand. Show me what I need to do." What would Randy experience as God's response?

RANDY: (*as God, responding to Randy*) "I will. I will. Live your life. Do what you know to do in each moment, and I will always be there."

GRIFF: Would you speak the words of the prayer as I sit in for God?

RANDY: *(as Randy, addressing God)* "God, I know you are there. And I am thankful and grateful. Help me to understand the things I need to do in these situations. Show me what is best. And give me the strength to do this."

GRIFF: *(as God, responding to Randy)* "I will. Do what you know to do in each moment, and I will be with you. . . . " And what response does that bring forth within you?

RANDY: *(reflecting on the conversation)* Gosh! I feel like I'm almost on my own!

GRIFF: Almost on your own?

RANDY: Yeah . . . yeah.

GRIFF: How do you mean?

RANDY: Like you are there but you aren't going to do anything. That's strange!

GRIFF: Did I speak God's words accurately? Was it close enough the way I said it?

RANDY: I think so. It was said with compassion.

GRIFF: And your sense of it is that "It is almost like I'm on my own"?

RANDY: Yes.

This interchange illustrates the impact of extending a conversation. Randy is astounded to discover that he feels abandoned by God's words, when the conversation is carried forward one additional speaking turn. This occurred without my making any interpretation or directed intervention. It then becomes possible to ask Randy how this discovery may change his sense of his relationship with God. During the next 11 turns in the conversation, Randy articulates a new sense of the meaning of relationship with his God:

GRIFF: Where would that then go in the conversation?

RANDY: *(as Randy, addressing God)* "You can't just leave me out here hanging. I need a little guidance. I need a little direction."

GRIFF: Okay. Let's switch back again. *(They switch places, with Randy assuming God's role.)*

GRIFF: *(as Randy, addressing God)* "I feel like I'm almost on my own, like you are not going to do anything. I need a little guidance. I need some direction." What is God's response?

RANDY: (*as God, responding to Randy*) "You are not on your own, because I've always promised I will be with you. But I won't tell you what to do every step of the way. You've trusted me in other things before, and I want you to trust me now. I won't make your decisions for you. You have choices. You know me to a great degree. Sometimes you make bad choices, but I've never let you down. I'll do everything that I can, but I will not make your choices for you."

GRIFF: Let's switch back. (*They switch roles.*) Can you speak just the last lines?

RANDY: (*as Randy, addressing God*) "I feel like I'm alone, like I'm kind of out here just hanging. I need some direction."

GRIFF: (*as God, responding to Randy*) "I said that I will be with you, and I always have been. You have choices, and I won't tell you what to do on each choice. You may make some bad choices. I still will be with you. You have trusted me before, and I ask you to trust me now."

RANDY: (*as Randy, responding to God*) "This is hard. Why did our parents bring us up to think that it would be so easy?"

GRIFF: Switch. I'll just give you those last lines. (*They switch roles, and Griff, as Randy, speaks to God.*) "This is hard. Why did our parents bring us up to think that it was so easy?"

RANDY: (*as God, responding to Randy*) "Perhaps for them it was. Perhaps they were brought up in a simpler time when things were more black and white, and now they are not. Maybe, too, they did the best they could."

GRIFF: Switch. Could you just speak those lines? (*They switch roles.*)

RANDY: (*as Randy, responding to God*) "This is hard. Why did our parents bring us up to think that it would be so easy?"

GRIFF: (*as God, responding to Randy*) "Maybe for them it was easier. Maybe they were reared in a simpler time. And maybe they just did the best they could."

RANDY: (*as Randy, responding to God*) "Well, so this is my life. Whatever I get, whatever I have, has got to come through my own struggle. I think that is what I hear you saying."

GRIFF: Okay, let's switch. (*They switch roles.*)

GRIFF: (*as Randy, addressing God*) "Okay, this is my own life, and this is my struggle. Whatever I have comes out of my struggle. I guess that is what I hear you saying."

RANDY: (*as God, responding to Randy*) "I guess you hear well. It is your life. It is your struggle. But I am still here and I am not going away. I love you. I want the best for you. I will not make it easy, but I will not desert you."

GRIFF: Let's switch. Speak those words. (*They switch roles.*)

RANDY: (*as Randy, responding to God*) "So I guess what I hear you saying is that this is my life and whatever comes, comes through my struggle."

GRIFF: (*as God, responding to Randy*) "You heard right. It is your life, and it is your struggle. And what you get will come through your struggle. But I am still here, and I am not going away. I love you."

RANDY: "Sounds scary. . . . Do life."

GRIFF: (*Steps out of role to address Randy.*) Is that like an ending point in the conversation?

RANDY: Yeah. That's the end of the conversation.

RANDY'S EMBODIED TRUTH,
OR AN ABSTRACT IDEA?

Is the new meaning that has emerged from Randy's extended conversation an embodied truth that resonates within him or an intellectualized musing that is merely an interesting idea? This will be the test of utility for the new meaning. If it is to serve Randy as a usable tool for managing future dilemmas, it needs to effect a felt difference in the paralysis he experienced. Together, Randy and I assessed the significance of this new meaning by examining how it freed his body from the binding dilemma he showed at the beginning. My questions focused on his bodily experience, rather than an analysis of the idea:

GRIFF: Where has this conversation taken you in your body? Where do you experience it?

RANDY: I feel it from here (*points to center of chest*). I feel relaxed. I feel extremely relaxed. I feel peaceful . . . like I've encountered some major obstacle or truth or entity, and I've made peace with it. . . . It has always been important for me to understand circumstances or conditions or boundaries. Once I understand those, I live within those, or learn to adjust. . . . I feel that I have just acted out the boundaries and found them. . . . And because I know the boundaries, I can function within them.

GRIFF: When we began, you described three different things: one, like having two horses pull you apart, then another like almost being crushed, then finally as if bearing the cross, burden-like. How has that changed from the beginning of this interview to the present moment? What were the main changes you have noticed inside yourself?

RANDY: With God's hand on my shoulder, I immediately felt relaxed—my spine relaxed, the muscles in my back relaxed. Then, moving my body so I actually was sitting in a more relaxed position caused me to open up more in an emotional or spiritual sense. . . . I had no struggle making the connections in the role play. . . . It was role play, but I felt like I was really connected. . . . Physically, I felt almost like I had been to a masseuse. Not quite that good, but relaxed.

It was my sense that, for Randy, this was his bodily experience of a spiritual moment. It was the discovery of an embodied truth for his life. In this state of being, he could know his life and its circumstances in a different way. It would be my assumption that he can make the wisest, most thoughtful decisions about dilemmas involving his child if he can make them from within this state of being.

SPIRITUAL SKILL: LEARNING HOW TO REACCESS EMBODIED TRUTH IN THE FUTURE

Randy needs to know how to reaccess this state of being in the future when he again is faced with similar dilemmas. There are a variety of methods that individuals employ in order to reaccess reliably important emotional postures. Some of these methods, such as spiritual practices and rituals discussed in Chapter 8, can be largely nonverbal. However, finding language that fits well the state of being that Randy located during this exercise would help him to be able to talk about this embodied experience with others. Finding language that anchors this state of being is the last step of the interview.

GRIFF: If you were to take this relaxation—the place where your body is right now—and were to think of it as a readiness of your body to initiate some action or to express something, what do you think that would be? If this were a bodily predisposition toward some path of action or path of expression, what would that be?

RANDY: It would be a calm and peaceful approach to life, yet confident. Hopeful . . . and the term "holistic" comes to mind, where you translate that into every aspect of your being. I wouldn't be rushing around. I might still hurry and do these things. But the inner wheels wouldn't be turning as fast. I would be living my daily life with a relaxed, somewhat deliberate, spirit.

GRIFF: I see.

RANDY: I would walk upright with confidence, but not haughtiness . . . like a person who is at peace with himself.

If instead of a research study this interview had occurred within a formal therapy, subsequent sessions might well have focused on Randy's practicing how to access this "holistic" state of being. Learning reliable ways to enter such states of being when facing life's problems can be considered a form of spiritual competence.

FOSTERING THE SPREAD OF INTIMACY ACROSS RELATIONSHIPS

This chapter has followed a dialectic between language and relationship. When new uses of language enter a relationship and transform monologue into dialogue, other changes commonly ensue. The new language and conversational practices tend to spread. In case studies, we have documented how this cross-fertilization can occur between human relationships and relationships with God. In some cases, change in a relationship between person and friend or between family members led to similar changes in relationships with God. In other cases, a change in relationship between person and God catalyzed changes in relationships with friends or family members.

Jane, for example, was a middle-aged woman who had made repeated suicide attempts in the months following a motor vehicle accident. Injuries to her brain had left her so cognitively impaired that she could no longer work as an accountant. Jane's grief over her inability to read and to do math seemed unending. "You do reading, writing, and arithmetic all the time and never think about it. You never know what words mean until you can't read anymore. Then you realize how important they are." She was certain that she did not desire life if these were the conditions.

I (Griff) knew that Jane had attended church regularly prior to the accident. I asked her where she experienced God in her situation. She said she believed God to know everything that will happen in every person's life from the their moment of birth, which meant that her suffering was in some way planned by God or had some purpose in God's eyes. However, she described God as now "like an old man, far away." She felt guilty that "I haven't put God number one in my life," and believed that God had given up on her because of her doubting him. She could not imagine God feeling compassion for her. She feared God's judgment if she were to commit suicide. "Why is it that it doesn't matter what Bill and Janet [husband and daughter] think, but it matters to me what God thinks?" Her wish at that time was to reach the point where she did not care what God thought so she would be free to die.

Over the next 2 years, Jane's situation worsened. Medications for anxiety and depression only partially buffered her distress. She could make only limited use of psychotherapy because her concentration, memory, and capacity to think abstractly were so limited. After yet another serious suicide attempt, her frustrated husband divorced her.

Several months later, Jane came for an appointment looking surprisingly content. She described how she could feel gratitude now for the first time in years and felt glad to be alive. After her husband left her, she had felt more empty and despairing than ever. Yet she was now remembering words that her grandmother often told her as a little girl: "Prayer changes things." She had decided to go with her parents to their church, a traditional rural Protestant church. After the first visit, she felt nothing, became angry, and refused to return for a month. However, she eventually returned and joined an adult Sunday School class. In the

Sunday School class, she met a man, Roger, who was divorced. Roger was a thoughtful, gentle man whose wife had abandoned him and their child. Roger and Jane became close friends. He was interested in the small moments of her day and her accomplishments as she struggled with tasks of daily living. She felt comfortable talking with him, unembarrassed about her obvious neurological problems. In time they married.

Jane's transformation was remarkable. She was going into stores alone to shop, unashamed of mistakes she made attempting to write checks or trying to remember what items she came to buy. For the first time in the 4 years I had known her, she was entering willingly into family and social gatherings where her mistakes with language had previously brought unbearable humiliation.

She also talked about a transformation in her relationship with God that had happened spontaneously after she married Roger. She began feeling God's presence. She no longer felt deeply alone. Whereas she had once characterized prayer as "empty as praying to those pine trees outside the window," she now felt comforted by God. With other family and church members, she began helping some of the poorer families in the community. "There's been a lot of prayers answered," she said. "It feels so good to be back in church. I didn't realize how important it was."

Jane thus was able to use relationships with human beings to bring life to what had been a stale and empty relationship with her God. First her relationship with her dead grandmother, then her relationship with Roger brought her into a new state of relatedness from which she could meet God in a new way. Her neuropsychiatric symptoms had fluctuated little during the previous 4 years. Although psychotherapy, family therapy, and a complex psychopharmacological regimen had partially ameliorated her mood and cognitive symptoms, their effects had been limited. There was little else to which such change in her relationship with her God plausibly could be attributed.

By what processes does such change occur? We have been curious about two processes that we believe to influence this kind of change: the addition of new language to the pool of words and ideas available for making relationships with others, and the role that embodiment can play in opening fresh possibilities for relationship.

First, language serves a tool-like function in human life apart from its use in representing objects and entities (Vygotsky, 1978, 1986;

Wittgenstein, 1958). What often matters most about a person's language is not the ideas it expresses but whether that person can use the language effectively to build relationships with others. In this sense, words and phrases are tools for building community. Innovations in talking and relating in one relationship always seem to be spilling over into other relationships. New metaphors, ideas, and stories birthed in one relationship can have cross-usages in building other relationships. As Shotter (1993a, p. 9) has stated, "To talk in new ways is to 'construct' new forms of social relation, and to construct new forms of social relation (of self–other relationships) is to construct new ways of being (of person–world relations) for ourselves." For Jane, the new relatedness with Roger gave her new tools with which to fashion a relationship with God, and possibilities appeared that had not been previously witnessed.

Second, a close relationship exists between a person's physical state of being and what it is possible for that person to know and to experience. We elaborated this proposal in Chapter 1 in our discussion of emotional postures. During the years after her accident, Jane had spent most of her waking time tensed, agitated, poised to shrink back whenever her cognitive deficits were noticed by others. The aloof detachment that accompanied this tension she also brought to conversations with her God. Within Roger's warmth and acceptance, she relaxed into a tranquil state that was physically visible during her therapy sessions. In this tranquillity she became more open to receiving new ideas not only from Roger, but from other people, from me, and from her God.

Kaethe Weingarten (1994, p. 178) has written: "I think of intimacy as something that people can create with each other at any time, if they are open to sharing what they truly care about and open to trying to understand what the other finds meaningful. This can happen in any relationship—with children, friends, clients, or strangers—but it surely doesn't always occur. In order to grasp what another person means, you have to really *listen* to that person." Our clinical encounters with Jane and others suggest that this notion holds no differently for relationships with God as with human relationships.

NOTES

1. I (Melissa) had an interesting and instructive chat with Priscilla soon after she had completed the interview and read the transcript. She immediately noticed

the word "him." "Did I say that?" she asked. "That's strange. I know it's not true to my experience, and not even how I talk inside my own head." She and I looked again at the videotape and found that, indeed, she did say "him." I wondered if she wanted us to change it for our writing. No, she decided, write it like she said it, but note that she misspoke herself. Her pronouns had not caught up with her experience. It was a good lesson to us, a reminder to hear words as we hear stories. Stories may be fluid and changing even as they are spoken, and words may not always be adequate, not quite caught up with the story that wants to be told.

2. The appropriateness of a therapist standing in the place of a person's God psychodramatically during a role-played enactment is heavily conditioned by the particular religious tradition. Protestant Christians whom we have engaged in such a role play generally have entered into this exercise with interest and curiosity. Some Jewish colleagues who have viewed our videotapes have expressed discomfort with the therapist stepping into the role of God. In Judaism and "high church" Protestant Christian traditions, the placing of an image on God is experienced as irreverence and a violation of their God's holiness. By contrast, many other Protestant Christians and those from the Twelve Step tradition experience their God in the casual manner of a friendship. Other religious traditions may have other responses. Using psychodramatic techniques in order to enact a person–God relationship requires a sensitive collaboration with the person and an accurate understanding for how the form of the exercise is likely to be experienced within the particular religious tradition. An example in which my (Griff's) failure to attend to these considerations resulted in therapeutic failure with an Orthodox Christian man was discussed in Chapter 2.

Chapter Six

Spiritual and Religious Beliefs

In the beginning of our conversation, Mr. Ali only wept. Then he began to speak about what he had endured at the hands of the Soviet soldiers in Afghanistan. With the Mujaheddin, he had fought guerrilla warfare against the Soviet invasion. The Soviets had captured him, imprisoned him, and tortured him for months. "They put me in prison and hung me up by my thumbs ... then they would put me on the floor. ... " He paused, casting his eyes downward, "for no reason ... except that I am a man." The tears continued to roll quietly, constantly, down his face. He looked up at me (Melissa), and, perhaps to allay the worry he might have seen in me, paused to explain his tears. "In my country we have a saying: One asks the candle, 'Why do you burn?' The candle says, 'I must burn to give off my light.' For me, I must let the tears fall from my eyes, to give off my light. How else can I live?"

> "The guards came to me in prison. They came up to me and screamed in my face, 'Now we will cut off your hands, then we will cut off your arms, then ... ' I knew they would do it. They had killed many of my friends. Earlier I had sat in my cell and despaired, but as my body was hurt, my spirit grew stronger. I knew that they could kill my body, but because of God, nobody can kill my spirit. Now they came to me again. I stood up. I thrust out my hands and said, 'Here, do it, cut them off and drain my blood. You may put

my body in the grave, but I am still alive.' And they just looked at me and walked away."[1]

Mr. Ali called the spirit of his God "the Light." His conviction that the Light could not be extinguished enabled him to stand up to his torturers, even to be ready for death. His belief that the Light was within him, and that his weeping would allow him to give off the Light enabled him to endure the separation from his homeland and to do the work of healing.

As a research interviewer, I had already been informed by Mr. Ali's therapist that he was a follower of Islam. I asked him more about how his spiritual and religious life had been important through his suffering and healing. "Yes, the spiritual," he said emphatically, then went on to make a distinction between the two. "The spiritual is different from the mind. The mind is philosophy, whether you follow Moses or Mohammed, whether you are Hindu, Muslim, Buddhist, Jewish, Christian. These are philosophies. They are only like ladders to put your feet on and go to God. There are many ladders. The spiritual is in the Light—you cannot see the Light because it is so bright, but you see the reflections of the light in people. I know the spirit of God because I feel the power in my body, and it endures."

Ancient teachings, metaphors, stories, relationships, and the experience he identified within his body anchored Mr. Ali in beliefs that supported him through his imprisonment, sustained him through separation from loved ones, and steadied him through the difficult therapeutic work for symptoms that were sequelae of the torture. This work was made easier and more effective because his therapist appreciated the centrality of Mr. Ali's spirituality. "All therapists should know about the body and about the spiritual if they want to help people," he told me.

Mr. Ali had a clear conviction about what mattered most for his life: the power of God that he felt in his body, the everlastingness of the Light through pain and death, and the sovereignty of the Spirit apart from any particular religion. In our meeting he held a well-worn book from his religion teacher on his lap. For him, these and other religious teachings, or "philosophies," were merely rungs on one of many ladders to climb to reach God. For others though, the rungs are more essential, and some believe there is only one ladder.

Richard was a 24-year-old graduate student when he was referred for treatment of severe anxiety. It had the effect of obstructing Richard's completion of course projects, and now he was being threatened with dismissal from his program. In the first sentences of our (Griff) meeting, Richard identified himself as an "immature Christian" who was in a crisis of faith. He feared that he might become vulnerable to the influence of professors who were religious skeptics. He felt that one of his professors in particular "attacked the Scriptures." He was angry with this professor, but guilty that he felt so angry. Guilt and anger had escalated to a point at which he was unable to complete classes or do his academic work. At the heart of his crisis was a dilemma that he could acknowledge: He valued intellectual honesty too much to pretend that he believed a doctrine if he were to find that the evidence was too weak to support it. On the other hand, he was terrified at the possibility of losing his faith. He could find no way to both be faithful and to examine the evidence.

Like Mr. Ali, Richard's beliefs were central to his experience of spirituality. Unlike Mr. Ali's beliefs, however, they were not shielding him from an abusive world. His beliefs fostered helplessness and despair, rather than agency and hope. They created a psychological walled city, an austere world into which few could pass and in which he suffered alone.

BELIEFS: STATING WHAT IS
REAL OR WHAT MATTERS

Beliefs are propositional statements asserting "truth"—what is real or what matters. Beliefs differ from metaphors and stories in their abstractness and in the propositional form of their language. Beliefs operate differently in human affairs than do metaphors or stories. Most people can find a way to live alongside others even when their metaphors and stories differ. This is not always so with beliefs. When beliefs are discovered to differ, conflict often is near at hand.

In therapy, it may be more risky to inquire about a person's religious beliefs than about his or her metaphors or stories of spiritual experience, unless a solid sense of trust and safety has been already established in the relationship.

BELIEFS ARE DRAWN FROM
OR JUSTIFIED BY STORIES

Often it is useful to regard a belief as if it were the label for a file drawer of stories. Beliefs are often drawn from personal, family, or cultural stories. A belief can abstract an idea from one or more stories. For instance, when Mary, in Chapter 2, was asked how God would protect her if another storm were to come, she imagined a story in which God pushed her into a ditch in order to shield her body with his own. Then she abstracted from it her statement of belief: "I don't really know exactly what he would do. Maybe I don't have to know, but I *do* know that *he* would know what to do."

Sometimes stories are recollected or composed to justify a belief. When I asked Mr. Ali about the development of his beliefs, he explained to me that he had learned these things as a child, both by formal instruction and by the way people in his country lived. "My people, mostly, live very simply, just in small cabins. Because they live so basically, they do not have such trouble with giving up materialism. They more know what is essential. They more know God." He then told me stories about how his neighbors and relatives had lived.

Beliefs are not reducible to stories, however, in that the same story for different people can give rise to quite different beliefs. Edward Bruner and Phyllis Gorfain (1984) illustrated with the Jewish story of Masada how divergent and opposing beliefs can be drawn from a single story. According to the Masada legend, the Romans in 70 A.D. crushed the Jewish revolt, conquering Jerusalem and burning the Second Temple. However, 960 Jewish fighters escaped across the desert to the mountaintop fortress of Masada, from which they continued guerrilla attacks on the Roman army. The Romans laid siege for 3 years, finally penetrating the Jewish defenses by building a stone ramp up to the mountaintop. When the Romans finally broke into the fortress, however, they found all the Jewish fighters had committed suicide.

The Masada story has been held passionately by the Jewish people and is central to the national identity of Israel. Yet Bruner and Gorfain detail how varied the beliefs are that different Jewish political factions have attributed to the Masada story:

- The Jewish warriors at Masada provided for modern Jews a model for heroic resistance to oppression (a belief of Jewish nationalists, and the dominant, "official" interpretation in Israel).

- The Masada story illustrates how an irrational armed struggle can end in needless loss of human life and suffering (a belief of political liberals).
- The Masada story illustrates what happens when Jews rely on fighting rather than prayer in order to survive (a belief of religious conservatives).

A narrator holding any one of the preceding three beliefs tells the story differently than a narrator holding one of the others, by varying what details are emphasized or omitted. A belief thus alters in reflexive fashion how the story from which it emerged is subsequently heard and retold. All stories have a semiotic openness that permits multiple tellings under the influence of different beliefs.

Several years ago, I (Griff) learned concretely that no story, or set of stories, necessarily implies a particular belief. I was experimenting during therapy with suggesting to some people that they view movies that were particularly evocative along some particular theme of their psychotherapy. At the time I hoped this homework would have a therapeutic impact because the movie plot would portray a character struggling with a dilemma similar to that of my patient. However, it too often seemed that whatever "lesson" was drawn from the movie would paradoxically support beliefs that only seemed to bury the person deeper within his or her problem. I recall the occasion when I learned the lesson that I needed to learn and ceased my efforts to try to teach in this way. Melissa and I had recently seen the 1993 film *The Joy Luck Club* and were inspired by the stories of women who prevailed against extraordinary sorrows and hardship to find love, compassion, and a robust sense of self. At the time, I was seeing a woman in therapy who had suffered greatly and was struggling to save her life. To this end, she was working to set limits on an adult child who was sapping her strength. Hoping that she, too, would be inspired and emboldened by at least one of the women's stories in the film, I suggested that, between our sessions, she go to the movie and see which stories she most resonated with. At our next meeting I asked what she had learned from her experience of watching. She was indeed captivated by the movie. However, the story with which she identified was the mother who committed suicide in order to further the well-being of her child. What she said she learned was that sometimes parents need to give up their lives for their children. I learned that one can never predict or control what beliefs a particular person will derive from the stories available to them.

SCIENCE, RELIGION, AND POLITICS AS SOURCES OF BELIEFS

Beliefs are sometimes transmitted as ideology or doctrine, as part of a cultural discourse not tied so closely to stories of personal, family, or community experience. Three major sources of such beliefs are science, religion, and politics. In Western cultures ever since the Enlightenment, the authority of science as a primary source of beliefs has gained ground in comparison to either religious or political ideologies. Today, medically ill people are likely to consult first a scientific textbook of medicine, Internet Website, or physician to learn about the diagnosis and possible treatments for their illness. Although some also spend money freely on homeopathic or alternative medical remedies, beliefs derived from medical science more commonly hold the greater authority.

In cultures organized around religious fundamentalism—whether Christian, Jewish, Islamic, or other religion—sacred scriptures and the clerics who interpret them provide the primary sources of beliefs. In totalitarian societies, statements of a ruler, or ruling political party, are sometimes imposed as the only permissible source of beliefs, as in "the sayings of Chairman Mao" in the 1960s. The 20th century in North America has been a pluralistic one, in which religion, science, and political ideology have competed with one another, each waxing and waning in its relative influence from one decade to the next, and from one subculture to the next.

THE ROLES THAT BELIEFS PLAY IN HUMAN AFFAIRS

Whereas metaphors and stories largely function to orient a person as an experiencing self, beliefs serve a different role in human discourse. They position a person in relation to his or her surroundings—to individuals, society, the physical environment. Beliefs denote rights, privileges, and entitlements, both for self and others, that constitute the "politics of daily life" (Shotter, 1993a). As such, beliefs more easily become topics of debate and commonly are the medium for political action and the exercise of power.

The role and significance of beliefs, of course, varies widely among different religious groups. Christianity and Islam are characterized not only by the importance they attach to beliefs about God but also to beliefs about their holy scriptures—the Bible and the Qur'an. Judaism, by contrast, focuses little on beliefs, as Lovinger (1984, p. 135) has noted: "Because Judaism does not depend on belief, there are no core doctrines, creedal statements, or confessions of faith, although certain basic concepts obtain. . . . Definitions of God really state what God is not rather than what God is, and visual symbolic representations are sharply avoided." In some Eastern religions, such as Buddhism and Hinduism, beliefs serve a lesser role than spiritual practices and rituals.

We have found it important to emphasize the distinction between *convictions*, as passionately held commitments to what is regarded to be of ultimate reality or ultimate in its importance, and *assumptions*, as more loosely held beliefs that are adopted strategically and only so long as they serve useful purposes. We often separate them according to their differing roles in human affairs, rather than lumping both together as "beliefs."

Convictions so strongly organize a person's life experience that they are unshakable in the face of contrary evidence. They provide autonomy and facilitate self-organization by enabling a person to sustain a particular posture vis-à-vis others despite what might be compelling arguments to the contrary. Assumptions, unlike convictions, are intended to be malleable. A person adopts different assumptions to position himself or herself flexibly in relation to other people or to the world, often in order to further a particular agenda.

Some religious beliefs are best considered as assumptions and others as convictions. The distinction between the two does not lie with their contents but how each is employed. The same statement can serve as an assumption for one person but a conviction for another. For example, a therapist might adopt as a plausible, working assumption that "religiously conservative families usually follow specific gender roles in marriage." If, however, this assumption were to prove more a hindrance than a help with certain couples in therapy, it should be easy for the therapist to drop it as a belief. On the other hand, a therapist holding a conviction that "God has ordained specific roles for men and women in marriage" would have difficulty letting go of that belief, even if it were obviously hindering clinical work with some couples.

BELIEFS BRING FORTH
SPECIFIC EMOTIONAL POSTURES

The practical differences between assumptions and convictions outweigh their similarities because each brings forth different *emotional postures* in relationships. As we discussed in Chapters 1 and 2, an emotional posture is the dynamic configuring of one's being, including perceptual, cognitive, and motor systems of the brain, into a state of readiness for action. Emotional postures are reflected in the following:

- Body posture and muscle tone, such as a physical posture that is poised, withdrawn, expressive, dejected, and tensed or relaxed muscles.
- State of activation of the autonomic nervous system, with its secondary effects on heart rate, blood pressure, and blood sugar.
- Settings for the span and focus of brain systems for vigilance and focused attention.

Mammals, including humans, show two broad repertoires of emotional postures. *Emotional postures of tranquillity* are those associated with grooming, grazing, and most parenting behaviors. These emotional postures are displayed similarly among all mammals. For humans, who possess language, this repertoire is expanded to include those that support care of self, maintenance of relationships, and creativity—musing, playing, nurturing, reflecting, listening.

Emotional postures of mobilization are associated with exploration of an unknown environment or with attack and defense. These include stalking, threatening, attacking, and hiding, behaviors displayed by all mammals. Emotional postures that support such behaviors as blaming, scorning, and flattering are available to humans who have access to language.

Beliefs recruit the body into particular emotional postures by employing specific metaphors, stories, and idioms in particular contexts. Among Israelis, the conviction *Tov la-mut be'ad artzenu*—"It is good to die for the sake of our country"—brings to mind the story of Masada as a metaphoric image of a mountain fortress that will not be moved, and the idiom "Never again!" (Bruner & Gorfain, 1984) brings forth an emotional posture of defiance. Due to these links between belief and emotional posture, a belief does not exist only as an abstract idea but also is embedded in specific physical states of the body.

The role of beliefs is important in regulating the emotional postures within which a person lives. Mr. Ali pointed to this importance with his assertion: "Therapists should all know about the body and about the spiritual if they are to help people." Although his beliefs formed the center of his religious faith, he could say, "The spirit is God. It is in the body, not in the mind."

The creation and sustenance of spiritual life is dependent upon emotional postures of tranquillity. Convictions and assumptions both serve this role when they facilitate reverence, reflection, and concern for others, which are central to spirituality. Adopting particular assumptions fosters emotional postures that lead to a desired relatedness with self, others, or a personal God. One of the most famous religious assumptions was the wager with which Pascal sought the emotional posture of certainty: "Either God exists or He does not exist; if you wager that He exists, and He in fact does exist, you gain all; if you lose the wager because He in fact does not exist you lose nothing. In wagering on God's existence, your stake is zero, your reward, if God exists, is infinite." That emotion rather than logic was driving this wager was understood by Pascal, who noted, "The heart has its reasons which reason does not know" (Thilly & Wood, 1957, p. 318). Such assumptions as "In the end, all will be well" or "Everything happens for a reason" are similarly adopted not primarily as hypotheses to be tested for their veracity, but because such assumptions (which cannot be proven or disproven) promote postures of tranquillity—hoping, opening to the other, accepting, expectant waiting—even when the weight of the evidence at a particular historical moment might not otherwise support such emotional postures.

Convictions, on the other hand, are generally used to sustain programs of action intended to remake the world into "what ought to be." In this manner religious convictions have helped focus the passion over time of a Mother Teresa or a Joan of Arc. The Mahatma Gandhi articulated well the spirit of conviction when he said: "I know this cannot be proved by argument. It shall be proved by persons living it in their lives with utter disregard of consequences to themselves" (Merton, 1965, p. 25). This spirit was echoed in the United States when Martin Luther King (1963, pp. 16241–16242) encouraged those who had been jailed and beaten to "Continue to work with the faith that unearned suffering is redemptive."

Tightly held convictions come with a risk, however. Because they are not checked by empirical evidence, there can be no "wrong" conviction. Even when evidence mounts that religious convictions are doing harm, they often persist until such non–reasoned measures as a more potent political argument or brute force counters them. Historical illustrations include the burning of religious martyrs, the hanging of accused witches in Salem, and the biblical justifications for slavery in the American South and apartheid in South Africa. Still pervasive in many groups are the oppression and silencing of women justified by beliefs about a divine order appointing men as the leaders of the family.

Moreover, convictions tend to arouse emotional postures of mobilization. More than assumptions, they foster a readiness to manage, to control, or to attack those who hold different beliefs. Emotional postures of certainty can as easily threaten a spirituality of relatedness and accountability as they can support it. As Pascal put it: "One never does evil so openly and contentedly as when one does it out of principle."

EMOTIONAL POSTURES
AND THE VALIDITY OF BELIEFS

In therapy, the two of us think about assumptions and convictions—both our own and those of individuals who consult us—in terms of the emotional postures fostered and the fruit borne. That is, we collaborate with those in therapy in examining, not so much the rationality or plausibility of their beliefs, but what real-life consequences the beliefs bear. Beliefs bringing forth emotional postures that *violate* relational interdependence and personal accountability are challenged; those bringing forth emotional postures that *nurture* relational interdependence and personal accountability are supported. Does a belief that "We are God's people" foster acceptance or contempt for those from other groups? Does a belief that "All life is sacred" lead to reverence or disdain for those who differ? Does a belief that "God controls everything" promote caring concern or neglect of others?

CONDUCTING THERAPY AROUND BELIEFS

The way we work with a belief is to listen for whether it facilitates emotional postures that sustain relationships with others and a hopeful, active involvement in the world.[2] We do not treat beliefs as if they were testable hypotheses. This point is sometimes missed by therapists when encountering the passionately held beliefs of religious people who consult them. Because a belief bears the form of a propositional statement, it can seem that the belief, like a scientific hypothesis, ought to be tested by empirical data. Can scientific evidence determine whether good health is a reward or that illness could be a punishment from God? Does marital therapy research show whether or not two people are bonded for life by sexual union? An examination of the ways that people employ beliefs in their daily lives suggests the contrary—that religious assumptions are selected or discarded according to their pragmatic utility in everyday life, and religious convictions are held according to their power in sustaining a vision that is vital to one's identity.

A belief does not need a demonstration of truth, or even a high probability of truth, to be usable. When a religious belief runs directly counter to scientific evidence, a person typically finds a way to reconcile the belief and the scientific facts, rather than changing or discarding either. This reconciliation is rarely difficult, as most spiritual and religious beliefs are both plausible and logical if certain scientifically untestable assumptions were to be granted.

REASONS FOR CAUTION
WHEN WORKING WITH BELIEFS

The two of us have emphasized more caution when addressing religious beliefs, compared to working with other aspects of spiritual experience. This may seem counterintuitive because the question "What are your beliefs?" is often the first one asked, at least among North Americans when inquiring about the spiritual life of another person. Our reasons for not leading with this question have been threefold.

Therapy is about solving problems through dialogue in the context of an open and trusting relationship. Beginning the talk of therapy around beliefs is often not a good way either to begin dialogue or to create an open and trusting relationship, for the same reasons that is wise when initiating conversation with new guests at a dinner party not to start with a discussion of politics or religion. Too often one gets debate rather than dialogue.

Second, focusing on beliefs often has become problematic for novice therapists we have supervised because skill in working directly with spiritual and religious beliefs is largely a maturational issue. Experienced, skilled therapists usually have acquired perceptual acuities for noticing subtle signs of discomfort, and know how to make quick, compensatory turns when necessary so as to keep a generative dialogue flowing. Novice therapists often are both less skilled and more preoccupied with their own thoughts about what to do next, such that unintended affronts can be made during discussions about beliefs that shut down openness and trust. Moreover, less experienced therapists often fail to attend to openings available with forms of spiritual expression other than beliefs. It has been an agenda of this book to highlight what useful options exist for work with other forms that express spiritual experience, in addition to beliefs.

Discussion about beliefs may not be useful for many persons who follow spiritual practices or a particular religion for which beliefs can play a minor role, as described in the examples of Judaism, Buddhism, and Hinduism. However such a discussion might be quite useful in working with a Protestant Christian, because beliefs are central to most of the Protestant groups.

Having stated these reservations, we assert both the importance of spiritual and religious beliefs in human life and the usefulness of clinical work with these beliefs in a well-conducted therapy. There are indeed situations in which addressing beliefs explicitly is not only an option, but essential for the success of a therapy.

Ample clinical methods have been developed for focused psychotherapy with beliefs that can be usefully applied to religious beliefs. Much of cognitive-behavioral therapy involves revising beliefs that engender illness or suffering, although the collaborative approach we promote here may not mix well with a more hierarchical one that emphasizes the diagnosis of psychopathological "cognitive distortions" or "overgeneralizations." Family therapists Lorraine Wright and colleagues (1996) have provided a broadly conceptualized, systematic approach for working with individuals' and families' systems of beliefs. Their text, *Beliefs: The Heart of Healing in Families and Illness*, is recommended reading for therapists working with religious beliefs. Narrative therapy, in externalizing problematic beliefs and their discourses, offers a whole repertoire of methods that can be applied to problems involving religious beliefs (Epston, 1993; Freedman & Combs, 1996; Roth & Epston, 1996; White, 1989a).

The illustrations in this chapter show some of the methods that we have employed in our work. Other illustrations in Chapter 9 discuss how beliefs with destructive consequences can be addressed in therapy. Cases in Chapter 10 show how beliefs can be addressed therapeutically in the context of a medical or psychiatric illness.

ONCE SPOKEN, A BELIEF IS "IN PLAY"

The initial step in working with beliefs in therapy is an inquiry that helps a person or family members to articulate beliefs they regard as important. While this step may sound like a preliminary, or "setting the stage" maneuver, the process of articulating just what a person's guiding assumptions and convictions are can provide the most potent of steps toward therapeutic change.

Beliefs commonly exist in the background of awareness only as prejudices and biases, that is, loosely connected thoughts, images, and associated emotions that have provided a background sense for "how the world is." Such unspoken beliefs exist more in a vague bodily sense of the world than in sentences (Shotter, 1993b). Ironically, a belief often holds most power over a person, family, or community when it has not yet been fully spoken in language.

Drawing a propositional statement out of this amalgam fixes the disparate parts within a coherent pattern that then can be addressed as a whole. The belief then takes on different, more flexible meanings when a person openly states it in the presence of others, particularly when it can be reflected upon in conversation.

Once spoken, a belief is "in play," accessible for challenge or revision. For example, Elaine was referred for evaluation of panic attacks. She had suffered them several times daily, and was on the verge of being fired from work due to her frequent early departures home. Despite her severe distress and possible job loss, she had refused to take the medication, clonazepam, that her primary care physician had prescribed. I (Griff) asked whether she had any particular beliefs about panic attacks—what they represented, what treatment was needed, what were the pros and cons of treatment—that had led her to refuse the medication. She told me about her mother, who had abused alcohol and benzodiazepines—Valium, Tranxene, Ativan—during her childhood. More recently, she and her mother both had begun participating in a Twelve Step recovery program. Her mother now had achieved nearly a year of sobriety.

In keeping with their Twelve Step program, Elaine and her mother believed that ingesting any mood-altering drug, including the clonazepam that her physician prescribed, violated the teachings of Alcoholics Anonymous. After Elaine articulated this belief, however, new options could be discussed: reconsidering her view of clonazepam based on scientific information (it rarely has been a drug of abuse), considering treatment with an alternative medication that would have no addictive potential (there could be several choices), or engaging others from her family or AA group in a collaborative monitoring of her use of clonazepam so that no insidious pattern of misuse would develop. As Wright and colleagues (1996, p. 189) have noted, "The very act of uncovering the core belief and saying it out loud . . . invites the [person] to examine the belief."

ASSESSING THE ECOLOGICAL
IMPACT OF A BELIEF

After a belief has been fully articulated and named as a belief, the therapist and the person can then collaborate in studying its ecological impact in the life and relationships of the person. They then can judge whether the belief sustains relationships and active involvement in the world. This provides the person with greater clarity in choosing whether this is a belief he or she desires to hold.

A person often is more aware of the immediate impact of a belief than of its consequences over time. Once it has been accepted as an operating premise, a belief often slips into the background of awareness and is no longer noticed as a chosen path. Its influence over the person's life then becomes hidden.

Assessing the ecological impact of a belief consists of a collaborative inquiry that systematically examines real-life consequences of holding the belief in order to learn how it makes a difference. For example, Richard, discussed earlier, was able to articulate during early sessions his belief that "Things must be done correctly or I unravel." After several conversations in therapy, we settled on "perfectionism" as a name for this belief. Perfectionism led him to take reasonable ideas and actions to such extremes that he was alienating friends, teachers, and family members. He noted how it fostered conflict with his parents, whose religious practices he considered to be lax. It led him to be critical of his wife, whose feelings were hurt by the judgment in his words. His criticisms had alienated him from his professors. He had felt more fearful and distant from God as he sensed that he was too flawed himself to meet his own high standards.

Richard had not fully realized how far-reaching was the influence of his convictions over the expanse of his life. As he became more mindful, he began working in therapy to counter the extent of this influence. Once named and spoken, the belief was externalized so that he could exercise choice in determining his relationship with it (Epston, 1993; Roth & Epston, 1996a; White, 1989).

DECONSTRUCTING A BELIEF

Therapy can also help deconstruct beliefs. Deconstruction consists of a systematic inquiry that makes explicit the interpretive assumptions out of which a particular belief emerged. This inquiry seeks both to identify these interpretive assumptions and to delineate their cultural and political origins. This process places the belief in a particular historical context and situates it within a particular cultural discourse (Madigan & Law, 1998; White, 1993).

A discourse, as discussed in Chapter 2, is an institutionalized manner of using language and nonverbal communications that characterizes a particular social group. There is thus a medical discourse in which physicians engage, a legal discourse in which attorneys engage, and a parenting discourse with which parents engage their children. Each group that is organized around some shared form of spiritual or religious experience has its own unique discourse that provides for its members a way of being in relationship with one another. Each of these discourses tends to validate certain ways of experiencing, expressing, and acting, while invalidating others. Beliefs are important instruments through which a discourse constructs the life-worlds in which people live.

Deconstruction can help a person to understand better his or her relationship to a particular belief, because a belief is often stated as if it were an objective fact, its historical and discursive contexts forgotten. Deconstruction is not intended to and should not destroy the belief, but rather enrich understanding and provide choice as to the role the belief ought to play in the person's life. The meaning and influence of the belief can be transformed once a person understands its historical and social contexts. With this shift, new openings often appear for resolving old problems.

Here are some illustrations of deconstructive inquiries:

1. *What personal and family experiences occurred such that this came to be an important belief?* Allison was spending her college spring break in the hospital to try to get her diabetes under control. A semester of eating and drinking with her friends, combined with failure to check and respond to her blood glucose levels, had been nearly deadly for her. The endocrinologist who consulted me (Melissa) warned that the parents might be impossible to work with, especially because Allison's father was "a rigid fundamentalist." When I had spoken with Allison privately, she said she admired her father, even though she did not have the close relationship with him that she had with her mother. He had always been very religious and very strong, and she thought he probably could not comprehend her situation or her choice of friends When I sat down with Allison and her parents, the worry and the sense of helplessness these parents felt was obvious. Allison expressed her regret and also her own helplessness to change her health-destroying behaviors. Rather than criticizing her, her father said gently, "Realizing your helplessness is the best place to start, Honey. Now the Lord can help you." Still harboring my colleague's warning in my thoughts, I feared this father's empathy might turn into a fruitless lecture. I asked him whether he knew anything, personally, about helplessness. He said he knew quite a lot. Allison looked startled, but her father did not elaborate. He returned to his main thesis: "She just needs to pray and the Lord will help her." Not responding, Allison averted her gaze. Wanting to respect her hesitation, I turned to her parents, asking, "I suppose you pray about Allison often."

"Almost constantly," her mother said. Her father told about their weekly Bible study and prayer group, and mentioned that their friends were praying for Allison also.

"If it would not be too intrusive, could you tell me what you pray, and how you sense the Lord responding?" As they each spoke the room became quieter, for they were not only speaking their prayer to me but, in that moment, to their God.

Allison looked flat and tense. "I'd like to pray, too, but I can't." I asked why. "I just can't. I used to be able to, but I can't anymore."

"But you can always pray, Jesus is always waiting for you to just come," her father implored.

"No, I can't," Allison protested. "I know that I can't. You don't understand. God does not want me to come to him this way." Her tone was final.

I asked Allison how she knew this. Had she tried to go to God and felt turned away by God? "No," she said, "It's just something I know. I've been taught the difference between right and wrong. I know right from wrong and I am still doing wrong. I can't go to God when I know I am doing wrong. I have to get right first."

Her father reached his arm out to her. With grief in his eyes, he said, "That's not from God. That's from me. I made you believe that. I'm sorry, so sorry, because it is not true. Those are my hang-ups and I gave them to you, before you can even remember." He went on to tell Allison what he had never told her, about the alcoholism from which he suffered. Sober for 15 years now, he still regretted his harsh and drunken days when she was a very young child. He told of his own stubbornness in this belief of needing to get it right before asking for help, and of the grace, both of God and of Allison's mother, that allowed him to "let go and let God." He confessed that he still got caught in it, that he had been a poor father, but that God was a good father. He welcomed you no matter how you came. He asked Allison's forgiveness.

Tears were streaming from Allison's eyes. "Oh, Daddy," she said, and hugged him tightly.

We met only a few more times. Allison did get her diabetes more in order. She realized she had more to talk about with her father and more to forgive. He continued to affirm her. Even though she did not organize her life in the way her parents would have wanted, and kept much of it private, she became more connected to both parents. She and her father instituted a weekly practice of going out to dinner together.

In most of our experiences, it has been the therapist who encourages the examination and deconstruction of a belief. It is usually not a once-and-forever act. As Allison's father said, we all "get caught" again in beliefs we do not believe. I cannot help but think, though, that because her father, rather than her therapist, offered Allison a way out, to walk alongside her out of the entrapment of her belief, she will be less vulnerable than most of us to getting caught again.

2. *For what group of people is this belief important? Who "has a stake" in continued adherence to this belief?* Greg was a man in his 20s who had sought therapy in large part over his conflicted sexual identity. He had been in several gay relationships. He had not dated a woman since his early teenage years. However, he believed that homosexuality was wrong, a violation of biblical teachings. "I have feelings and desires toward men, but that's not what I want," he said. "That's where the double standard comes in. My lifestyle is a big lie."

I (Griff) asked him at one point, "Who else in your life holds this belief? If you were to believe differently, from whom would that difference separate you?" He told about his large extended family who, over three generations, had lived a life of simplicity that traditionally centered around their church. Although Greg now lived a different lifestyle in a large city, it was with his parents, grandparents, and cousins hundreds of miles away that he felt he most belonged. His conviction that his homosexuality was intrinsically a violation of God's commandments was part of that sense of belonging.

The dilemma with which Greg struggled was a difficult one, for which he had not reached a final resolution by the time he ended therapy. By that time, his questioning appeared to have become more complex. In addition to asking "What does the Bible say?" there was another question: "With whom do I choose to identify?"

3. *How it is decided who should be an arbiter of beliefs? Who speaks for God?* In our (Melissa) initial meeting, Sandi, a graduate student, concluded her list of what needed to be different in her life by adding: "There is one more thing—I am desperate to get back to God again."

"Desperate?" I asked.

"Yes," she said, "I used to be very close to God and now I can't go to church at all."

It was not hard for Sandi to pinpoint when things had changed. Her friend, Emma, had called few months ago and had lectured Sandi on how she was sinning, displeasing God, by having sex with her boyfriend. Sandi had felt so bad that she could not bring herself to face her God.

"Is this your belief, that you are displeasing God?" I asked.

"Probably . . . maybe . . . I don't know! I'm confused," Sandi responded.

I asked her how she imagined God was responding to her confusion, both to her desperateness in wanting to come back, and to the bad feelings that were keeping her away. She said she believed in an accepting God, not a mean one, as Emma described. Still, though, she had been so upset by what Emma had told her that she could not bring herself to go back to Mass.

Our conversation had shifted now from the question of whether having unmarried sex was sinful to whether a fear that one was displeasing God should keep one from drawing close to God. Unlike Allison, Sandi was unreservedly certain that God would not want her to hide away in fear. I asked Sandi how she came to have this belief about God that was so different than her friend's belief. The source was her mother, whom, Sandi said, "is more like a saint than anyone I know. It's all about love with my mother. God is and she is. Rules are there, too, but they are way down the list after love." Her mother had taught her about God when she was a little girl, to rely on God and not to be afraid of him. She trusted her mother's knowledge of God. Besides, she said, that is how she had experienced God herself. Just not lately.

"Gee, with your experience, and with your trust in your mother's teaching, how do you suppose Emma got to be the spokesperson for God?"

She said she would have to think about that. She didn't want it to be the case.

At our next meeting she had already made several changes to put her relationships in line with respecting and taking care of herself, including researching a church that was associated with her university, a place she imagined she might find like-minds, friendship, and possibly a closeness to God again. She was planning a visit. I asked her what, if anything in our meeting had contributed to this. She said it was thinking over "that question about the spokesperson for God." Once the question was posed, she knew clearly that she would not choose Emma for this, that her words did not deserve such power.

ATTUNING TO AND HONORING
THE BELIEFS OF THE OTHER

I (Melissa) had not seen Leslie for a few months. She had consulted with me two summers ago, when she was recovering her identity and her strength after she had been systematically harassed and tormented by a clique at drama school. She was now reporting some successful recent months, telling stories of feeling appreciated, taking care of herself, and making good, trustworthy relationships. It was all great news, the culmination of hard work. I felt celebratory along with her.

"That's not exactly all," she said. "You're not going to believe this, but I told Tom that if he needed a place to stay in the city, there was an extra room at my house."

I was indeed surprised to hear this, because Tom had been the ringleader of the group who had treated her so cruelly a couple of years ago. This sounded risky to me. My thoughts must have been obvious to her.

"I know that was bad; I can see it in your face," she added. "He didn't come, which is just as well. But that's what I did, and I'd do it again."

"No, I couldn't say it was bad. How could I make such a judgment? I am surprised, though. How did you decide to make this offer?" I inquired, wanting to suspend my assumptions so I could understand hers.

"I believe . . . I hope . . . that Tom has changed, that he could be a better friend now. I've told you before that I believe, if at all possible, people should never just disconnect. I just believe that at heart people are basically good."

I did recall hearing her articulate those beliefs 2 years before. These convictions had been a mainstay in her struggle against becoming cynical and detached. At that time Leslie had given me a window into her spiritual life. She was Jewish, and celebrated holidays with her family, but she drew wisdom from many sources, including the character of her grandmother, reflective moments in a Quaker meeting, and the support of a nun friend in college. She believed in and allied herself with those who were willing to struggle with forgiveness, tolerance, and a commitment to connect. Perhaps it was not only Leslie's persistence in hope in the face of injustice, but also her Jewish heritage that made her words echo to me the words of Anne Frank. I told her that a passage of the diary kept coming to me. "Do you know it?" I wondered. " 'I still believe, in spite of everything, that people are still truly good at heart.' "

"Yes, that page is on the wall of the house in Amsterdam where she was hidden. Did you know that? I have seen it. . . . That is what I believe."

Through this process, I was moved to a position of deep respect for her belief. Earlier in the conversation my wish to see Leslie protect herself might have pulled me, at least inwardly, to contradict her belief that "people are good at heart." I could have considered it naive for her to act as she did, offering hospitality to Tom. But a desire to understand Leslie's conviction and honor it guided my thoughts to *The Diary of Anne Frank*, locating her conviction in a noble, wise, and courageous lineage. In making this connection, I, and certainly Leslie, would never want to imply an equation of her suffering to those who suffered and died in the Holocaust. It would dishonor them. We hope that we bring honor to them when we let their words and lessons permeate our thoughts, inform our beliefs, and open our hearts.

Working with beliefs means that therapists examine not only the beliefs of the other, but our own beliefs and how they influence relationships with self and others. Sometimes the belief systems of clinician and client collide. One can be drawn into paternalism when a person articulates a belief or plans a belief-based course of action that seems to be against his or her best interest or to run counter to "known" psychological principles. Avoiding that, we want to be honest about the difference, yet open to dialogue and change. Perhaps we will come to understand that the belief works well for that person. If we listen broadly and deeply, perhaps we will hear wisdom from other cultures or religious traditions.

Another situation in which I (Melissa) moved from differing with to accepting a belief of the other occurred in the couple work with Frank and Mary (Chapters 3–4). They had abstained from sexual relations for nearly a year. Mary was not ready, and was unsure that she would ever be ready. Frank assured her that he would never push. He knew he had hurt her and said that he could wait forever, knowing that this might even mean never. I held the belief that it would be difficult to repair their marriage without physical intimacy, and I wondered if their conversation had become a cycle of avoidance. Could it really be okay never to have sex? I even doubted the authenticity of this position, or, if authentic, how long could it last and what might the effect be. I had approached this question with them on more than one occasion. After the third or fourth time I mentioned it, Frank gently offered me a 3" × 5" notecard at the next session containing notes on the question of abstinence within marriage. He had taken my concerns seriously. He searched his heart for honesty and the Scriptures for the truth. He now wanted me to take his convictions seriously. Here is the notecard, which, at my request, he read aloud:

ABSTAINING FROM SEXUAL ACTIVITY: I CORINTHIANS 7:5

In answering questions posed by the Corinthians about sexual activity between a husband and wife, Paul explains that they may mutually agree "to
refrain from the rights of marriage for a limited time, so that they can give
themselves more completely to prayer."

Obviously, if we belong both to God and to our spouse, we will want to act
in ways to please both. Our challenge is to not seek only for our personal
gratification. We must be patient and content in our period of reconciliation with each other. God will let us know when the marriage has been
healed.

Frank concluded that while sex was touted by the culture as the "be
all and end all" of a relationship, it was not central. As partners they
could be reconciled, joined, and intimate in many ways as he matured in
the faith and as Mary healed. His words were reassuring to Mary. She
had been worried that he would grow tired of waiting and of the time
she needed to heal. These words were also settling to me. I was convinced that their decision was right for them and I never tried to push
against their convictions again. I was also prompted to let go my own, in
retrospect, rigid beliefs about sexual intimacy and marriage.

REVISING BELIEFS CAN REPOSITION
A PERSON IN RELATIONSHIP WITH GOD

As in human relationships, a relationship with a personal God has dimensions of both power and intimacy. Beliefs help regulate each of these
dimensions. When a person–God relationship fails to operate as a generative dialogue, the reason sometimes is that hierarchical aspects of the
relationship have become too imbalanced (e.g., "God is so powerful and
I am so weak") or emotionally distant ("God does not know or care
about me") for a fruitful dialogue to take place between the person and
God.

When asked about her experience of God, Anne, a 35-year-old
woman who was participating in our research study (Griffith et al.,
1992, 1995), responded: "In the last year or so, I've done a whole lot of
questioning, so that right now God feels more remote than he had previ-

ously. I used to experience him as more gentle, more personal . . . more the stereotype of what Jesus was . . . a more interactive kind of God." She went on to describe how her beliefs about God had changed little over the past 20 years, until the past few months. She had become a Christian at age 15, and she had held a faith since that time that God was putting together the puzzle pieces of her life into some coherent pattern. She felt comforted and cared for by God, trusting that "there was something beyond me greater than me that was guiding things a little bit."

During recent months, however, Anne had experienced tragedy in her life and had witnessed tragedies in the lives of two close friends. She began noticing more often than before the suffering of abused, oppressed, and disabled people. "How can God permit these things to happen?" she wondered. She now felt uncertain who God was and what God's participation was in the world. As her beliefs became more riddled with doubt, God also became emotionally distant and inscrutable. Anne asked: "What do I do? What do I believe in? What was all that stuff the last 20 years? Why were you there then, God, and what's happened now? What's changed?"

Two vignettes, one of Katherine and another of Daniel, illustrate ways that therapeutic dialogue about beliefs can help a person reposition a relationship with his or her God. A person's beliefs can sometimes point to more possibilities for intimacy and freedom with one's God than the person has as yet discovered in the relationship. When this is the case, the therapeutic task is to highlight the belief as a bearer of hope.

Katherine articulated her goal at the beginning of our meeting, "I feel like I'm a wimp. I want to gain more courage. I feel so fearful and fragile, and I don't want to be that way. I want to be more sturdy." I (Melissa) asked if the harsh standard by which she judged herself, and the habit it engendered—berating herself as a wimp—was impeding her progress. Not accepting her fear, it seemed, was keeping her from noticing her courage. "Maybe what I really need is to become patient with myself as I get sturdier," Katherine said. Attending to this revised goal, we began an interesting and fruitful conversation.

Near the end of our session I realized that, while I knew from her profession that spirituality was central to Katherine's life, we had not brought it to bear on this issue. I asked a final, very general question. "In your desire to be more patient with yourself as you continue to get more sturdy—It is hard to hold to that, right?" Katherine nodded, and I continued. "I was just wondering, is there anything from your spiritual life, or relationships, or beliefs that will help you hold steady to being more patient and becoming more sturdy? You may not wish to answer this question now, but just to take it with you."

Katherine thought for a moment. "Well, yeah," she slowly began, "I do want to answer that question. You see, I believe that God gave me all my feelings—my fears and fragilities and desires—God gave us all our feelings, so even though I have problems with them, God doesn't, so they must be okay. So there's room for them. They don't have to be hidden or chased out. But his love is so much bigger than they are. I guess if I just lean into his big love," she laughingly said as she heaved her body to the side into a big imaginary something, "I can just lean into his big love and bring my little fear along with me." She was holding the imagined fear as if it were the size of a small doll. "There is room for it there and he can hold all of us. Yeah, I need to remember this."

My intent in asking that final question was to shore up her preferred story of patience with herself and hold it in place over time. Indeed, Katherine's belief that all that she was struggling with was created by God, and thus accepted by God, as well as her perspective of God's big love enveloping her little fears did seem to deepen the changes brought about during our meeting. When she had begun the conversation, she spoke of her experience of fear and of the oppression of an exacting standard. Katherine expanded her view of herself, loosened up and accepted herself more as she talked. Finally, it was when she articulated her belief that she seemed to connect with the most liberating experience, that of leaning into God's big love.

For Daniel, his beliefs promised a greater intimacy with God than his experience had yet provided. He and Diane were in couple therapy. Though we had never talked about anything spiritual, I (Melissa) knew from the way they talked about their week's schedule that they were actively involved in a local Protestant congregation. The couple work had been progressing slowly but steadily, until Daniel had another verbally explosive tirade at home, reminding them of their former distress and creating serious doubts as to whether things would ever get better. Daniel immediately took full responsibility for his behavior and acknowledged with regret the hurt he had caused Diane and their children. Daniel was ashamed, Diane was sad and resentful, and both were discouraged. We set the first priority as ensuring safety and preventing future destructive outbursts. I suggested taking "time-outs" as a procedure that had been helpful to many couples. They developed their own signal system and agreed to practice during the week by calling one time-out each. Daniel then voiced his concern that things might be no different when they rejoined after a time-out. He wanted to come back cooler and more reflective, but said he feared that he would only use his time away to fume and build a case against Diane, making matters only worse upon return. He wanted to know, when he felt that tense, how could he change to a reflective mode? Did I have any ideas that might help to prevent this?

I told them that I had recently read an article in a professional journal (Butler et al., 1998) in which the author discussed some couples using their time-outs for prayer. "Would that be something that might appeal to you?" I asked.

Diane looked interested, but Daniel said no. He just couldn't imagine praying at a time like that. "That's when I think the Catholic prayers are helpful," said Diane, "As prayers that are memorized, rather than having to come up with words of your own when you are upset."

"It's not that," said Daniel, "I've always felt that I need to be more composed, more presentable before I pray. I can't fathom going before God when I am such a wreck."

"Is that your experience of God, that you must be composed and presentable to go before God?" I added, " I am not asking about what you believe, your theology, but your experience of it."

Daniel responded with a statement about his belief. "I don't believe God needs me to be that way. It's my pride that keeps me from going at those times. I'm just too ashamed of myself."

"Can you recall any experiences with God that confirmed that, that God didn't need you to be that way?" I asked him.

"No," he said, "Never. I have always been held back by my pride. I'm the one who needs to change, not God."

"But how can you be so sure about God's willingness to accept you, if you have never experienced it?" I was really curious.

Daniel looked directly at me and spoke with clear intensity. "Every human soul," he emphasized, "*Every* human soul belongs to God, and he accepts it, no matter how deplorable its state."

I repeated these sentences to Daniel, asking him if we could wait, so that I could record them in my notes, word for word. Daniel and Diane left the session with a commitment to try the time-outs. After they left, I glanced at the clarity of Daniel's words in my notes, recalling also how difficult he said it was for him to think clearly in periods of anger. I decided to give his words back to him in the form of a letter. On a small, blank business card I wrote:

"Every human soul belongs to God, and he accepts it,
no matter how deplorable its state.
It is I who needs to change, not God."

I enclosed the card with a brief note:

Dear Daniel and Diane,

Daniel, this note is primarily for you. That seems right because you took full responsibility for the anger outbursts. And that alone is a hopeful sign. I wrote down the words you said that expressed your conviction, though not yet translated into your experience, of God's acceptance of you even during and after an angry and destructive outburst.

I wanted to send these words back to you, perhaps to keep in your pocket, to have at the ready when the practice or real time-out comes. I believe I have your words down right. Will you let me know? As I understand you, you do desire to live into your belief.

I will be curious and hopeful as to what difference this might make. The shame that leads to blame must be a terribly isolating experience. Could this acceptance in which you believe break through that isolation? If so, it seems it might alter the whole cycle.

I know things cannot go on as they are. I will hold the memory and possibility of what has and can happen and hope for the lasting change you both desire.

Sincerely,

Melissa

Several weeks had passed before I saw either Diane or Daniel again, though I had heard from both about how much better things were. Diane was too pressured at work to come, but she encouraged Daniel to come alone and he did. He said he had carried the card I had sent and had pondered it often. I said it had made an impression on me as well and recollected the beginning phrase. "That's a strong word—*deplorable*," I said.

"Yes," he agreed, "it's strong, but it's reality, at least in some ways." There are inescapable reasons that I say that. It's all right, though. It doesn't engender self-denigration, because it is combined with the acceptance. It does, however, allow me to be poor in spirit and that allows me to pray, though not in the way that you might think prayer would sound. This allows me to know compassion for Diane. She really deserves that because these have been hard days for her at work, you know. My job now is finding a way to express the compassion. It can't be in that old paternalistic, patronizing way I used to do it. I can't fall back on that. It's too easy and it's not fair. My job is learning to express it a the new way, a way of creative, respectful listening."

NOTES

1. Mr. Ali's account is drawn from an ongoing project studying whether engagement with spirituality provides resilience to destructive effects of political torture on those who have survived it (Gaby et al., 2000a, 2000b).
2. We of course assert a particular value in stating this criterion, that sustenance of relationships and a hopeful, active involvement in the world is good. Other individuals, spiritual traditions, and cultures might view this differently. Their summum bonum could be utter detachment from the world. The relationship to be sustained might be the one with God, through a life dedicated to prayer and contemplation.

Chapter Seven

Rituals, Ceremonies, and Spiritual Practices

On a few wonderful occasions Jewish friends have asked us to join them for their Shabbat meal. We stand with them around the table as they light the candles and sing the blessings, and it seems that we are standing on the edge of a body of people that extends over the world, into the past and the future. Simultaneously, I (Melissa) am listening to the explanations our friends so cordially provide and recalling a movie scene from *Fiddler on the Roof,* which I saw as a child. Tevye and his humble family are gathering around their table. As he sings blessings for his daughters, in the glow of the Shabbat candles, one can imagine other families, their remembered grandparents and great-grandparents, their neighbors, and Jewish people throughout the land, all enacting the Shabbat ritual, filling our minds with their fidelity and enduring strength.

As a child watching this movie, I did not understand the significance of the ritual, but I was still inspired by it; inspiration is often not related to comprehension. This was before the days of VCRs, so I saw the movie as many times as I had money to go and then purchased the record. I wrote down the words to Tevye's Shabbat blessing in my diary, memorized them, and determined that this would be a song sung at my table when I grew up. What I did not realize then was that the ritual did not create a magical connection; it was instead an affirmation of a mystery, a connection to the Holy, to the body of a people, and to their history. I could visit, honor, and appreciate it, but it could not be appropriated by me. It drew its power from the Jewish community from which it came. It belonged to them, and they to it.

RITUALS, CEREMONIES, AND SPIRITUAL PRACTICES

What is often striking about rituals, ceremonies, and spiritual practices is their stereotyped character: The same actions are repeated sequentially, over and over, at regularly prescribed times. From one celebration to the next, and from one generation to the next, the words and actions of a Passover Seder, a Ramadan Fast, or a Christian Eucharist are repeated.

Rituals, ceremonies, and spiritual practices share some other similarities. To perform each of them, a person must participate with body as well as mind. Each of the three goes beyond language to engage the body through physical action and bodily experience—specific posturing, gesturing, speaking, hearing, eating, drinking, touching, smelling. Whether it is the filing of teeth in a Balinese initiation rite, the tasting of wine and bitter herbs in a Jewish Passover, or the sweltering heat in a Native American sweat lodge, avenues are opened to unique psychobiological states, fostering experiences that might be difficult to access through language alone. Wittgenstein (cited in Monk, 1990, p. 578) observed that "we reach the end of doubt, rather, in practice: 'Children do not learn that books exist, that armchairs exist—they learn to fetch books, sit in armchairs.' " Through the actions of rituals, ceremonies, and spiritual practices, there is a direct encounter of bodily experience with culturally shaped stories, myths, and sagas.

Rituals, ceremonies, and, in some cases, spiritual practices signal to others messages about "to whom I belong"—that one is a member of a particular family, culture, or people for whom that ritual, ceremony, or practice holds special meaning. They call to memory the idea that "we belong together" and remind us why this is so. They also bring about an attunement of bodily experience among members of the group, so that,

for example, "We are Muslims" is not just an idea but the shared physical experience of bowing toward the East five times daily.

RITUAL AS SYMBOLIC PERFORMANCE

A ritual represents the public enactment of *synecdoche*, such that the
form of ritual also embodies its symbolic meaning. Synecdoche is a complex trope, built by integrating two simpler tropes: metaphor and
metonymy. Metonymy points to a relationship of contiguity or proxim-
ity—that which matters is that which touches or is close to. Metonymy
can be contrasted with metaphor, which maps a pattern of similarity between a source and a target domain. A metonym states a relation between parts of the same whole ("He's a chip off the old block"); a metaphor states a relation between aspects of different wholes ("He's as
dense as a block"). Roman Jakobson showed how the two traditional
classes of magic are dependent either on metonymy as a relationship of
contiguity (sticking pins into someone's nail clippings in order to harm
him or her) or on metaphor as a relationship of similarity (sticking pins
into someone's carved image in order to harm that person) (Friedrich,
1991). For a Jewish person to touch the Wailing Wall while speaking a
prayer or for a Muslim to turn toward Mecca to pray denote metonymic
relationships. Jesus' statement "I am the true vine . . . you are the
branches" articulated a metonymic relationship that has remained one
of the most powerful symbols in the Christian religion (John 15:1, 5,
RSV).

Synecdoche merges a metonym with a metaphor. In synecdoche a
part of a whole (a metonymic relation) also replicates the pattern of the
whole (a metaphoric relation). It is a part that appears as a microcosm,
much like a fractal image in which any part of the image also replicates
the form of the whole. For example, the Mahatma Gandhi, in an act of
civil disobedience, picked up a handful of salt and began his walk to the
sea, refusing to submit to the law that gave England a monopoly on the
salt trade. As the multitudes poured into the streets to follow him,
Gandhi's act of breaking even a tiny part of English law (metonymy) embodied the form of civil disobedience (metaphor). Ritual can convey
powerfully symbolic meaning by drawing from these dual sources simultaneously. Gandhi's use of synecdoche was so powerful that it birthed a
new nation. Rituals, such as the Jewish Seder, the Christian Eucharist, or

the Islamic Ramadan, typically are performances of synecdoche conducted publicly within a social group.

Symbolically, a ritual permits entities that appear as separate totali-
ties in everyday life (e.g., "nature" and "society," "God" and "humankind," "people as individuals" and "family") to be recognized as inter-
dependent parts of a whole, in a unity that the ritual action creates. In a
wedding, there is presented not only the abstract idea that two individuals should now become a spiritual unity, but the wedding participants—
family members as well as bride and groom—physically experience this
meaning as the bride and groom enter the chamber from separate ends
of the building, are joined, then walk out together, and the members of
the two families separated in their seating on either side of the aisle during the ceremony are then mingled during the celebration that follows.

Rituals and ceremonies serve a special role in human life by punctu-
ating experience into meaningful chunks of time. They highlight and illuminate important occurrences, while pointing to transition and future
change. The positioning of a series of graduation ceremonies in the edu-
cational system—kindergarten, middle school, high school, then college—segments childhood into discrete regions of time. A baptism or a
Bat Mitzvah points backward toward what has happened in the past,
while also pointing to a future of new possibilities. This backward-and-
forward looking character of ritual and ceremony also serves to join the
known and the not-yet-knowable. As Evan Imber-Black and Janine
Roberts (1992, p . 3) have put it: "Rituals surround us and offer opportunities to make meaning from the familiar and the mysterious at the
same time."

Rituals and ceremonies thus provide a way for human beings to address that which existentially must remain ambiguous, uncertain, or inchoate. When a relationship breaks up for reasons that cannot be understood, tragedy strikes the life of one who is blameless, or an immigrant
grieves silently for his or her lost home, then life presses the realization
that destiny can be neither logical nor just. Ritual and ceremony can
provide a capacity to bear that which cannot be understood.

RITUAL DEFINED

Turner (1982, p. 79) defined ritual as "prescribed formal behavior for
occasions not given over to technological routine, having reference to

beliefs in invisible beings or powers regarded as the first and final causes of all effects." From Turner's perspective, ritual always has a referent in transcendent experience. He viewed the performance of ritual as a process by which a culture adapts both to internal changes, such as group conflicts over relationships or values, and to external changes, such as erratic weather patterns or natural disaster. Unlike theater, where one watches the action from a distance, ritual provides a direct way to participate in symbolic expression.

Across different cultures Turner noted how a major function of ritual is its staging of a direct encounter between the person and the numinous—God, or other primal forces that surpass human understanding. This encounter brings a participant in ritual into a direct experience of that which lies beyond the superficial order and predictability of everyday life. In the awe and wonder that are felt, an expectation of new possibilities builds, supplying opportunities for creative change and new beginnings. The sequence of words, movements, and singing in observance of the Jewish Shabbat is a ritual honed over thousands of years of history. It articulates a relationship between God and humankind and establishes a bond among Jewish people that is central to their identity.

RITUAL AND COMMUNITAS

Communitas is a social process that is an important aspect of a ritual experience. As discussed in Chapter 1, communitas describes the pervasive spirit of unity among those who participate together in the performance of a ritual, when the awareness of connection with the other is so strong that any sense of differentness according to wealth, social status, power, race, or culture evaporates. Turner (1982) quoted from Malcolm X's *Autobiography* (1966, pp. 340–341) to illustrate communitas as it existed within a hajj, a Muslim pilgrimage to Mecca:

> You may be shocked by these words coming from me. But on this pilgrimage, what I have seen and experienced has forced me to *rearrange* much of my thought-patterns previously held and to *toss aside* some of my previous conclusions. . . . During the past eleven days here in the Muslim world, I have eaten from the same plate, drunk from the same glass, and slept in the same bed (or on the same rug)—while praying *to the same* God—with fellow Muslims, whose eyes were the bluest of blue, whose hair was the

blondest of blond, and whose skin was the whitest of white. And in the *words* and in the *actions* and in the *deeds* of the "white" Muslims, I felt the same sincerity that I had felt among the black African Muslims of Nigeria, Sudan, and Ghana. We were *truly* all the same (brothers)—because their belief in one God had removed the "white" from their *minds*, the "white" from their *behavior*, and the "white" from their *attitude*. I could see from this, that perhaps if white Americans could accept the Oneness of God, then, perhaps, too, they could accept *in reality* the Oneness of Man—and cease to measure, and hinder, and harm others in terms of their "differences" in color. (pp. 168–169, original emphasis)

RITUAL AND LIMINALITY

Communitas characterizes the liminal stage of rituals and other ritualized social processes. Liminality was first described in the writings on "rites of passage" by the French anthropologist Arnold Van Gennep (1909). As the 19th century ended, Van Gennep was noting that rituals nearly always accompany transitions from one situation or stage of life to another, and he described rites of passage as those rituals accompanying change from one place, state, social position, or age to another. He found each rite of passage to be marked by three phases: (1) a first phase of separation in which the person detaches from the former place or situation, as when a young man in an initiation rite is taken by older men in the tribe into the bush; (2) a liminal phase in which the status of the person is ambiguous, during which the young initiate is subjected to ritual acts that can be either degrading, such as ritual beating or cutting, or uplifting, such as being entrusted with secret language and knowledge; then (3) a reaggregation phase in which the person performing the ritual reenters society as belonging to the new position and stage of life. These three phases can even be seen in remnant form in modern weddings, in the separation of bride and groom by respective male and female groups of relatives and friends through bridal showers, bachelor parties, and forbidden contact during the hours immediately before the ceremony (separation phase), then their meeting again at the altar before the minister, priest, or rabbi (liminal phase), and finally, their walking out of the ceremony into the reception as husband and wife (reaggregation phase). As a ritualized social process, the three phases can also be seen in the United States when teenagers journey to college, often attending school away from their homes for the first time (separation phase); while in college often experimenting with roles and values (sexual behaviors, alcohol and drugs, political movements, religious conversions) that challenge or critique those of their families or society at large (liminal phase), and then returning to structured society after school as adults who are often more similar than different from the parents and culture that birthed them (reaggregation phase).

What interested Turner about the middle, liminal phase of ritual was its frequently intense association with communitas. Liminality and communitas brought a moratorium on the usual rules structuring society that permitted a playful ambiguity. Experimentation about rules, roles, and values was often condoned. Turner (1969, pp. 167, 133) noted: "If liminality is regarded as a time and place of withdrawal from normal modes of social action, it can be seen as potentially a period of scrutinization of the central values and axioms of the culture in which it occurs," and "Structure tends to be pragmatic and this-worldly; while communitas is often speculative and generates imagery and philosophical ideas." Turner hypothesized that liminality and communitas were the fundamental social processes through which the genres of symbolic action—ritual, myth, tragedy, and comedy—came into being.

CEREMONY

A ceremony is an occasion of prescribed social behavior that is choreographed to proclaim order in the face of life's uncertainties and chaos. To the extent that a ritual emerges from encounters with the numinous, a ceremony more often is inspired by its own human society. As anthropologists Sally Moore and Barbara Myerhoff (1977, p. 16) noted, a ceremony is a "a declaration against indeterminacy. Through form and formality it celebrates man-made meaning, the culturally determinate, the regulated, the named, and the explained. It banishes from consideration the basic questions raised by the made-upness of culture, its malleability and alternability. . . . [Every ceremony] seeks to state that the cosmos and social world, or some particular small part of them, are orderly and explicable and for moment fixed."

Rituals have only participants; all are drawn into participation in the symbol. When there is an audience for a ritual, the meaning of the performance is better considered as theater. With ceremony, however, an audience may play a critical role as witnesses who impart meaning to the ceremony. The transfer of office during a presidential inauguration is intended to be witnessed by the citizens of the nation and would otherwise hold little meaning for the politicians participating in it.

Ceremony Indicates; Ritual Transforms

Whereas rituals stir emotions of wonder, reverence, awe, and openness to new possibilities, ceremonies tend to stir certainty and conviction. These differences in associated emotional postures enable ritual and ceremony each to address a different side of an important ambivalence that humans share: whether to open oneself to transformation by new and not-yet-revealed possibilities, or whether to seek security in the already familiar and stable. Participation in the Christian Eucharist, as a ritual, is an encounter with mystery. Ceremonies of state that presidents and prime ministers conduct serve primarily to give assurance to their citizens that there is stability and security in the governance of their society.

A ceremony lacks the liminality that is so characteristic of ritual. As Turner (1982, p. 80) noted: "Without taking liminality into account ritual becomes indistinguishable from 'ceremony.' The liminal phase is the essential, *anti*-secular component in ritual *per se*, whether it be labeled 'religious' or 'magical.' Ceremony indicates, ritual transforms." Social structures established by power, wealth, or social status disappear during the communitas evoked by the liminality of a ritual, whether it be a Christian Eucharist, a Japanese tea ceremony, Ramadan, or Passover. Ceremonies, on the other hand, tend to reinforce societal distinctions of power and position. An awards ceremony in an organization, a school graduation, or the installation of officers in a club all restate and reinforce the structures of their social groups.

Understanding Ritual and Ceremony in a Therapeutic Context

If these differences in meaning, emotion, and social relatedness are the distinctions that matter between ritual and ceremony, then a particular occasion of prescribed social behavior can serve a ritual function for some members of a group and a ceremony function for others. Some participants in a Catholic Mass experience the event as a moment of mystical encounter with God (a ritual), while others experience it as a public statement that "I am a member of the family of Catholics" (a ceremony). For some, a wedding is a moment when two persons become one being, joined in a mystical union that will last throughout eternity (a ritual). For others, participation in a wedding seals a legal merger between two persons and their possessions, social positions, and social networks (a ceremony).

In dealing with rituals or ceremonies in therapy, this distinction can help a clinician generate reflective questions. For instance, a therapist might wonder:

- Does this person or family find emotions of openness—awe, wonder, reverence—or emotions of certainty—assurance, conviction, zeal—by participating in this performance?
- Does this performance function to reinforce a social status quo, or to open the status quo to the possibility of transformation and radical change?
- [If a couple or a family] How is this meaning different for the different partners or family members?

Such questions can open new understanding for the therapist, the individual, or the couple partners, particularly when partners have become entrenched in repetitive, fruitless exchanges over differences in religious preferences.

SPIRITUAL PRACTICE

A spiritual practice is a method for transforming one's being—mind and body—to expand its openness to spiritual experiences. What is important is not the symbolic meaning of the enacted behaviors but the change in consciousness that ensues. Examples of spiritual practices involve dietary disciplines, physical exertion, quieting of body arousal, or chanting, which religions throughout the world have employed to facilitate a desired state of consciousness.

Spiritual practices differ from rituals and ceremonies in several ways. They are less an experience of "living into" a symbol. Ceremonies and rituals are usually social events among a community, but spiritual practices often can be enacted by individuals in solitude. A spiritual practice usually places more emphasis than either ritual or ceremony on direct engagement of physiological processes. While spiritual practices can include traditional practices of a religious body, like fasting, chanting, or dancing, they may also represent practices tailored to fit unique life circumstances.

The story of Antonio shows how a person can also craft a personal and unique spiritual practice to meet the demands of a specific situation. Antonio had been sexually abused as a boy. He was distressed that in his sexual relationship with his spouse, Isadora, he sometimes found himself objectifying her, relating to her body first and to her as a whole person secondarily, an attitude he considered to be violent. When this attitude would predominate, it saddened and disappointed both Antonio and Isadora. He wanted to be physically present with her in a way that was more reflective of their loving connection. Both partners knew their marriage and intimate life had been and would continue to be intruded on by the pervasive cultural influences that have long urged men to objectify women, and sometimes vice versa. They wanted to work in couple therapy to restore and protect their relationship from the damage wrought by Antonio's abuser, and from the sway of the unwanted messages from the larger culture. Antonio crafted a simple practice for his moments of intimacy with Isadora: "I say to myself over and over, like a mantra, 'My body is a channel of peace. I love and respect her. My body is a channel of peace.' And I am able then to be present, gentle, and connected." When inquiring later whether I (Melissa) had understood the meaning correctly, I commented: "My notes read that you say to yourself: 'My body is a vessel, filled with peace. I love and respect her.' " Antonio responded: "There is one difference. You said the word 'vessel'—I say 'channel.' " I asked him to say more about the word "channel." He explained that a channel, unlike a vessel, is open on both ends. The channel was himself, yet it also held a capacity to be filled with something greater than himself—a peace that he could feel flowing through him. His mantra moved in a circle, continually connecting him to something greater than himself, to his own body, and to Isadora in an attitude of love and respect.

Because spiritual practices help modulate physiological states of the body, they can play important roles, not only in mediating relationships, as with Antonio and Isadora, but also in preparing the body to be resilient in the face of a medical illness, a discussion that will be elaborated in Chapter 10.

RITUAL, CEREMONY, AND PRACTICE:
BODILY FLOW OF SPIRITUALITY

The relationship of ritual, ceremony, and spiritual practice to the body is a more important commonality than any resemblances they share in symbolic form. They each extend beyond language to involve the body directly. As the body is reconfigured under the influence of ritual, ceremony, or spiritual practice, constraints are loosened as to what can be experienced. This nonverbal, bodily experience of meaning is added to the verbal meaning that is expressed in ideas. This is one reason why experiences can be so profound when encountered within ritual, ceremony, or spiritual practice.

A contrast between the bodily experience of ritual and the intellectual experience of ideas can be seen in one of the most beautifully articulated descriptions of therapeutic ritual in Western literature—Sonya's confrontation of Raskolnikov in Dostoyevsky's *Crime and Punishment*. In this passage, Raskolnikov has come to Sonya to confess his murder of two women, a crime committed only to demonstrate that he had the daring of an exceptional man, a Napoleon whose will to power would be unfettered by the common morality of the masses. Now he wants to confess to end his torment, and is even willing to accept the price that his confession would exact, hard labor in a Siberian prison. His confession is elaborated through a rational analysis of his reasons for killing. Sonya hears the tearful confession, but does not let it end with that. She asks him to make a ritual confession to the earth, its people, and to God, by placing a cross around his neck, bowing to the earth in the middle of the city Haymarket, and confessing his sin to all present in this public place. He at first refuses, then returns to perform her request:

> He walked into the Haymarket. It was unpleasant, very unpleasant, for him to encounter people, yet he was going precisely where he could see the most people. He would have given anything to be alone, yet he felt himself that he could not have remained alone a minute. . . . He suddenly remembered Sonya's words: "Go to the crossroads, bow down to people, kiss the earth, because you have sinned before it as well, and say aloud to the whole world: 'I am a murderer!' " He trembled all over as he remembered it. And so crushed was he by the hopeless anguish and anxiety of this whole time, and especially of the last few hours, that he simply threw himself into the possibility of this wholesome, new, full sensation. It came to him suddenly

in a sort of flame, engulfed him. Everything softened in him all at once, and the tears flowed. He simply fell to the earth where he stood. . . . He knelt in the middle of the square, bowed to the earth, and kissed the filthy earth with delight and happiness. He stood up and then bowed once more. . . .

Without looking back, [he] went straight down the side street in the direction of the police station. On the way an apparition flashed before him, but he was not surprised by it; he had already anticipated that it must be so. As he bowed down the second time in the Haymarket, turning to the left, he had seen Sonya standing about fifty steps away. She was hiding from him behind one of the wooden stalls in the square, which meant that she had accompanied him throughout his sorrowful procession! Raskolnikov felt and understood in that moment, once and for all, that Sonya was now with him forever and would follow him even to the ends of the earth, wherever his fate took him. (Dostoyevsky, 1992, pp. 524–526)

The language of bodily sensation stands out throughout Dostoyevsky's story. Through early chapters, it is notable how Roskolnikov experienced the world from a detached intellectual viewpoint, observing it from a distance, witnessing and analyzing the sensations of his body—its hunger, dizziness, pains, fatigue—with such detachment that they could well belong to another person. Murder was measured as an idea, not for what it might mean in either his experience or that of his victims. When Raskolnikov performed the ritual confession, however, "Everything softened in him all at once, and the tears flowed." From this point of redemption forward, Roskolnikov's body, mind, and spirit starts moving together as a unity. Such is the power of ritual for transcending language and ideas.

While distinctions between rituals, ceremonies, and spiritual practices can serve useful purposes in clinical work, in daily life the three flow together, merging and separating, as symbolic forms are inclined to do in any aesthetic work. A specific episode of spiritual experience might employ each of them, much like different instruments harmonizing while performing a piece of music. In some Christian cultures, a prayer vigil on Good Friday (a spiritual practice) prepares the participants for the experience of the Mass (a ritual), which might be followed by an Easter Sunday parade with its brightly colored dresses, baby carriages, and ribbons celebrating new birth and the coming of spring (a ceremony).

On the whole, the mental health disciplines have been slow to incorporate clinical work with rituals and ceremonies. Clergy and pastoral counselors have utilized their roles as officiates for life-cycle rituals—

births, marriages, deaths, and such rites of passage as Bar Mitzvahs and baptisms—to integrate personal and family therapy with ritual performances (Friedman, 1985). Some strategic therapists have used the assignment of family ceremonies as a method for leveraging change in the family system (Madanes, 1984; Palazzoli et al., 1978). With *Rituals for Our Times*, Imber-Black and Roberts (1992) have provided what is perhaps the most accessible, readable guide for therapists and families seeking creative ways to draw from the healing potentials of rituals and ceremonies.

RITUALS AND CEREMONIES CAN BE DISTINGUISHED FROM PSYCHOPATHOLOGY

Confusion between psychopathology and the normal rituals and ceremonies of everyday life has diminished the interest of some clinicians in utilizing them. The stereotyped behavioral sequences in rituals and ceremonies have led to comparisons with phobic or obsessive-compulsive behaviors ever since the writings of Sigmund Freud. However, the resemblances are superficial.

Authentic rituals and ceremonies are in most cases qualitatively different from "rituals" in the clinical literatures of psychiatry and behavioral psychology. Repetitive behaviors associated with anxiety disorders, such as compulsive cleaning rituals or checking-the-locked-doors rituals, have an urgency and drivenness that is lacking in the important rituals of a culture. The dominant affect in a compulsive ritual is that of fear, and even the person performing the behavior often regards it as a mindless, irrational act devoid of meaning other than relieving anxiety. Authentic ritual stimulates creative expression and personal growth; rigid, obsessive "ritualized" behavior functions only to bind anxiety.

Participation in the choreographed behavior of authentic rituals and ceremonies also is voluntary and closely tied both to the person's values and to the meaning experienced during the performance. This intense association of rituals with meaning and values, as well as their religious connotations—"beliefs in invisible beings or powers regarded as the first and final causes of all effects" (Turner, 1982, p. 79)—have been too much ignored by Freudian psychiatrists and Skinnerian behavioral psychologists, who have viewed them as psychopathology.

RITUALS AND CEREMONIES IN THERAPY

The therapeutic possibilities that ritual and ceremony present in psycho-therapy differ according to the position of the therapist within the social structure of the person's religious tradition. A therapist who also serves as pastor, priest, or rabbi is in a different position than a therapist who is a secular psychotherapist or family therapist. Edwin Friedman (1985), drawing from his rabbinical experiences, has provided illustrative examples of how clergy can use the occasion of such life-cycle rituals as christenings, Bar Mitzvahs, weddings, and funerals to effect healing transformations in families. As a spokesperson for God, clergy can at times utilize a privileged position to structure how rituals and ceremonies are to be conducted or to declare what is spiritual truth, while at other times asking the same questions of curiosity that a secular therapist might ask.

As secular therapists, the two of us have usually found ourselves in a different role. We help people to notice, honor, and make space for important rituals and ceremonies in their lives, staying curious about what the person's experience is and how that may be relevant to the work of the therapy. Our role is to support the person in "holding the mystery" as he or she participates in, learns from, and draws strength from a ritual or ceremony.

Laticia, for example, was an accountant rising through the ranks at a large firm. Articulate and sophisticated, she moved easily through her professional and social circles. She was engaged to marry Phil, a senior partner in another accounting firm, but could not bring herself to tell her family. She hesitated because it often seemed that the more success she achieved in her professional life, the more distant she felt from them. Her parents had been immigrants from a Caribbean island a generation earlier, and she had grown up in a large family where daily life was dominated by family traditions and their Catholic faith. Not only had she been the first college graduate in the family, but she had attended an Ivy League college and graduate school. She seldom traveled home and felt a world apart from her family. Now she was marrying a man—white, wealthy, and older than she—who represented the antithesis of her African Caribbean family and its values. She feared that the marriage might widen a gulf that could never be bridged with her family.

In an early session, I (Griff) commented, "From what you have told me, it sounds like coming to therapy to sort out a problem like this is not how such a problem would have been dealt with in your family while you were growing up?"

There never would have been anyone around to marry who was rich!" Laticia laughed.

"At home whose opinion would have mattered about it?" I asked.

"My father—my parents, although my mother died when I was 12—and my family, friends in the community . . . our priest."

"As you and I have been talking here, have there also been ways in which you have continued to draw from the wisdom of your family and culture as you weigh what to do about Phil?" I wondered.

Laticia looked thoughtful. "I have started going to Mass again— every day. For years I had left the church. The rituals seemed like so much superstition. But now sitting there in the quiet . . . I feel peace."

I was surprised by her revelation. She had never before spoken about her spirituality. "What happens when you go to Mass?"

"I empty my mind. I listen and feel God's presence," she said.

"How long has it been since you began attending Mass again?" I asked.

"I began about the same time I started coming to see you. . . . I also want to show you this [lifting an amulet from around her neck]. This was passed to me from my mother when she died. It was said that it held special powers. . . . I am very intuitive. It is a West Indies ritual that the midwife feeds the newborn infant some of its mother's placenta, so that the mother's wisdom will enter the baby's body. I was always told growing up that I had special powers of discernment."

I was curious what she was able to know differently as she experienced the Mass and the amulet. "During the Mass . . . and when you feel the presence of the amulet on your chest . . . it's a different sense you have of your being, is it not, than when you are caught up in the guilt and obsessing over what to do? How do you experience your dilemma differently from that state of being?"

"All will be well," she spoke softly. "I don't know how, but that is what I sense . . . 'All will be well.' "

"What is your best sense for how the conversations we have here should stand in relation to your experience of the Mass and the presence of the amulet on your chest? . . . Where does your worship in Mass fit, and where does therapy fit?" I asked.

She paused, then reflected, "They are different. . . . In a way, talking with you is a part of my world here in Washington, and the Mass is a part of the world I came from."

It is important that the voice of each be a part of the conversation that goes on within you?"

"Yes," she said assertively.

As her therapy progressed, there were periodic questions about her experience of Mass and the amulet, usually along the theme: "When you are in that state of being, what are you able to understand that is hard to understand in the press of daily life?" The process of therapy became that of sustaining a dialogue that could contain both discourses, that of her professional Washington culture and that of the island culture from which she had come. My task as a therapist was one of attending to, respecting, and expressing curiosity about what could be revealed from her experience of ritual.

As the two of us view it, a clinician standing outside that tradition is not imbued with the authority to change the form of the ritual, nor would we have the wisdom to do that effectively within the whole context of the person's life. Rituals and ceremonies have implications beyond their influence in a psychotherapy. However, therapy can be conducted in a manner that is informed by participation in a ritual observance.

A clinical context in which North American therapists commonly encounter ritual is with people in Twelve Step recovery programs. Like the rituals of the Mass or a Seder or Ramadan, an AA meeting is embedded in its tradition, meaning that each meeting is constituted by a community joined in the language and actions of the ritual. Such questions as the following can be asked:

- When you sense the presence of your Higher Power and the presence of the other participants in the AA meeting, how does your dilemma then appear differently?
- How does your participation in AA support your coping? What seems to matter most in how that works?
- How is your participation in AA similar to or different from the role of therapy in your life?
- How does therapy fit within your broader spiritual life that is reflected in your attendance in AA meetings? In this context, is

there anything we should rethink about how we are conducting
the therapy?
- How does what we do in therapy stand in relation to AA? Where
  does each fit?

Lawrence Kirmayer (1994), in his research on primary care medicine, showed how a typical patient seeking medical care for illness is simultaneously pursuing a multitude of therapies outside mainstream
medicine, ranging from vitamins to yoga to chiropractor visits. He found
that most of these alternative therapies lay outside the awareness of the
medical physicians, making it difficult for the physician to have ascer-
tained correctly what had been healing as the patient improved. Similarly, people in therapy are often participating in rituals intended to heal
troubled lives and relationships, often while meeting with professional
psychotherapists and family therapists who are unaware that these rituals exist, as I was for many weeks of Laticia's therapy. The task of the
clinician is not to refine these rituals as they exist within their traditions,
but to sustain a dialogue between ritual or ceremonial life and the work
of the therapy.

SPIRITUAL PRACTICES IN THERAPY

Some of the ways spiritual practices differ from rituals and ceremonies
make them more accessible to the process of therapy. Rituals and ceremonies are governed by the traditions of which they are a part. While
the same holds true for some spiritual practices—a chant or dietary practices might be strictly specified by tradition—they more often assume the
character of a personal tool. As with a chisel, it is not the act of chiseling
but the beauty of the sculpture that is important.

When and how a spiritual practice is employed are usually preroga-
tives of the individual practitioner rather than the dictate of a church or
religious group. This when and how often can be integrated smoothly
into a therapy alongside secular exercises and homework.

The task in therapy is first to clarify the meaning and appropriate
form of the spiritual practice according to the tradition or circumstance
from which it arose, then to clarify what the consequences are of performing the practice. For example, a daily routine of reading passages of
Scripture for 15 minutes followed by private prayer would be a spiritual

practice that is common among Protestant Christians. If a Protestant Christian in therapy were to mention "my daily devotion," it might be important to learn in detail what it is comprised of, what has been its history in the life of the person as well as in the church tradition, and what the changes are that have ensued when this daily devotion could be practiced consistently over time.

Some clinical vignettes can illustrate the range of possibilities for incorporating spiritual practices into therapy. These examples do not illustrate therapies that are centrally organized around a singular spiritual practice so much as ways in which spiritual practices can be integrated into the fabric of an ongoing therapy.

Chanting

Ruth was an attorney who struggled with traumatic memories from her adolescence. Ruth followed spiritual practices of Buddhism. One day she described how she had meditated in silence for 3 days. She felt filled with joy:

"These were the most wonderful 3 days I have ever spent! I could feel the presence of God!" she exclaimed.

"Can you still feel this presence now?" I (Melissa) asked.

"Yes! It's like I am still there," she responded.

What do you mean?"

"There is such a sense of peace within me," she said.

I wanted to learn what had been her bodily experience of this sense of peace and what emotional postures were associated with it.

"What exactly do you feel within your body?" I asked.

"Warmth."

"Where? Where in your body do you feel the warmth?"

"Inside my chest." She motioned with her hand over her sternum.

"You know, we have been talking for a while about the violent images that haunt you . . . but you haven't mentioned them today." I gathered that the violent images that tortured her were not a felt threat in this state of being.

She paused. "It's like they are far away. I've not thought about them."

"The state of your body that you are experiencing right now . . . this state of being . . . do you suppose that it can be protective against those thoughts and images?" I asked.

"Yes, and it has always worked that way . . . but this doesn't last. It lasts for a time, but then my closeness to God eventually fades. I have been wondering whether I should quit my job and move to a monastery, to devote my life to worship."

I knew from our past conversations that this was her dilemma, whether to follow her spiritual practices while attempting to live within mainstream society or whether to abandon society for a monastic life. I wanted to know what might be the possibilities for her to sustain an intimate sense of God beyond the time that she had been accustomed to its fading.

"Do you have any idea what sustains this physical experience of closeness to God? What keeps it going even as long as it does?" I wondered.

"I think it is the chanting," she responded. "For each person it is different, but for me it is the chanting more than anything else. I get sloppy about setting aside time for meditation and chanting every day. Then I begin slipping away from God."

This was a surprise. While she had described earlier her chanting during meditation, it had not occurred to me that the chanting was so central to her accessing God's presence. It followed naturally that our therapy should examine what happened when, against her intentions, she would become slack in her chanting and meditation.

"Perhaps then this needs to be an aspect of our conversations here—to notice carefully what happens to take you away from your daily meditation and chanting," I suggested.

She nodded.

Meditation

During the course of our therapy Michael mentioned that he wished he could enjoy sexuality more in his marriage. Although he did not feel conflicted in his religious beliefs about sexuality, he had difficulty experiencing physical desire. Michael's spiritual life centered on daily meditation. One conversation that began on an unrelated topic eventually touched on both his spirituality and his sexuality. It began with a passing comment that he made—"I believe in God." While I (Griff) realized that his comment had been no more than an idiomatic expression dropped into the middle of his sentence, it often is the case that such timeworn phrases are like geodes, dull stones on the outside but containing exotically beautiful crystals on the inside. From his words, I followed with a question:

"You say you believe in God. Do you sense the presence of God?" I asked.

"Oh, yes!" he responded quickly.

"How do you sense God's presence?" I wondered.

He seemed puzzled by my question.

"Can you tell when God is present or not present? . . . What do you sense inside your body that tells you God is present?" I waited to hear what would be his language.

"It is like waves passing through me," he said, reflecting on the question. "I can feel it."

An important question for the therapy likely would be whether this sensuous experience of God's presence was circumscribed and walled off in a private domain, or whether he could carry this felt presence into his daily life as he interacted with humans.

"Do you sense that presence when we are here in this room together?" I asked.

"No . . . not at all," he responded cautiously.

Such a boundary was likely to be important, I thought. It suggested that the regions of his life-world in which he could be richly expressive were delimited.

"What hinders it here?" I inquired. "When you talk about your daily life, it sounds like this flow of waves comes and goes naturally and comfortably. But here something excludes it?"

"No, I don't think that," he said, disagreeing with the interpretation I had placed on his statement. "I don't feel God's presence all the time. . . . When I meditate regularly I sometimes can feel it all the time, everywhere I go. . . . And when I am meditating, I always do feel it. . . . But I don't usually feel it at work . . . sometimes I do with my children."

I understood him to be describing certain contexts in which he could experience God's presence within his being, and others where he could not. It was my operating assumption that differences in emotional postures between these different contexts would govern what was possible for him to experience. I would like to learn more about them, but I knew from his wariness that I was treading on ground that felt sacred.

"I have the idea that it may be important for these spiritual moments—I know there are no words, but when the waves come—to somehow inform what we are doing here in this therapy, to give us some guidance," I said, attempting to make my thinking transparent. "As best you can tell, what is the place of the therapy within this larger process?"

"I wasn't ready to face things before. I feel that the therapy is a part of this process, a place where I look in a mirror and see what is true," he answered.

His comment provided both a metaphor—"a mirror that reflects a true image"—to which we could periodically return in subsequent sessions and guidance to me for how I could be positioned most usefully in his life.

"It may be important for us to get the best sense we can of what metaphor for this work best fits the work of your spirit. From what you just said, I will hold on to this: that our work needs to be 'a mirror in which you can see truth.' "

"Yes," he nodded.

I paused, then asked, "How do you experience the waves within your body? Where do you experience them?"

"Through my head and upper body, kind of from the waist up."

There would be two ways to hear his response, not necessarily exclusive of one another. The first would be within the meaning of his Hindu religious tradition, that he was describing energy states within particular chakras, a series of energy centers extending downward from the head in a manner approximating the physical anatomy of the body. However, his description could also be understood psychobiologically as demarcating a portion of his body held inert by dissociative numbness. I wondered, might his capacity to feel and express freely, which seemed to accompany the touch of God flowing through his upper body, also release the numbness in his lower body?

"What about your lower body? . . . Would it ever be possible to experience God's presence—the waves physically passing through—your pelvis, your sexual body?" I queried.

"I love Phyllis. But when we are together I feel tension in my solar plexus," he said, frowning and placing his hand on his abdomen.

"Are you feeling some of that tension now as we talk?"

"Yes."

My sense of his religious convictions was that he would not have wanted any area of his life, or body, shut off to God. However, it sounded as though he were unable to make this belief real in his bodily experience.

"Have you ever thought about love-making in your marriage as if it were a sacrament, as something sacred?" I asked.

"I know that Scripture says that everything is sacred, but sex has always felt profane to me."

"Suppose you were to focus during meditation on an awareness of the waves flowing through all of your body, to include your pelvis?"

"I'll think about it. . . . I don't know if I'm ready for that yet."

I would follow his sense of timing and readiness to change. Notably he had not questioned my proposal that this be a direction of therapy—that he begin to open all of his body, and bodily experiences, to the felt presence of God. His practice of meditation would be the vehicle of this change.

Dietary Practices

Chris studied Taoist philosophy and traditional Chinese medicine with its dietary practices. He struggled with his experience of God. Although he believed God was loving, he usually experienced God as a distant, judgmental figure. He could not name any evil act he had committed other than "impure thoughts" from time to time, yet he felt as though he deserved punishment. After a spiritual retreat that centered on meditation, he returned stating "I was able to feel compassion for myself. . . . I know that God does not punish, but sometimes I torture myself."

I (Melissa) knew that Chris was describing an achievement for which he felt some jubilation. At different moments during the therapy I had asked him whether he could feel compassion for himself as he had articulated the painful binds in his life. He could imagine that I might feel compassion for him, and he could imagine feeling compassion for someone else, but his sense of shame was so strong that it deprived him of compassion for himself. The question today would not be how to change, but how to sustain this change he had made.

"The question, then, is how you can stay in this position, how you can sustain this sense of peace and compassion that you are experiencing right now," I offered in response to his news.

"When I am away from my daily life on a retreat—meditating and sharing with others—I feel compassion from God. But when I'm away from it a long time, I can't. I can't get that sense from studying Scripture and just believing," he said.

I felt he was acknowledging an important distinction. While his study of Scripture and the strength of his religious faith held special value in his life, it could not sustain the quality of relationship with God for which he yearned. He wanted intimacy with his God but had usually found God removed and distant.

"Are there some things in your daily life that can facilitate what you are right now experiencing within your being?" I asked.

"Eating the right foods in regular meals makes a difference. A bad relationship with food will screw up my connection with God. When I get careless with what I take into my body, it feels like God begins slipping away, like I am not honoring God."

While I had been aware that Chris followed dietary practices drawn from his spiritual beliefs, I had not realized until that moment how they mattered in his life. His dietary practices were key to his sustaining an emotional posture of honoring and revering God, which reflexively attuned his sensibility for compassion from God. We agreed that part of our work would be to attend to the effects of the state of his diet and what secondary routines in his habits and lifestyle supported or distracted him from following his dietary practices.

Words as Liturgy

Gina Rhea and I (Melissa) were talking about the difficulties she encountered steadying her emotions while searching for employment. She had finally determined that her present job was detrimental to her mental health. So she had given notice, but with no other possibilities at hand we both were alert to the new dangers this created for her. Reentering the job market, riding out the rejections, emotionally taxing for anyone, was especially treacherous for Gina Rhea. She had suffered from severe depression in the past, so severe that it had nearly killed her. She had to stay out of its clutches. She also feared that her sobriety, maintained for 2 years, was now at stake.

"I've got to change jobs," she said, "but *I've* got to change, too. . . . Gotta get a new me."

"What do you mean?" I asked her. "What do you think needs to change?"

"People tell me I am too negative, and I think it is true; I tell them they are right. I *am* too negative. But what I want to tell them is 'If you knew my mother, or even if you knew how I used to be, then you'd know 'negative.' You just don't know how positive I am! But it's not enough. Not even for me. I want to be more positive. Do you think you can help me with that?"

"Well, let's start with what you know. So you already have made a huge shift in your life, away from the negativity of your mother and even from how you used to be. So you know lots about this. How did you do that?"

"You know, it was when I became a Bahai. That's when it all started to change."

"When you became a Bahai? What was it about that?"

She was quiet. I did not want to intrude. I said softly, "That may be private, but if you would like to speak about it here, I would like to try to understand, especially since that was what generated this change that you want to keep going, that I want to support you in."

Gina Rhea inhaled, slowly and deeply. Her shoulders moved back as her chest expanded with her breathing. She looked up and off into the distance, " 'Oh, Son of Man, Noble have I created thee,' " she quietly recollected. " 'For if.' . . . something about if you don't love yourself . . . 'in no wise can I reach thee.' I used to know those words by heart. I kept them on little cards and said them to myself through the day. But I do remember this one: 'Oh Son of Man, Noble have I created thee.' " She savored these words. Her body was relaxed and she was smiling.

"It looks like you really like thinking about that. Do you?" I observed.

"Yeah, I love that word, 'noble.' I mean, think about it. People don't know they are noble. They'd act differently if they knew."

"The other one, the commandment to love yourself. . . . " I stopped myself, realizing "commandment" was my word, not hers. "Is it a commandment or more of a plea?"

"Neither," Gina Rhea said. "It's called a *hidden word*. These words were given to Mohammed's daughter, Fatima, in her grief after his death. An angel came to help her and gave her these words."

"A hidden word"—I was fascinated. "These words were first given to Fatima in a time of despair and now they are given to you in a time of despair."

"Yes, they comfort me. I want to be immersed in them." She paused to check with me: "I don't want you to think I am being an evangelist here or anything."

Although I did not experience her in this way, I was not surprised at her qualification. People often check, or almost apologize, when speaking with enthusiasm about their spirituality. "Oh, no," I assured her, "I just think that you are telling me about something that is very important to you. I feel you are honoring me when you tell me these things, and you are certainly teaching me. Earlier, when I asked you what had made a difference in moving away from negativity, I remembered your saying that you had been in therapy back then, and were moving into recovery. I thought you might say those things, but your answer, at least your first answer, was that it was when you became a Bahai. So it seems to me that it's quite relevant to talk about it here."

She said that, indeed, AA had helped, therapy also, and that her husband had helped, but that her faith was the foundation on which the other helps were built. I wondered with her how this foundation could be more available to her during this time. She thought she might make the little cards again and keep them with her, so she could repeat them several times a day while she searched for a job.

My conversation with Gina Rhea, like the one described earlier with Antonio, served to remind me how important it is to grasp the specific language, in these situations the specific words, of a spiritual practice. In each of these conversations I was unfamiliar with the language and stories. In searching for a common language, I fumbled, inadvertently substituting a word from my own faith tradition: "commandment" to Gina Rhea and "vessel" to Antonio. Their respective corrections, "hidden word" and "channel," helped expand our conversation. I hope that teaching me also served to clarify and deepen their own experiences. These language lessons reminded me again that, as in other aspects of spirituality, curiosity serves better than certainty.

Chapter Eight

The Community
in Spirituality

Many years ago in Mississippi we were drawn into working with a spiritual community, not because of our own planning but because of the persuasiveness of Mrs. Carver. Her husband had been admitted to our inpatient psychiatric unit for "bizarre sexual behavior." Known to be a courteous Southern gentleman during his previous 64 years, he cavalierly had propositioned several women who lived near him in his suburban neighborhood. The families involved in the situation had mixed reactions of confusion, shock, and outrage. Mrs. Carver was distraught.

In the hospital, a neuropsychiatric evaluation rapidly produced an explanation for what had happened: Mr. Carver's diabetes had been unstable in recent years, with his blood sugar elevated at some times, then dipping dangerously low at others. These repeated bouts of hypoglycemia had left brain damage in their wake. His capacity for abstract thinking was limited. He had poor control over his impulses, and his memory was so impaired that he had no recollection of the events that had been disturbing to his neighbors. Through family meetings during Mr. Carter's stay on the unit, Mrs. Carver came to understand his impairment. Viewing this aberrant behavior in the whole context of their years together, with practice she was able to respond in a helpful and

189

nonreactive way when Mr. Carver made inappropriate sexual remarks, reminding Mr. Carver of who he was, effectively limiting the behavior, and preserving their dignity. But now the problem was bigger than the couple. It had become a community problem. While Mr. Carver was in the hospital, Mrs. Carver spoke to some of her neighbors. Though some were satisfied with the medical explanation, others continued to view Mr. Carver as a lecher. There were heated exchanges, neighbors arguing and making accusations, with Mrs. Carver caught in the middle. Caught between her husband and neighbors, she was at once sympathetic to their plight and exasperated with their behavior. Moreover, Mrs. Carver needed both her community and her husband and was fearful of what might happen when she took him home. She told us she wished that we could explain Mr. Carver's medical condition to their friends as we had to her. So with Mrs. Carver's urging and Mr. Carver's consent, we arrived at the idea of going to their home and having coffee with a few of the neighbors to provide explanations that would prepare the way for a successful homecoming.

To have this meeting go as well as possible, Mrs. Carver wanted it to take place when their pastor, Reverend Phillips, could attend. We agreed and met with him to request his leadership in the meeting. Years ago, we would have seen this as an astute strategic intervention, due to the authority that Rev. Phillips held in this group, mostly Southern Baptist Christians, many of whom attended his church. With his involvement, those who were fueling the gossip would be more likely to behave well. But in the meeting that occurred, and on present reflection, it became apparent that much more than an invocation of religious authority was occurring. His quiet, compassionate presence and words called these people together as a spiritual body and a healing community.

He must have also spread the word to encourage people to attend the meeting to support the Carvers. Mrs. Carver seemed as surprised as we were that on that evening her living room could not contain the group. They spilled over to the hall and kitchen. Thirty-five neighbors and church members had come! And many bearing coffee cakes. When we had received their hospitality, Rev. Phillips began the meeting with a prayer for Mr. and Mrs. Carver and for the community. He then made some brief comments, reminding those gathered of their long-time relationships both with each other and with "the spirit of Jesus who dwells among us." He introduced the two of us to the group. Melissa assumed the role of family therapist and Griff the role of neurologist. Griff gave the biological explanation for Mr. Carver's behavior, drawing analogies from medical illnesses familiar to the group members. He responded to questions from the group until their understanding was clear. Melissa asked those gathered about the kind of man they had known Mr. Carver to be during their years of relationship. Stories were told and they in turn elicited other stories. The affection and laughter in these fond and funny memories of him and their times together lent a tone to the gathering that was of the wholeness of life over time and of community.

After all points of view had been expressed, there was a consensus that those involved should try to support Mrs. Carver and to address Mr. Carver's actions as an illness. We still needed to make a plan for responding to his disturbing behavior. Drawing from an approach that had been effective on the inpatient unit, from Mrs. Carver's helpful responses, and from the wealth of stories that these friends had provided, we arrived at this plan. It was designed to help him reaccess his identity and previous internal controls on his behavior: If he were to make an inappropriate sexual comment, they should say, "Bill Carver, this is not the husband and father I have known all these years," followed by a specific, positive recollection about him that would lead into a conversation about shared memories of good times.

Rev. Phillips enjoined the gathering in a benediction, thus bracketing the conversation from beginning to end as not only a problem solving meeting, but a sacred gathering. Mrs. Carver graciously served more cake and coffee. The evening ended as neighbors expressed their good wishes to her and departed. Mr. Carver subsequently was discharged and returned successfully to his home. In the occasional contacts we had with the Carver family over the next 2 years, no further complaints about his behavior were mentioned.

As with the Carvers, there are times when a therapist's most useful role is one in which he or she helps a person to maximize the healing potential of relationships within a spiritual community. This is particularly important when the cultural gap between the life-world of the person and the therapist is so great that it cannot be bridged. From our personal experience of growing up in the Deep South, we in a sense knew quite a bit about the local culture of such Southern Baptist neighborhoods as the one where the Mr. and Mrs. Carver lived. Yet as mental health clinicians, we were also part of a professional community whose ideas and values were viewed skeptically and suspiciously by some members of that subculture. Acknowledging this, we came as outside consultants to their community, respecting this community as their primary relationships, rather than presenting ourselves as either part of this community or as an alternative to it.

THE MEANING OF COMMUNITY

Interventions involving a person's community offer a unique set of options. In the chapters of this book thus far, we have considered therapeutic options available for a series of expressive forms—metaphors and other tropes, narratives, beliefs, practices, dialogue, rituals, and ceremonies—that differ both in their complexity and in the roles they play in human life. Community is a form of symbolic expression that provides a structure within which all other symbolic forms can be implemented and exercised as human beings live their daily lives.

Community is above all about belonging. It is about belonging to a neighborhood, family, clan, tribe, or the fluid postmodern substitute for all of these—a social network. Being in or out of community with those with whom one belongs is the fundamental distinction upon which the notion of community rests. Those who are included in a community are entitled to both the physical and emotional resources that are shared by members of the group. The deliberate withdrawal of community—as in shunning by some religious groups as a spiritual rule, by military academies as a disciplinary measure, and by teenage cliques as a method for enforcing group conformity—can create such anguish and grief that suicides sometimes result. Whether or not Mr. and Mrs. Carver would continue to be included as valued members of their community was the question being raised by the discussions and arguments among the neighbors while Mr. Carver was hospitalized.

Clinical work with community centers on five sets of questions:

- *Community identity.* What constitutes community for this person? That is, to whom does he or she belong?
- *Community expectations.* What is required in order to be included within this community? Are these requirements problematic or not, given the character of the problem that brought this person to therapy?
- *Community access.* Does he or she have access to this community? What kind of access is essential to make real the experience

of being in community? That is, must it be physically present, or can it be experienced through telephone or e-mail contact, written letters, or even imagined images or memories?

- *Community provisions.* What is provided by this community for its members? How can these be utilized as resources for the work of the therapy?
- *The role of a guest.* How does a clinician enter the community as a respectful—and respected—guest of the community?

COMMUNITY AS PLACE

The story of the Carvers illustrates one sense of community and its meaning. Their community consisted of several dozen families nested together in rows of contiguous homes. The relationships among these families were largely organized by the structure of place. In daily life, their business, school, and recreational activities brought these families into scheduled contact with each other where conversations could occur, from social greetings to mundane chatter to serious discussions. Daily routines throughout the neighborhood gave a sense of order and expectation to the relatedness that had developed among the families.

As with many such communities, the local church was integral to this structure. A knitting together of lives occurred within the church activities—Sunday School classes, home visits to the ill, Sunday worship services, midweek prayer meetings—that defined a spiritual community for Mr. and Mrs. Carver. When we decided to include the community in Mr. Carver's treatment, it was important that we physically went to the community and entered it according to this structure.

Drawing from her studies of survivors of war, migration, natural disasters, and other disruptive events, Mindy Fullilove (1996, p. 1517) concluded: "The sense of belonging, which is necessary for psychological well-being, depends on strong, well-developed relationships with nurturing places. A major corollary of this proposition is that disturbance in the essential place relationships leads to psychological disorder." This governance over possibilities for community by place and place-dependent structures raises an unwelcome warning for postmodern societies in which families migrate regularly, following jobs and careers with the expectation that relationships and other psychosocial processes will be equally fluid and portable. Pauline Boss (1999) has conducted research on ambiguous loss, as the psychological cost in numbness, detachment, emptiness, longing, and an inability to engage in new relationships that often occurs when losses are ambiguous. There is a high risk for ambiguous loss when a loss cannot be "made sense of" by the person or is unacknowledged or not validated by the surrounding culture. Dr. Boss (1999, p. 58) tells the story of her own grandmother, Elsbeth, who migrated with her husband to the United States from Switzerland:

> Physically cut off from her mother, siblings, friends, and the Alps she so loved, Elsbeth never adapted to her new surroundings. "Her mind was always back in Switzerland" my mother would say. . . . When I asked my mother, Verena, how she coped, she told me this story: "I could never reach her. . . . When I'd come home from school—I was in the third or fourth grade—Mother would be standing by the window in the door, motionless, always looking east. In her dialect, she said she was looking toward the "Heimatland." . . . As I got older, I noticed often that my mother wasn't all there. You could tell when her mind was in Switzerland.

The reality of ambiguous loss among those who, perhaps for the best of reasons, leave behind the landscapes, houses, friends, and family members of home tells us that there may be more to the material limits of our lives than many of us in the postmodern age commonly assume.

COMMUNITY AS RELATIONSHIP

A different sense of community—as quality of relationship—is expressed in the writings of Martin Buber. According to Buber, community does not exist in any particular place, but wherever persons as whole persons directly encounter one another, in I–Thou relatedness, while sharing experiences in the back-and-forth, speaking, listening, and reflection of dialogue. In similar language, the Christian New Testament quotes Jesus: "For where two or three are gathered in my name, there am I in the midst of them" (Matthew 18:20, RSV). This is community as communitas; in this sense, community is not a place but a state of being in relationship.

In our interactions with Mr. and Mrs. Carver, we did not clarify this distinction between community of place and communitas. Had a therapy continued with them beyond Mr. Carver's hospital discharge, however, we certainly would have needed to learn who they considered to be not only "neighbors we see at church," but those who shared with them both their sorrow and their faith in God.

THE POLITICS OF BUILDING COMMUNITY

Dialogue and relationship are the mortar and bricks of community. One helps a person build community by creating contexts in which sustained dialogue and committed relationships can exist among those sharing common concerns. Success in this endeavor demands that one pay focused attention to power relations that may bear upon the participants. These power relations are exercised both through the organizational hierarchy of the group with its laws, rules, and regulations, and through the informal methods by which group members employ charisma, kinship, prejudice, customs, and collective fears and desires to render some group members "more equal than others." Dialogue is exquisitely sensitive to the influences of culture and politics. As we discussed in Chapter 5, culture and politics dictate whether dialogue can exist at all and how it evolves over time (Anderson, 1997; Griffith & Griffith, 1994).

Suggestions for how one might attend to power relations when working with a spiritual community can be drawn from family therapists' clinical projects that, because they have been implemented in public settings, have placed a premium on attending to power issues in order to create the possibility for relationship and dialogue. Two such projects have been the work of Imelda McCarthy and Nollaig O'Reilly Byrne with incest victims and perpetrators in Dublin, Ireland, and the work of the Public Conversations Project with highly polarized political debates in the United States. Both groups have informed the methods we have adopted for clinical work with community. We will present briefly some of the salient aspects of these projects.

McCarthy and Byrne have worked as a treatment team in a Dublin university hospital with families referred for family therapy due to the discovery of incest. Their clinical work has been made difficult not only by its tragic dimensions in the personal lives of the involved daughter, father, and mother, but also by the extent of shaming and outrage stirred within the community. Responding to this outrage, legal authorities and social agencies step in to impose protective measures on the daughter's behalf. In some cases, a daughter would be placed in foster care; in other cases, the father would be required to leave the home; in still others, family members would continue to live under the same roof but with regular monitoring by agents of the legal system.

While protective of the daughter's safety in the short-term, the Dublin team found that this external regulation of the family's inner life also skewed family relationships in ways that made healing among those injured nearly impossible. The usual societal discourse surrounding cases of incest tended to create personas of "bad father," "good mother," "bad marriage," and "damaged daughter," and a disempowerment and negation of the father's fatherhood. In such a climate, family therapy could not be conducted. Showing empathy for the pain of individual family members would put the therapists at odds with the social authorities, while siding with the social authorities would alienate one or more family members.

The Dublin team sought a position of statesmanship in a chamber of partisan politics, where trust and cooperation were lacking, with each party pressing its moral agenda of vindication or vilification (McCarthy & Byrne, 1988, p. 189):

> When we mistakenly stressed "family," it merely served to activate even more monitoring, control, and vigilance of the family. However, if there was an unqualified acceptance of these actions, then the family's definition of itself as a unity was lost. If we affirmed the parents, the young girls and their "protectors" were angered; if we sided with the daughters, we undermined any possible affirmation and understanding of the parents and the circumstances that had made it "necessary" or possible for them to act as they had.

The Dublin team adopted as a starting premise that healing transformation for the family would need to begin with creating a "domain of consensual understanding" that could replace a discourse based on blame, shame, punishment, and negation. The guiding beacon for their work became a metaphor drawn from Irish mythology—the existence of a "Fifth Province of Ireland" as a meeting place where "there can be a neutral ground where things can detach themselves from all partisan and prejudiced connection and show themselves for what they really are" (McCarthy & Byrne, 1998, p. 189). They then sought a way to create a conversational space in which all participants could be affirmed and consensual understanding could appear. Therapies of the Dublin team have been characterized by a "politics of listening" that has several notable characteristics (McCarthy & Byrne, 1998):

- *An inquiry that seeks multiple discourses about the problem and its needed solution.* In addition to the dominant discourse of "bad father, bad marriage, damaged daughter," they invite with their questions other ways of describing and discussing the problem.
- *Encouragement of family members to speak from their positions in the discourse.* For example, "This is the bind I am in as I speak . . . " or "I have been afraid to say X, because it might have the effect of Y."
- *Questioning at the extremes, that is, asking questions intended to extend family members' expressions beyond the detail that has been customary.* If the daughter were to say that her father "ought to leave the family," she might be asked how far should he go away? For how long? How would his leaving be understood—as his punishment or his seeking penance? Should he maintain any contact with family members? If so, in what form? How often? Opinions of the other family members, including the father, would be sought for the same questions.
- *Positioning of the therapist to a "Fifth Province dis-position."* The therapist actively listens and responds in ways that prevent one dominant discourse or one dominant speaker from dominating the conversation.

Across the Atlantic from the Dublin team, another experiment in creating community has taken place in the middle of the "pro-life" and "pro-choice" fratricide over legalized abortion in the United States. The Public Conversations Project in Boston has made a committed effort to opening dialogue and building community among people who have been divided by politically polarized positions (Becker, Chasin, Chasin, Herzig, & Roth, 1995; Roth, Chasin, Chasin, Becker, & Herzig, 1992). The Public Conversations Project began as an effort by family therapists at the Family Institute of Cambridge to bring to public political forums their skills for resolving family conflicts. Although it has applied its methods to other kinds of polarized conflicts, its most sustained efforts have been toward building relationships and dialogues between pro-life and pro-choice proponents in the abortion controversy. It has sponsored carefully structured social gatherings that bring pro-life and pro-choice advocates into a respectful, reflective dialogue in which stereotypes can

be explored and difficult dilemmas examined. Newspaper columnist Ellen Goodman (1992, p. 79), has described such Public Conversations as
a "demilitarized zone in the abortion war." Although the project has not
sought for participants to change their stances on the issue, some groups
nevertheless began creating joint projects—the physical signs of new
community—instead of renewed conflict.

Addressing issues of power has been central to the success of the
Public Conversations Project. In each conversation, emphasis has been
given to ground rules that protect participants from being shamed, attacked, or silenced. These ground rules are vigorously enforced by the
group facilitator so that each participant can trust the safety of the process. Other measures are used to block some of the common ways in
which power plays are commonly exercised in public forums: Participants initially meet each other over an evening meal during which they
talk openly about their personal lives but initially are not permitted to
disclose to the others their political position; during the subsequent dialogues, participants are instructed to speak from stories of their personal
experiences, not their political beliefs. They are encouraged to describe
not only their convictions, but also their dilemmas and doubts. Participants are restrained from asking questions rhetorically or as veiled attacks; instead they are asked to restate them as questions of curiosity
about the other. Finally, participants are invited to explore areas of common ground, to imagine projects they might engage in together, work
that would be best conducted when representatives of both perspectives
were participating. Sometimes people have collaborated to reduce teenage pregnancies and to provide public support for single mothers choosing to bear their babies so other families might adopt them.

The lessons of the Public Conversations Project can be usefully applied within a spiritual community. In 1992, for example, a Public Conversation was conducted within a church in Mississippi by Sallyann
Roth and me (Melissa). Unlike other Public Conversations, which involved strangers meeting for the first time, this one brought together
people who shared a history and commitment to Christian community
with one another, however much they might have differed about legalized abortion. Friends I had known, and who had known each other for
years, spoke from their hearts to tell not-yet shared stories of tragedy
and wonder, of struggle with God and with life born and aborted, stories
that had formed their deeply held convictions. Those women with opposing convictions listened, leaning in attentively toward their friends,
their very postures reflecting the fragility of the situation. At the conclu-

sion of one of the conversations, Gloria Martin, one of the participants, expressed these words: "What I will carry with me from this time is the knowledge that if ever my daughter were faced with this dilemma, I now know that I could have friends from both sides available to counsel her."

The Dublin Team and the Public Conversations Project demonstrate that proactive steps can be taken to open possibilities for dialogue where historically it has been precluded. These proactive steps focus on establishing power relationships among family and group members that make space for multiple perspectives and enable and protect speaking, listening, and reflecting among the participants. These steps set the stage for community to come into being and can bring fresh communitas into an established spiritual community.

COMMUNITIES WITH SPIRITUAL
OR RELIGIOUS IDENTITIES

Community provides the stage, props, and audience for enacting life. It also protects from danger and provides sustenance for physical needs of daily life. It is difficult to survive as a Robinson Crusoe on a proverbial deserted island. If one were to endure for long, it would be difficult to find that kind of life worth living, due to all that would be missing for the lack of community.

A spiritual or religious community can offer a physical and emotional infrastructure for scenarios of daily life. Indeed, the role of church, temple, or synagogue as social network has assumed increasing importance as nuclear and extended families have lost dominance as centers of communal life.

Jo Anne was a young single woman who was accompanied to her initial consultation with me (Griff) by an older woman, a member of the church that Jo Anne attended. Jo Anne had moved to Washington, DC, from the home of her family 2,000 miles away. Before arriving, she knew no one here. Her pastor from home suggested she attend this church based on its reputation as a caring community. Due to her anxiety symptoms, Jo Anne might well not have come to her appointment had she been alone. In the context of this support, Jo Anne's symptoms responded relatively quickly to a combination of antianxiety medications coupled with psychotherapy. In this new city, her church was her primary community.

The loss of a spiritual or religious community can result in a "crisis of the spirit." This can occur as an experience of loss that is keenly felt even though religious beliefs or spiritual practices are maintained. Mr. Milton, for example, was a middle-aged man who sought treatment for depression. He had been a successful Capitol Hill lobbyist for a group of manufacturers for a decade. In his social circles, he was known as a charming dinner host and an entertaining hand at poker. Privately, he felt contempt for himself and his work, despairing that "no one could live with me because I am so hard and demanding." He described his typical mood as "lost and lethargic."

I asked him who knew about the emotional pain he suffered. He thought one friend might have an inkling, but no one else. He talked about how much he hated Washington. He had lived in Washington for a decade, but felt he would be leaving nothing of himself behind if he were to move away. It still did not feel like home. He was tired of the intrigue, pretense, and grasping of the politics that pervaded the city. He wistfully remembered the town where he had lived until he left for college, yet he knew that a return now to his boyhood life could not work, either.

I asked Mr. Milton from where he drew direction in trying to discern what to do with his life now. How did he understand its meaning? "I just pray. I pray every day." I asked what words he prayed. "Lord, help me to know your will for my life and to accept it," he responded. He had grown up in a family in which life revolved around their United Methodist church and its Sunday services, youth groups, picnics, and volunteer community projects. I wondered whether there was any community with whom he shared his faith and experiences in Washington. He did not regularly attend any church. The only community religious gatherings in which he participated were prayer breakfasts with some of the congressmen. I wondered whether in that setting he could open himself to others with his doubts and worries. He said he could not. He was yearning for a community he could not locate or bring himself to try to create.

A SPIRITUAL COMMUNITY CAN
EXTEND BEYOND THE RELIGIOUS GROUP

While churches and other religious groups provide important and unique resources as social networks, a person's spiritual community generally extends beyond that which has been organized around his or her religious group. A spiritual community is constituted by both human and spiritual beings—God, angels, saints, spirits, ancestors, an animated world of nature—who are engaged in concerned dialogue around the problem and goals of therapy. It refers to a community whose definition extends beyond human beings to encompass the relatedness of spirituality as we have discussed it throughout this text.

The presence of spiritual beings as active community participants expands the therapeutic power of a spiritual community. Spiritual beings can be what human beings cannot—always present, available, and interested in conversation. Two brief examples illustrate how nonhuman presences can be active agents in a person's spiritual community.

In Maya Angelou's production of the 1998 film *Down in the Delta*, a silver candelabra—named Nathan—is central to the life of an extended family of African Americans. The great grandfather in the story had been a slave during the Civil War. As a small boy he had witnessed his father, Nathan, sold on the auction block in return for a silver candelabra that then was set on the mantle of the family home of the slave owner. When war came, Union soldiers were looting houses as they passed through the territory. During the chaos, the great grandfather secretly took the candelabra from the slave master's home, buried it, and set out to search for his father. He never found his father. But, in time, he retrieved the candelabra from its hiding place. Thereafter he kept it close, hidden under his bed, taking it out at special times and talking to it, as Nathan, when he was troubled. In time this became a family ritual. When a serious discussion needed to occur, the doors would be closed, the family would gather, and the silver candelabra, Nathan, would be placed in the midst as the focus around which the conversation would take place. As the years passed, a tradition was established such that Nathan would be placed in the safekeeping of the eldest child of each family generation. Generation after generation, Nathan remained the spiritual center of the family: Whenever there was serious trouble in the family, Nathan would be brought into their midst, and family members would talk with Nathan and with each other. Nathan—to outside observers only a silver candelabra—was perhaps the most significant member of the family's spiritual community.

Within this movie, the meaning of the candelabra, the history of Nathan, unfolds slowly, his identity revealed to the moviegoer late in the story, not to heighten suspense, but because one must come to know this family in order to honor the sacredness of Nathan. It was so within the family of Nathan's descendants, as well: Children saw the candelabra and knew that it was special, but were only told the whole of the story when adults deemed that they were able to understand it and honor it. And so it often is in therapy, that we can be introduced to unseen members of a spiritual community only when the person speaking with us perceives that we know him or her well enough to honor those they honor.

Thus I (Melissa) believe it was no accident that it was only at the end of a fruitful series of meetings with Julia that she spoke with me about her Committee. In a planned conclusion to our therapy, we were conversing about the changes Julia had made that helped her to manage the difficult circumstances in her life. She said that one of the most important changes was that she thought now of the gifts of even her most difficult family relationships. "I have begun to realize and receive the gifts," she said.

"When you say gifts," I wondered, "does it imply a giver? Is that the important thing? Or is more about your keeping an attitude and a stance of a receiver?"

"Both," she said. "Some people would say something like 'God is the giver,' but it's not that way for me. I do think of a giver, but it's kind of strange." She paused and I listened. "It's a group of women, of my ancestors, who are watching over me. It's like a whole committee looking out for me."

I was intrigued. "Who is in this group? People you know? People you have been told about?"

"Some I know personally," she replied, "and some just by the stories that have been told. I think of women like my grandmother and her sisters who came to this country, not knowing a word of English. They worked so hard! I think of how much they had to go through, their courage and their wisdom, and their longing for Lebanon. But it's not all ancients in this group. I think of my aunt of whom I've often spoken here. She is a model for me, including the way she divorced, and lives her life with such zest."

"So it's a collective, a whole committee of women, watching over you? Wow! What is it like to be under their watch?" I asked her.

"It's good. It is a gift. Among them there's pretty much wisdom. Perhaps I don't call on them enough. I really like thinking of my connection to them."

"So you can call on them? Ask them for help? Like for an answer to a question? Or just to be with you?" I wanted to understand.

"Sometimes I think to myself, 'I'd better ask the Committee about that,'" Julia elaborated, "and sometimes I just send up a question, and let it be. Maybe I don't get a specific answer, but I get to release the question."

The opportunity, as Julia said, "to release the question" captures what community is about—a place in which one can know that questions and needs can be released, even when not perfectly fulfilled. By contrast, a community that through transformation of the group or individual has become a place in which questions cannot be released can be experienced as counterspiritual. "I have to admit that I am both sure and unsure of God. I am sure that there is something which is spiritual. I am not sure about what it is or what it is limited to. . . . I am not sure about the very foundations which were at the heart of my faith 5 years ago. I feel I do not know anymore about the Father, Son, and the Holy Ghost. I am left only with grace. I have no room in my heart for the God that separates people by good and bad, sinful and righteous," commented Ellie in the e-mail she had sent me (Melissa) following our session. She had been giving serious thought to a question I had raised. During our session, Ellie had mentioned how important and often how nurturing the church had been in her former home. She said she had long weekends alone now, and I had wondered if she wanted to connect with a church. "I feel differently now about God, about life, about love, about loss. But, I have no idea how I will live out this faith I have. The church will always be HOME to me, but I want to worship alone. Ruth [her former priest] would tear that apart in a minute. Worshipping alone is almost a paradox. But having to swallow what I do not believe is truth only widens the chasm further and makes me more and more isolated from feeling spiritually alive." In the writing of the e-mail, though, Ellie became aware of the longing for both connection and authenticity, so she wrote another letter, this one to a friend in her church back home who would keep her confidence and to whom she could release the questions.

As with other kinds of communities, a spiritual community includes both its aspects as communitas and its aspects as place and structure. Both are vital. Communitas without structure can be intense but ephemeral, dissipating rapidly. For example, the sudden diagnosis of a dread disease may bring about an immediate, spontaneous outpouring of friends who want to express compassion and encouragement to their ill friend. However, there may be no one there over the ensuing weeks unless someone helps organize this spontaneous "spiritual community" so that there is a scheduling of its members to help with such mundane tasks as meal preparation, transportation to medical visits, and help with finances. In the opposite case, a social organization whose purpose is to provide assistance to the medically ill can operate according to such overorganized, bureaucratic procedures that it can feel like a lifeless machine both to those it serves and to those who work within it. A spiritual community may build structures—buildings, organization, policies and procedures—that order the material aspects of life so as to sustain I–Thou relationships and dialogue, both among its members and between the members with their God.

Both communitas and structure are evident in spiritual communities that operate successfully over an extended period of time. The African American church in the American South provided a center where families met weekly for fellowship with each other and to worship God with prayers, songs, and sermons. With the civil rights era of the 1950s and 1960s, the same structure became the organizing center for voter registration drives, boycotts of businesses, and rapid community response to aid victims of racist violence. Without the dual role of the African American church—both in sustaining communitas and in providing a structure for political action—the civil rights movement may well have foundered. Similar stories can be told about the labor union Solidarity in Poland, as a secular spiritual community, and the Desmond Tutu-led Anglican Church in South Africa.

A contemporary example of clinical work that is particularly apt for psychotherapists is that of the The Family Centre in Lower Hutte, New Zealand. The multicultural group who constitute the Centre have made a conscious attempt to integrate spiritual traditions from Maori, Samoan, and European New Zealanders while addressing the struggles of poor and disenfranchised New Zealanders. The interior life of the Family Centre community revolves around reverence—for all people, the earth, the ancestors, and God. Each person's story is regarded as sacred. This communitas is balanced by an organized political effort to establish culturally informed approaches to therapy that honor the stories of nondominant cultures, lobby the government on behalf of the poor and powerless, and press the legal case for honoring historical government treaties with the Maori. The Family Centre approach is one that integrates therapy with community development—a "Just Therapy" approach, as they have named it (Waldegrave, 1990).

DRAWING FROM SPIRITUAL COMMUNITIES

An initial step in therapy is learning who are the members of a person's spiritual community. Some members, such as a particular saint, ancestor, or God, likely hold permanent seats. Others members become involved depending on the specific problem of the therapy. A spiritual community is above all a community of concerned presences.

Some helpful kinds of questions for identifying who participates in a person's spiritual community include the following:

Aspects of communitas

- With whom do you discuss this problem? Do you discuss it in prayer or meditation with God, or other spiritual beings?
- Who helps you as you cope with this problem?
- To whom do you turn for support? This applies either to other persons or spiritual beings.
- If we work together on solving this problem, who are the others you would want to be involved with you in the effort?

Aspects of place and structure

- Where are the places you go to replenish your spirit?
- Where in your experience do you most commonly encounter that which is holy?
- Where, or in what setting, can you most easily feel God's presence?
- In your life is there a context, a place or a group of people who help you make space for prayer or other daily practices important for sustaining your spiritual life?

It can be important to determine the extent to which a spiritual community is place dependent. Devi's mother, as described in Chapter 1, was homesick for her temple in India. Had she gone there, she imagined, she might have been calm enough to guide her daughter out of her distress. A serious factor in demoralization among many Southeast Asian immigrants who recently have come to the United States has been their physical separation from the graves of their ancestors in Vietnam and Cambodia. A similar despair was articulated centuries ago among the Hebrew people when separated from their Temple, first when taken by forced migration into Babylonia, then later by the diaspora: "For this our heart is faint; for these things our eyes are dim. Because of the mountain of Zion, which is desolate, the foxes walk on it" (Lamentations 5:22). Confronting the loss of the Temple and their exile in a strange land, the Hebrews successfully refocused their attention on their rituals and practices as a way to sustain a communitas that could become portable.

Working with a person's spiritual community is directly related to learning how to enter it as an invited guest, as discussed in Chapter 2. This also means learning the structure, history, and customs of the spiritual community so that one can show appropriate respect for that which is revered by the members of that community. Entering as a guest means learning how the therapist's social identity, as it may have been constructed by race, gender, ethnicity, socioeconomic group, occupation, or religious affiliation, may give special meaning to his or her presence in that community. Sustaining such self-awareness is a delicate and demanding task. One must rely on ongoing consultation and collaboration with members of the community for guidance.

HELPING A PERSON
RESTORE A SPIRITUAL COMMUNITY

When a spiritual community has been fractured by conflicts over values and beliefs or by personal injuries in its relationships, the work of therapy often is that of restoring and rebuilding community. Key questions that must be addressed include the following:

- Which relationships can serve as the core of a new community because their capacity for dialogue has been preserved?
- Which relationships potentially can be healed if needed steps toward restitution, penance, or forgiveness are to occur?
- Which relationships will not be available for a foreseeable future because the trust, openness, and acceptance needed for dialogue, realistically, will not be present?

- Where is God or the Spirit positioned in this rebuilding process? What guidance for this process is available from God, or from one's sense of spiritual principles?
- What other steps in this process need to be taken to restore the structure of a participant democracy, in which all members have an assurance they will be respectfully heard, understood, and taken seriously in the dialogue?

When Melanie called for her first appointment, she told me that she hoped that I (Melissa) would engage with her struggle without pushing her back to the church or presuming to know what was best for her. She said she felt "pulled" by God, but unable to respond. She had spent her early years in the bosom of the Episcopal church, assisting in the Eucharist as an acolyte, serving as a youth leader, and even spending a brief sojourn in seminary to prepare for the priesthood. But an open-hearted friendship with a married student became too intense, leading to an affair. Melanie ended the affair before it was discovered. She confessed her wrongdoing to her own priest, who offered her grace. By her own choice, she left the seminary and the church. Now, 6 years later, she still struggled with a deep sadness and spiritual yearning.

"I still pick up the prayer book and read it at night when I cannot sleep," she said. "It gives me comfort, but when I imagine returning to church I feel acutely uncomfortable." I wondered if her discomfort was with the people at church or with God. She thought it might be both. When she imagined being at church, it was "like there is this coalition of people, a stadium full of them, and they are all looking down at me."

"And would they have words to say to you?" I asked.

"Not many words. It is mostly in the way they look at me. Their look says, 'You have a lot of fixing up to do.' "

"Now this stadium coalition," I inquired, "as you look up into the stadium, can you see individual faces or just a mass of people?"

"It seems like just one big group. I'm sure there are individuals—I even know who is there. They aren't bad people. In fact they are wonderful people, good friends. It's just that they can't imagine that anyone would ever entertain the thought of adultery, much less do it."

I realized along with Melanie that this Coalition was quite unapproachable. I wondered if its members had been very experienced in life. "No, they are mostly young people," she answered. I asked if there were any among her spiritual community who had longer, wider experience with life. "Yes," she smiled. "There is this group of middle-aged women—I call them the 'Wild Women'—several of them are my friends. And they are not up in the stadium." We both became curious about how they would receive her. She could imagine one of these friends welcoming her, saying, "Come and bring all your doubts and hold onto them and hold onto us." They would not be appalled by her past actions. In fact, she said, they would hug her and take her in. "And," she added, "they would let me be where I am, but assure me I would not remain there."

I thought to myself that if these Wild Women were able to hold both the paradox and Melanie, then maybe they could both hold and expand this conversation. I placed a notepad on the table between us. "Okay, can we look at this? If they are here (making a dot and labeling it "Stadium Coalition"), and if these others are here (locating another point, labeling it "Wild Women," then drawing a line to connect the two points), where is God?"

"Maybe here"—she put a point high above the midpoint of the line, making an equilateral triangle when the points were connected.

"And you?" I wondered.

"I am right smack dab in the middle." She positioned herself in the center of the triangle.

That seemed to be both an interesting vantage point and a position of entrapment. I was intrigued, but unsure what to do next.

"What do we do with this?" I inquired. "Could you imagine a three-way conversation, between the members of the Coalition and the Wild Women and God?"

"Oh, I think it is already going on, but it's something to think about," she said.

I gave her the notes, making a copy for myself as we prepared to conclude, but before we parted Melanie had a question for me. "Actually, I think of you as a part of the Wild Women. Is that okay?"

"Absolutely! I would be honored to be in with those women."

Many of our future conversations drew on the Wild Women, both through her intentional real-life contacts with some of them and also through responses she imagined they might make. The Coalition continued to appear also, but less as a powerful block of people and more as separate individuals, with varying degrees of openness to Melanie.

Melanie had not decided to return to the church by the conclusion of our therapy. However she had a sense of there being not one but many doors to that spiritual community, doors that she could choose to open or not to open, and a sense of what might be behind those doors— some hostility and some hospitality.

RE-MEMBERING

Of the therapeutic practices we have illustrated for restoring community, many resemble what Michael White has termed re-membering. This phrase comes from anthropologist Barbara Myerhoff (1982, 1986). White (1995b, 2000a) highlighted and elaborated her ideas for therapy. Problems "dis-member" people (Madigan & Law, 1998) by shame and isolation, separating them from nurturing communities, and even the knowledge of their identities, skills, and abilities. As a counter to this process, White points us to re-membering, providing a forum to identify those who have and might contribute to one's desired identity and the knowledge and skills needed for one's life. White points us to Myerhoff's (1982, p. 111) words, that re-membering calls "attention to the reaggre-gation of members, the figures who belong to one's life story, one's own prior selves, as well as significant others who are part of the story. Re-membering, then, is a purposive, significant unification, quite different from the passive, continuous, fragmentary flickerings of images and feel-ings that accompany other activities in the normal flow of conscious-ness."

Re-membering practices have been quite fruitful in our experience, and are often initiated and embraced by the people who consult us. Ear-lier in this chapter I wrote about Julia's telling me about her guiding and supportive Committee. Julia had begun that conversation by referring to the Committee as "the giver," tying her identity to theirs, in a way that was the beginning of a re-membering process. Much later, we had an op-portunity to extend what she had begun. Three years after our last meet-ing, Julia called me, wanting to talk together just a few times to get through a seemingly impenetrable barrier of self-doubt and anxiety that were blocking the completion of her dissertation, a long-awaited achieve-ment in her life. "I'm afraid I can't do it. That I'm just not competent. I just keep hearing, 'Why did you ever think *you* could do this?' And I freeze." I was eager to be of help to Julia in getting through this barrier. I knew how persistent she had been, against the odds, keeping the vision of herself as an anthropology professor. She was the first in her family to pursue a doctorate, and events had occurred earlier in life that had obscured her own recognition of her intelligence and scholarly skills. I knew also that many people, with seemingly lesser obstacles, had deferred or missed their goals at the point of their dissertation. When Julia arrived it quickly became clear to her and to me that the physical symptoms of anxiety were nearly overwhelming her. They had taken on a life of their own, and she and I wanted to employ all avenues to end anxiety's sabotage of her goals. As we neared the end of our conversation, I recalled the Committee. I wondered aloud how they might be responding to her now. She said she knew they were in her corner and were supporting her, but she became curious, wanting to ask what they might actually say to her. Together, Julia and I made a plan that she would try to discover and write down their responses, so that she and our work together might be informed by them. She arrived at our next meeting quite enthusiastic, bringing with her two diagrams and a story. "I decided to also write my questions to the Committee. Then I wanted to think about just whom I was addressing, because I figured they would each have a different thing to tell me. When I visualized the Committee, I was surprised to see that my father is there! So it isn't just a group of women after all." She described the other members, some recalled from years past, some still living. I could see them all in the first diagram Julia displayed (Figure 1). They each held their place, making a circle surrounding Julia.

"I did my Committee," Julia said, "and I really loved looking at their words. Then I realized I also have a peer review! I have friends who love me, here now, who can say to me the words I need to hear. Some I could have imagined, but some I needed to hear. So I asked them. You know, the wonderful thing was they not only gave me their words of encouragement, but their presence. My Lebanese cousin even brought me some soup to keep me going. I wrote their words down, too, so the anxiety could not make me forget them. I'm keeping them right by my word processor, to read when I get stuck. "My Peer Review" was at the head of Julia's other diagram. Again, she was encircled in the drawing, in this one by her friends, who were saying things like "You can do whatever you set your mind to. You've proven it. You're so capable and a hard worker." "You've come so far. You work so hard. You've really got it together." "You rule! You're so thoughtful and nurturing. You're a great friend. You can do it." "I know it's hard, but you are so strong. Cut yourself some slack. Take care of you."

My Committee

Aunt Lena
You're capable.
You'll do it.   *Situ* & Grandma*
I'm impressed!   You need to go back to the basics.
                                       Eat more and dress warmer. You can endure.
                                       Look at our genes!

                    Me   *Aunt Sucena*
Aunt Larissa   You make your parents proud.
You're smart.   You make all of us proud.
You're good enough.
                    Dad
                    You know what's best, kiddo.
                    Trust your gut.
                    I believe in you.
                    I'm so proud of you.

FIGURE 1. Julia's Committee. *"Grandmother" in Lebanese.

Julia not only kept her friends' words before her, but, because she was not cowed by the critical, anxiety-making voices, she was able to ask for and receive their support until she met her goal. In retrospect, looking over my old notes from these sessions, I can see even more of the creativity and complexity in Julia's re-membering. Giving the usually intimidating academic status of "Peer Review" to the friends who mattered the most to her was a perfect antidote to the scrutiny of the world of graduate school, the expected evaluation that would qualify or disqualify her from that professional peerhood. Within the circles of her Committee and her community of friends she could again know herself and reach into the future.

We are keenly interested in how therapy works in fostering communities, in congregating voices, in establishing identities. Julia's comments on her prepublication review of this text were informative. "Prior to my disclosure to you that day, my Committee was an unnamed, underdeveloped idea. As I began telling you about it, however, the idea grew very tangible and real. I remember naming this group of women 'my Committee' in your office, and for the very first time I truly understood their potential."

White (2000, p. 70) says that "through re-membering practices, self and identity cease to be synonymous." The many voices surrounding Julia reach far beyond the either/or description of competent or not-competent student. She is described as nurturing friend, wise daughter, dedicated worker in all arenas, an already tested and well-proven person. The members of both her communities provided her with a multi-layered, multifaceted identity.

A SPIRITUAL COMMUNITY CAN FOSTER RESILIENCE TO TRAUMA AND LOSS

The unique role of a spiritual or religious community is graphic in some accounts of those who have endured severe trauma and loss. Mr. Kiem Le is a counselor with immigrants and refugees who tells his own story of survival and endurance in the face of prolonged imprisonment and abuse. As a South Vietnamese citizen, he first spent a year in a prison cell after the fall of that country, then 5 years in a forced labor "reeducation camp." During his imprisonment, he was interrogated daily for months. Working at hard labor, he and the other prisoners nearly starved, eating only three bowls of rice a day, occasionally with bits of fish added. He witnessed the execution of his cellmates by his captors, and suicides by others who sought to escape the physical and emotional abuse through death. He lived with a daily fear that he might be executed next. Some prisoners tried to escape, which was impossible due to the three fences surrounding the camp. They would be shot and their bodies left in the dirt for Mr. Le and others to retrieve the next morning.

Prior to his arrest, Mr. Le had regularly attended Catholic Mass, but this religious faith had been merely a "routine" aspect of his life. In prison, however, it became his central focus. "I kept thinking of God, asking him to give me strength," he recalls. On his work team, he met two Catholic priests. Secretly, he, the priests, and a few others celebrated a ritual Communion each day with the realization that they would be beaten or tortured if they were discovered. Through a process he called a "communion of feelings," the members of this secret church would look into the eyes of other prisoners to discern whether they also could be trusted to join in the Communion. When Mr. Le could feel this "communion of feelings," he sensed strength within him. He says, "I know I suffered. I had physical pain, but I didn't have psychological pain. I had to think that there was hope. The hope God gives compensates."

For Mr. Le, there was protection and sustenance within this community that organized around its ritual observance of Communion and by his belief that his suffering was somehow part of God's plan. When he eventually was released and emigrated to the United States, he did not suffer symptoms of posttraumatic stress disorder, as do many who have been abused or tortured in prison.[1] He has been able to create a new life in a new land and to engage with vigor in his work as a counselor serving others.

Others have commented upon the vital role that community appears to play in providing resilience to trauma, abuse, and torture. Henri Nouwen (1972, p. 66), studying the lives of men who survived long jail terms in brutal prisons, concluded that, "A man can keep his sanity and stay alive as long as there is at least one person who is waiting for him." Nouwen also concluded the converse, that "no man can stay alive when nobody is waiting for him." Etty Hillesum could not know who, if anyone, was waiting for her. News from the outside world was blocked from or distorted to her in Westerbork and then in Auchwitz. She kept the community in her heart, though by daily prayer for others and by fidelity to those who would come later. Though she was powerless over the circumstances that would eventually take her physical life, Etty was determined to stay mentally and spiritually alive as long as she had breath. This 28-year-old Dutch Jewish writer defied the prediction that she could not or would not think there. "I would like to be the thinking heart of the barracks," she stated. Through her diaries (Hillesum, 1984) and letters from prison (Hillesum, 1987; Seivers, 1995), we can feel the pulse of her thinking heart:

July 3, 1942

I wish I could live for a long time so that one day I may know how to explain it, and if I am not granted that wish, well, then somebody else will perhaps do it, carry on from where my life has been cut short. And that is why I must try to live a good and faithful life to my last breath: so that those who come after me do not have to start all over again, need not face the same difficulties. (Hillesum, 1984, p. 130)

NOTE

1. We are not suggesting that community guarantees protection against post-traumatic symptoms. We have proposed and are studying currently whether it may amplify resilience to the effects of extreme trauma (Gaby et al., 2000a, 2000b). A primary strategy of political torturers is to destroy relational bonds to others, and with them, spiritual community. This points to a potential power of community as a protective force against trauma.

Chapter Nine

When Spirituality Turns Destructive

Whether it is a large-scale horror like the Jonestown massacre or a local story about a husband who justified beating his wife by quoting scripture, disturbing reports regularly appear in newspapers and on television describing religion as an instrument that inflicts suffering or death. Most of us read these stories and recoil. We may be curious about how people could commit these acts, but cannot imagine ourselves in such a situation. It was different for us, though, as we took in the tragedy of the unnecessary death of 11-year-old Wesley Parker. His parents' dilemma was palpable. As we heard their story we wanted not to back off, but to draw close. The difference was that this account was not told by a horrified reporter, but by Wesley's grieving father, Larry. He and Wesley's mother, Alice Parker, hoped that his writing would honor their son, that his death might not be in vain, that other believers might be spared such heartache. The title of his (Parker, 1980) book, *We Let Our Son Die*, is in keeping with their acceptance of personal responsibility for this and their accountability to their family, their community, and their God. A movie—*Promised a Miracle*—was made from his book. It explicated not only the family's painful choices, but also the role of the cultural context in Wesley's death. These two titles of book and movie are emblematic of the therapeutic tension and task, to keep both cultural context and personal accountability at the forefront of our own minds when we work in situations where such exploitation is occurring, just as we must when we listen to the story of Wesley, his parents, and his community.

Wesley suffered from juvenile diabetes, a taxing illness from which his parents had always hoped God would heal him. Since his diagnosis, they had sought out excellent medical care for him, and had studied to become well informed about the illness. They had attentively cared for Wesley, assisting him with dietary management, glucose checks, and the requisite insulin injections. The Parkers' concerns were also borne by their church family, a lively Christian church in a desert town in California.

Together this church family shared home Bible studies, prayer circles, church baseball games, and concerns for the sick and suffering among them. For years community members had supported Larry, Alice, and Wesley by persisting with them in prayer for eventual divine healing of the diabetes. Then, one day, events were set in motion that turned the community support to scrutiny and turned patient prayer to deadly pressure.

A traveling evangelist came to the church to preach a revival. He preached a compelling sermon about how, through his faith, God had miraculously healed his ailment, and that God wanted to do the same for anyone who would show faith in him. In that service, Larry and Alice brought Wesley to the altar for healing prayer. Wesley believed he felt the touch of God's hand and declared to the congregation that he had been healed. His mother and then his father also believed they felt the hand of God and wept with gratitude. Their pastor and church family rejoiced in God's work and all came round to congratulate Wesley.

At home that evening, Wesley felt liberated from his illness and proud to have been chosen to show God's power. Through the night, however, Larry and Alice agonized, uncertain whether to question or to believe in the miracle, whether to give the insulin if his urine were to show sugar the next morning. The convictions of their community and the scriptural passages they studied convinced them to believe in the healing they felt God had given them. They feared that doubts could ruin not only their son's promised physical health, but also his spiritual health. To keep them from backsliding in their faith, the decision was made to discard the insulin. For the 3 long days it took the diabetes to kill Wesley, each escalation of symptoms was interpreted as a further test of faith for the family. During this time, Wesley did not ask for his insulin, only for more prayer. Repeatedly, as Wesley's cramping and pain intensified, Larry and Alice struggled and questioned their decision. But just as they would decide to abandon their belief and go for more insulin, friends would arrive at their home to arm them against Satan with strong prayer, or Wesley would slightly rally, or familiar scriptural passages would be recalled, like "What things soever ye desire, when ye pray, *believe* that ye receive them, and ye shall have them" (Mark 11:24, KJV) and their resolve to believe would be strengthened. Near the end, Larry pleaded to his good friend, Karl. "It's so hard to watch your son suffer like this, especially when you know that if you give him insulin he's going to stop suffering. Yet, if I do that, Karl, I'd be going against what God wants. I'd be denying the faith for Wes' healing, and then he'd lose it because I'm weak" (p. 57). His friend understood, as Larry knew he would, for Karl had had his own experience with illness, prayer, and recovery. Karl, too, then joined the group gathered for the vigil at the Parker's home.

A few doubts were voiced from the community after Wesley began to lapse into a diabetic coma. The pastor urged them to check with a doctor to validate the healing and another church member implored them to take him to the hospital, but these doubts were lost in the groundswell of the family and community's confident faith and yearning to prove to God their fidelity. In resistance to Satan and his temptations, Larry and Alice held out hope even after Wesley died. Surely, after all this, God would not let them down. Surely, this was the final test and their boy would, like Lazarus, be raised from the dead.

Many supporters joined them for the resurrection service, but Wesley was not raised and Larry and Alice finally recognized that they had let their beloved son die. In a court trial, they were convicted of involuntary manslaughter and child abuse. Their remorse was apparent to the judge, though, and he recognized that no sentence he could mete out could be greater than the heartache with which they would always live. He mercifully granted a probationary sentence and returned them to their other children to bind their family's wounds.

How do we understand the process by which prayers, beliefs in a caring and protective God, and religious practices led this family not to safety and comfort, but to death and agony? More immediately, how can we enter such tragedies to make a difference? As the two of us watched the film, we did not feel distant from Larry and Alice, not only because we could understand the spiritual and community dilemma, but also because as parents we could deeply connect with the desperation and loss of bearings one can have with a child who is chronically suffering.

ENCOUNTERING THE SACRED
CAN OPEN A DOOR TO HARM

An awful irony of human life is the recognition that spiritual beliefs and practices, intended as doorways into the wholeness of life and relationships, can as quickly become doorways to hell. In one cultural context, religious beliefs and spiritual practices provide resilience against suffering when all other methods have failed, but they become fashioned into instruments of torture in another context. The power of spirituality and religion must be respected but not idealized.

The accounts we have told through the chapters of this text have emphasized how spiritual life can provide comfort, protection, and healing. It is essential, however, that we look as closely at its dark sides. In the Parkers' story, the interpretation that some church and family members gave to religious experiences led to Wesley's death. In stories we have heard from people we have consulted, spiritual experiences have given rise to painful dilemmas, fractured relationships, the emptying of pleasure and meaning from life, or the obstruction of healing change.

As we consider the story of this family, we wonder how contact could have been made that might have averted this tragedy. We might hope that our profession could have offered help to this family, but we might be separated not only by religious differences, but also by other obstacles to relationship. Working-class people have often felt professionals accord little respect to the practical wisdom from their daily lives or to the religious wisdom of their traditions. Why should they turn to us or trust us? Acknowledging this concern allows us to be accountable for the part we play in the division between us, to question our taken-for-granted notions of how we offer consultation and help. We would guess that our cultural ceremony of scheduling an appointment with a mental health professional as if secular solutions were the answer to their problems might have set Mr. and Mrs. Parker at odds with their church community and with their own convictions. One could say that an intervention by a department of social services or child protective services would have been the appropriate intervention. Perhaps an earlier, less intrusive, more constructive way to assist these loving parents might have supported their faith and community, while also safeguarding the health of their son. Could home-based family therapy services have helped? Could a visiting nurse have mattered? Could a community member trained as a health promoter have made a difference? If there had been a helper who genuinely believed in divine healing working in concert with medical treatment, could he or she have formed a therapeutic relationship with the family? Might a professional have related to a concerned church member, deeming that member a link-therapist, in order to work within the church to support the parents yet still challenging the treatment of this child (Landau, 1981; Landau-Stanton, 1990)? What might have made the bridge that could cross the expanse between the either/or position of their religious convictions and medical science?

Only Larry and Alice could answer these questions.[1] We can be grateful for the gift they have made to us out of their loss, the clarity with which they have shown us how loving, attentive families can be decimated by the destructive power of religion. We can try to honor their dilemma and to accept and grapple with the dilemmas they offer us. We do know that in the end they remained both faithful to their God and accountable for letting Wesley die. They still believe in the Bible, but they believe differently now. They say they dwell now on the passage "faith, hope, and love, but the greatest of these is love" (I Corinthians 13), and know that faith works through—never against—love, that the worry and compassion they had felt for Wesley's suffering was a gift from God to be trusted, given to inform them, not to test them. "To maintain faith," Larry said at the trial, "we forgot love. I see now that that was a mistake. Our love should have overruled what we thought we were required to do." Larry and Alice Parker reconciled with their church and became teachers there. All of this tells us that whatever ways a professional helper might have earlier intervened, continuity, rather than cutoff, from their God and from their community would be central to health and healing.

HOW RELIGION AND SPIRITUALITY CAN BE DESTRUCTIVE

A simple maxim guides our clinical work: Expressions of religious or spiritual experience are harmful when they violate the relatedness on which spirituality is based. Spirituality comes into being as one's commitment to relatedness—to other people, the environment, one's God or the numinous, one's heritage, one's body—becomes the paramount concern that organizes understanding and action. Some metaphors, stories, and beliefs that are held sacred can nevertheless usher a person into paths away from relatedness toward practices of objectification of self or others, or, worse, toward their destruction. Many different religions have justified the labeling of people as "heathen" or "infidels," resulting in those excluded being treated as subhuman. More insidious is the exclusion by silencing that exists within many religious bodies when, under the name of establishing holy order, women can not openly question men, younger persons their elders, members their leaders, and people their God. Some religious and spiritual traditions have viewed the physical body so much as a repository of sin and degradation that acts of neglect or mutilation are virtuous. There are even forms of prayer and meditation that can alienate people from others or themselves.

Antispiritual sequelae of religious practices often present in ways more subtle than an inquisition or ethnic cleansing. They appear regularly in psychotherapy. I (Melissa) understood such sequelae to be driving a wedge between Will and Jean as they began a long-awaited evening, socializing with friends over dinner and a movie. Devout in his Christian faith, Will prayed each morning, night, and before every meal. As he and Jean sat down in a restaurant with their friends that night, his attention was captured by a private worry over whether or not to pray a public blessing before eating their food. He felt he could be true to his beliefs only if he were to bow his head and ask a blessing before eating. However, since the others in the group did not do so, he worried that he would be intruding and imposing by praying in front of them. He became so anxious over this conflict that he finally insisted that the two of them eat alone, away from the others, so that he would not have to deal with the issue. It was too awkward, then, to go to the movie together. The evening was ruined, with Jean furious, separated from friends, fun, and Will.

For many people daily prayers are a spiritual practice that deepens connectedness with God and others. But as Will listened to Jean during our session, he determined that the intensity and rigidity of his practice of prayer were damaging relatedness with Jean, with friends, and even with himself due to the guilt he was feeling for causing the problem. What mattered was not some intrinsic property of prayer as a spiritual practice but how in real life it influenced relatedness.

As another illustration, Janice struggled with conflicts over sexuality in her marriage with Ethan. She had been sexually abused as a teenager and now felt fearful during lovemaking. Even though she believed this fear was irrational, she could not dismiss it. Janice's spiritual life was organized around meditation. When I (Griff) interviewed her about her bodily experience during meditation, she described a process of leaving her body, experiencing it as if it were the body of another person. During lovemaking with Ethan, she entered this detachment, avoiding fear by experiencing the lovemaking as if were happening to another, with that person, not Janice, feeling pleasure. This psychological compromise, however, robbed her of the intimacy she desired with Ethan and left her feeling even more distant from him. A part of the therapy consisted in her working through small steps to remain within her body while she and Ethan slowly and gently collaborated in finding ways to talk and to touch that would quiet the alarm. Learning how to detach spirit from body can be a valued spiritual practice in some traditions, but it had become a barrier to intimacy for this couple.

Religious beliefs and spiritual practices that violate spirituality often do so by fostering despair, helplessness, meaninglessness, or isolation. Dana was a woman struggling with brain injuries after a blow to her head. She was seriously suicidal as she faced a future life with impaired memory and an inability to think abstractly. Searching with her for potential sources of hope and meaning, I (Griff) asked about her religious faith. She turned her head away bitterly; "I don't talk to God anymore." I gently pressed for the reason why not. "God made the world, and whatever happens, happens," she said. "Does God feel like he is close and present in your life, or far away?" I asked. "Far, far away," she responded. "Does God know that you suffer from this injury?" I wondered. "He knows but he doesn't care," she replied firmly. Such images and beliefs about God were only serving to amplify the despair and isolation that Dana's injury had already brought into her life. They separated her both from her God and other people.

The most graphic accounts of harm are those involving stories that are held sacred by a group. Treasured myths have justified rampant destruction, as with the Nordic-derived myths of the Nazis or the Christian-derived myths of North American European settlers, each of which has led to genocide. Part of my (Griff) childhood was being taught from the Bible in Sunday School that people of color were intended by God to serve white people because they were a race descended from

Ham, the son of Noah who was cursed by his father for looking at Noah while he was drunk and naked. These biblical interpretations helped support racism in the American South during the century prior to the civil rights movement. Even today biblical references are invoked to justify attitudes and actions of racist, anti-Semitic, and heterosexist hate groups in our country.

How is it that religious beliefs and spiritual practices, intending to be life giving, can become sources of suffering and destruction? A full response to this question no doubt would fill a book of its own. There are two groups of processes on which we have focused because they have such direct relevance to the work of psychotherapy. They corrupt our language in a manner that sets the stage for violence and exploitation under the guise of spirituality or religion:

- The symbolic language of spiritual and religious experience decays in its meaning as time passes. A path to evil is paved when language loses its power to move people to do good.
- Those who rely on predatory practices to accrue power, money, or personal gratification regularly use the rhetorical power of spiritual and religious language to exploit, just as they use the language of politics, slick commercial advertising, and any other rhetorical device.

DECAY OF MEANING IN RELIGIOUS LANGUAGE

Any important metaphor, story, belief, or ritual faces inevitable decay in its meaning as time passes. Sometimes this decay is due to the gradual disappearance of those witnesses who had firsthand knowledge of the human events that anchored the meaning of the language. Such an example is recorded as one of the pivotal events in Jewish and Christian religious history. The Biblical accounts in the books of Genesis and Exodus tell how generations of Hebrew people lived within the confines of Egypt in peaceful coexistence with the Egyptian people. The social bond in which this coexistence was embedded was a story of Joseph, the Hebrew leader who saved the Egyptians from starvation by his wise administration during a time of famine. But the Hebrew people were later taken into slavery when a new Pharaoh arose "who knew not Joseph." The power of the story of Joseph to organize social relations between

Egyptians and Hebrews had ebbed as those who could remember Joseph passed away. In a similar manner, the power of metaphors, stories, beliefs, and rituals that were formed around other moments in moral history—the waving red flag with hammer and sickle (marking the Bolshevik Revolution in Russia), the story of the invasion of Normandy (marking the defeat of Nazi Germany), beliefs such as "Better Dead Than Red" (marking the anti-Communist crusades of the Cold War)—have tended to wane by the time of the third-generation descendants of those who physically participated in or witnessed the historical events giving them meaning. As time passes, the same symbols that once stirred hearts, brought tears, and straightened spines become as matter-of-fact as the slogans of a television commercial.

Symbolic meaning also decays when social contexts that initially inspired the meaning undergo shifts and transmutations. For example, by the latter part of the 20th century it had become notably more difficult for labor organizers to use traditional slogans and images of 1930s labor solidarity to rally U.S. workers who were investing their retirement stock funds in corporate America. Similar kinds of decay affect the symbolic language of spiritual experiences.

CORRUPTION OF RELIGIOUS LANGUAGE BY PREDATORY PRACTICES

Less innocently, language of spiritual experience becomes corrupted when it is co-opted by those who are interested only in exploiting its rhetorical power. Religious language—powerful metaphors, stories, and beliefs—can slip past analyses by the rational mind to engage the body. By touching the body, this language can expand possibilities for spiritual experience, but that movement can be toward either good or evil. It is a testament to the power of such language that so many people with bad intentions are drawn to it.

In Tennessee Williams's *Sweet Bird of Youth*, the image of Boss Finley, a corrupt American politician who quotes Scripture to incite racial hatred, differs little from Slobodan Milosovic, who used Slavic myths to rouse his troops to commit genocide in Bosnia and Kosovë, while displaying their trinitarian Christian salutes. Stories of preachers who steal money from their churches, and charismatic spiritual leaders who have repeated, exploitative sexual liaisons with their followers are common. Fascist Spain and Nazi Germany produced stories of religious leaders who betrayed their church members by actively collaborating with their totalitarian governments. Such betrayals of communal trust have created for many people a gulf of distrust, not only for the involved churches and their leaders, but also for all spiritual and religious discourse.

Other corrupting influences are more subtle. When religious language is spoken as a clever device to influence others' behavior, not as an authentic voice of the heart, the language soon loses its resonance. Invoking images of the Holocaust or recalling Martin Luther King's "I have a dream" speech as trite rhetorical devices in political speeches risks accelerating the decay of meaning for either the Holocaust or King's speech within our culture.

An underground market commerce traffics in the language of spirituality and religion in order to influence, to control, and to exploit those moved by it. This is predatory behavior. It relies on deception and commits violence toward others in the guise of piety. Sometimes these marketeers exploit the language for the least complex of motivations, namely, money that can be lifted from unsuspecting believers, as with Sinclair Lewis's mythic tent-revivalist, Elmer Gantry, and some from the modern televangelism industry. However, other processes are more complex than simple avarice can explain.

SYSTEMIC EVIL

Processes are evil when they violate the relational interdependence of spirituality, whether by harming particular persons so that the society can prosper (a scapegoat), or by harming society so that specific persons within it can prosper (a privileged class). Each of the expressive genres we have discussed holds a potential for systemic evil.

Usually the initial step of systemic evil is the setting of a boundary, or a system of boundaries, to demarcate a special, circumscribed group who are afforded unique rights and privileges. Religious beliefs or spiritual practices can be invoked to justify these rights and privileges as necessary for the worship of God or the protection of the community. Among different cultures this special class can be represented by adherents to the faith, a priestly class, a racial group, a gender group, a political party, or a hereditary lineage.

As a second step, this special group becomes regarded as if it constituted the whole society. Nonmembers are made invisible, or relegated to an inferior status in regard to rights and privileges, with limited access to resources of the system. They become noncitizens or second-class citizens in the community. Some of the earliest steps taken by Nazis against Jews in the 1930s, and by Serbians against Albanian Kosovars in the 1990s, were restrictions on what forms of education and which professions could be sought by the oppressed group. For the special group, these two steps merge religion, identity, and privilege.

This systemic perspective on evil focuses not so much on evaluating the motivation of a single individual, as has been more traditional in Western religion, but on evaluating the impact of patterns of behavior on interdependence and relatedness within a society. In some ways, this analysis resembles Victor Turner's (1969, 1982) description of the evolution from communitas into structure, when the spontaneity and symbolic expressions of communitas within a culture are replaced by norm-driven relationships, cultural values, and a hierarchical social structure. Our interest, however, is in potential ethical and moral consequences of this process, rather than its sociological description.

A variety of different psychological and social processes help generate systemic evil. While none of these specifically characterize spiritual experience, the expression of religious beliefs and spiritual practices provide ground in which they often take root and flourish.

Malignant Narcissism of a Leader

Certain individuals are best characterized by their reliance on exploitation as a preferred method for supporting self-regard. Such individuals thrive only in nonreciprocal relationships. They crave praise, admiration, and submission from those with whom they are in relationship, while neglecting the wishes and needs of others (Kernberg, 1975). A relationship structured in this manner is the antithesis of spirituality. Ironically, such individuals commonly wrap their seduction in the language of spiritual enlightenment, righteousness, and the glorification of God because this serves as an effective strategy to gain submission, obedience, and adoration from others. Malignant narcissism puts into play systemic evil when it fuels destructive entitlement and scapegoating, or encourages idealization of the leader and neglect of self among members of the society.

Destructive Entitlement among a People

Destructive entitlement is organized by the idea "We have been wronged, therefore we deserve. . . . " Destructive entitlement as a response to perceived injury can lead to scapegoating (Boszormenyi-Nagy & Spark, 1973, p. 139). As a systemic process, it becomes self-sustaining when the society becomes focused upon its wounds, expressing its pain as moral outrage, and asserting a right to take freely from others as salve for the wounds. As Robins and Post (1997) have noted, a paranoid and narcissistic leader, such as an Adolf Hitler, Pol Pot, or Saddam Hussein, cannot orchestrate widespread destruction unless the society also has enough members who resonate with the leader's outrage from their personal sense of hurt and humiliation (Robins & Post, 1997). Religious myths, stories, beliefs, metaphors, and communities all can sustain and amplify a sense of destructive entitlement among a people. The Milosovic government in 1999 justified its assault upon Kosovë not only as a defense against threats to Serbian citizens but also as protecting sacred sites of the Serbian Orthodox Church within Kosovë. In an open letter to world leaders, Patriarch Pavle Ras-Prizren, leader of the Serbian Orthodox Church, turned to the Bible to support this invasion: "Our ancestors went to Kosovo to defend, rather than to take someone else's land, to defend their freedom and not to repress other people, to defend, and not to impose their faith, and they have taught us that Abel has the right and duty to defend himself from Cain." (Higgins & Block, 1999, pp. A1, A8).

Radical Fundamentalism

Either religious or political convictions can drive a social process that pronounces absolute truth while setting a rigid boundary between believers and nonbelievers. Those inside and outside the boundary are treated differently. Setting this boundary can permit zealots a guilt-free zone of aggression against those who challenge, reject, or violate tenets of the faith (Robins & Post, 1997). When a society becomes organized hierarchically by radical fundamentalism, there commonly occurs coercion, control, and exploitation of those who belong to excluded groups, as with the plight of people of color in a racist society or women in some religiously patriarchal societies.

The Political Targeting of Relatedness

Examples exist in which direct attacks are made upon relational beliefs and practices among a people because their inclusiveness and honoring of differences is viewed as inimical to a narrow political agenda. Stevan Weine (1999) has described how Serbian nationalists, in their campaign to destroy the Yugoslavian state, specifically targeted *merhamet*, the Bosnian moral practices and values that supported a multiethnic society. *Merhamet* has been translated from the Bosnian language as "mercy," "pardon," "grace," "alms," "charity," or "kindness." In the former Yugoslavia, *merhamet* was a core cultural value that supported Croats, Serbs, and Muslims living alongside one another. As one Bosnian survivor of the ethnic violence remembered (Weine, 1999, p. 13): "We called that the 'merhamet'—that you feel sorry for someone who has bad luck. Philanthropy. You like all people. You want to support everyone. If you can help, you help. You can even forgive bad things. You can find good in all religions. You will be good and decent to everyone." Two Bosnian Serbian psychiatrists, Jovan Raskovic and Radovan Karadzic, saw in *merhamet* an obstacle to a Serbian nationalist state. As Weine chronicled, they began utilizing for political ends both their knowledge of local Serbian culture and their psychiatric understanding of paranoia and wounded entitlement. They spoke and wrote to stir Serbian remembrances of traumas and injustices from World War II. Raskovic, in particular, collected and communicated stories of Serbian suffering, intending that they generate the outrage and fear needed to fuel nationalism: "Nothing is more successful at establishing a national collectivity and a national consciousness than genocide" (p. 94). Raskovic and Karadzic projected upon the Bosnian Muslims genocidal intentions to slaughter Serbs.

The violence that ultimately ensued against Bosnian Muslims had "betrayal by my neighbor" as its hallmark. Account after account told how Serb nationalists struck without warning against their Muslim friends, neighbors, teachers, and colleagues. A Muslim businesswoman's former employee, who was a Bosnian Serb, made her watch with him as he set fire to her house—"Well, boss—everything you had burned." (Weine, 1999, p. 43). Another Muslim man remembered: "After seven days in detention, my best friend came. We had to give everything we had. He took us to our house and burned it down and made us watch it" (p. 43). Still another remembered:

Many of our friends were Bosnian Orthodox. In April the Serbian army oc-
cupied Banja Luka. The Bosnian Orthodox agreed with the Serbian politics. Our good friends changed their behavior. They left us. All our friends,
our neighbors. They did nothing for us. One neighbor and close friend was
a secretary in the Republic of Serbia government. She could have helped us.
Her husband was in the police. They turned their back on us. My colleague
in the institute—a colleague of twenty years—dismissed me from my job.
Now he is the boss in the institute. I thought he was a good person. He left
me and my family without money. (p. 44)

There is no reason to think that the interethnic friendships and
collegiality existing prior to the conflict had been inauthentic. Rather,
primitive suspicions and fears were introduced that stirred emotions
capable of overrunning the generosity and good will that had long existed.

Religious Retreat from the World

Although the preceding processes also occur in many nonreligious contexts, "spiritualism" supports systemic evil in ways that belong uniquely
to religion. By spiritualism we mean the focusing of devotion upon
nonmaterial aspects of spirituality that are mystical and noumenal, while
detaching from the material world. In explaining why the Serbian
Orthodox Church did not take a strong stand against the Milosovic government's ethnic cleansing in Bosnia and Kosovë, Noel Malcolm (1999,
pp. 12–13) noted that "the Orthodox Churches withdrew from social
and political engagement into a realm of contemplation and liturgical
celebration. As a result, the cultures of their countries had fewer chances
to develop the bits of critical social and political thinking which were
generated in the West by the Catholic Church and its Protestant off-
shoots." The great Christian theologian Rudolf Bultmann (1960, p. 286)
explained why he remained on a university faculty in Germany during
World War II, while colleagues left the country or died in resisting Hitler,
by stating simply: "I have never directly and actively participated in political affairs." Much of my (Griff) upbringing as a Southern Baptist in
the American South was imbued with sense that the physical world in
which we live is doomed by its sin, that investing time and energy in bet-
tering it is pointless at best and hubris at worst, and that Christians
ought only to focus on personal righteousness and gaining a better life in

heaven after death. Such perspectives open space for processes of systemic evil to flourish without moral challenge.

A DILEMMA FOR A THERAPIST

What does a therapist do when feeling strongly, whether from personal or professional experience, that someone is expressing spiritual experience in a way that is destructive? What does one do when religious beliefs or spiritual practices vital to a person seem to support systemic evil? If a person believes that the Bible instructs the beating of children when they are disobedient, or senses God directing that abortion clinics should be bombed, or discerns it to be God's will that he or she should drop out of college and live on the streets in poverty, what does a therapist do?

These are difficult binds. If we as therapists use our professional authority to label certain beliefs or practices as immoral, misguided, or simply wrong, we impose our personal values onto others. Invoking professional authority is fundamentally a political act. It risks being oppressive or, at the least, violating a spirit of collaboration.

When the dilemma involves a direct communication from a person's God, a therapist's limited access to such a private experience poses an added difficulty. Communications among human beings have witnesses. Whether a political debate or a dispute among family members, human conversations can be described by different observers from various perspectives. Conversations with God have no external witnesses. Moreover, the person's account of the communication often consists of sparse words, phrases, and fragments of sentences, as one sees in relationships between two persons who are so intimate that few words are needed. Both the inaccessibility and nonverbal character of person–God communications are obstacles for a therapist who is equipped only with words as tools.

When a person–God encounter lies at the center of a clinical problem, it can be difficult—more so than with human relationships—to bring God into the therapeutic dialogue as a participant. A therapist can consider referring the dilemma for a religious specialist—a chaplain, priest, rabbi, or pastor—to resolve. Such professionals can speak with the authority of God, or, at the least, with the authority of the church or religious tradition. Sometimes a religious professional can convince a person that destructive beliefs are misinterpretations of the scriptures or doctrines of the religious tradition. However, the authority of religious professionals is often least effective with those who do the most harm in the name of religion, who often are beyond the perimeter of a mainstream religious organization and zealous in their pursuit of a mission issued directly from their God. The shootings, bombings, and mass suicides by religious groups in recent years have all been instigated by group leaders outside the mainstream organized religions, whether Christian, Jewish, Islamic, Buddhist, or Hindu. Were a new Abraham to appear today, declaring that God had ordered him to slay his son as a human sacrifice, it is questionable whether a religious professional could sway his judgment otherwise.

FURTHER DIFFICULTIES FACED BY POSTMODERN THERAPISTS

How to respond when religious beliefs seem destructive can be problematic in a different way for therapists who emphasize a collaborative relationship.[2] They privilege the wisdom that people bring from their lived experiences, and they draw primarily from this personal, practical, and community wisdom to fashion solutions for the problems people present. These therapists encourage people to make mindful choices about which narratives they do and do not wish to guide their lives.

How to honor a personal narrative is confusing when the stories, beliefs, and traditions that are the core of a person's spiritual life are ones that seem intrinsically destructive. In such situations, a commitment to honor the wisdom of the person's lived experience and one's ethical accountability as a professional can seem mutually exclusive. This is gut wrenching for a therapist who most wants to respect people's stories, beliefs, and traditions.

Such clinical dilemmas arise regularly. Terry was a patient hospitalized for pneumonia. Terry's internist had asked me (Griff) to "evaluate for depression." Although Terry had known that his partner had been HIV positive for the past 9 years, his partner had never shown signs of AIDS. They had carefully followed safe sex guidelines for the past 3 years, and Terry's HIV status, checked repeatedly, was never found to be positive. On this hospital admission, however, Terry had been diagnosed with pneumocystis pneumonia, a telltale sign of AIDS. Further blood tests confirmed that not only was he HIV-positive, but that AIDS and its medical complications were full blown. Terry became so despairing that his medical team worried that he could become suicidal.

When I met with Terry, I told about him about research studies suggesting that the body's immunological competence may be supported by resolving conflicts in one's important relationships. I wondered what were his important relationships and their state of well-being. To my surprise, he began talking not about his relationships with other persons, but about his recent decision to start attending church again.

Terry said that he was the son of a minister, and that he knew from the Bible that homosexuality was a sin. He had never been able to acknowledge to his family that he was gay. Although he had been promiscuous and had abused drugs at earlier times in his life, he had never stopped feeling the pull of his family. He had stopped the drug use and settled into a long-term, committed relationship with his gay partner, yet he had never felt peace about their relationship. Six months earlier, he had decided to cease having a sexual relationship, believing that to continue doing so was against God.

In talking with Terry and his partner at his bedside, I asked questions intended to open possibilities for some resolution in these important relationships, both with his partner and with his God. "Do you ever experience God in any other way?" I asked. "When you closely feel the presence of God, do you ever sense a different perspective about God than you find in the Bible verses you've told me about?" In my previous clinical experiences, the answer to this question has nearly always been "Yes," as people begin describing very different experiences they have of their God in different contexts. As Terry described his experience of God, however, there was no margin for interpretation—Scripture was authoritative and absolute: Homosexuality was evil, and he was evil as long as he engaged in it. He had no sense that God might understand or have compassion. He could not imagine it otherwise. I knew that it was not my position to recommend whether or not Terry should have a sexual relationship with his partner. However, I was accountable for helping him enter into a dialogue in which possible perspectives and paths for his life could be thoughtfully considered. In this I felt I had failed.

As another illustration, Ronald and Judy were referred for couple therapy. Ronald had entered the mental health system seeking treatment for depression. The psychiatrist who evaluated his complaints felt that the primary source of his depression was his troubled marriage and referred the couple to me (Griff). Ronald and Judy had spent a 21-year marriage rearing two children who were maturing into happy and successful adults. The corporate culture in which Ronald worked had provided the family a substantial income, a large home, travel, and private colleges for the children. However, it had also meant that Ronald was largely absent from the parenting and, emotionally, from Judy. At midlife, the children were in college, and Judy, now two decades out of college, was returning to graduate school. The marriage was overtly in trouble, with Judy threatening to leave. I knew this scenario to be a not-uncommon experience for marriages at midlife, one in which some couples, with or without professional help, can right the relationship, while others cannot. The unique aspect of Ronald and Judy's story was the way the conflict was mediated by Judy's relationship with her God.

Judy told about the dreariness and emptiness that for years she had accepted in her marriage. Two years earlier, she had begun volunteering for a program tutoring inner-city schoolchildren that was conducted by a Catholic organization. As she made new friends there, she began attending Mass and became involved in other church activities, including a charismatic prayer group. During one of the prayer meetings, she experienced a powerful mystical experience in which she felt the embrace of Jesus. He spoke soft words of comfort directly to her. Her prayers and work in the Church became the single passion of her life, and she entered social work graduate school to gain professional skills for serving the impoverished families she had come to know through her volunteer work.

Judy's blossoming vocational and religious awakening coincided with Ronald's growing awareness of how much he had missed from the lives of both his now-grown children and Judy. He began looking earnestly for ways to spend more time with her and was showing new interest in the college careers of his son and daughter. For Judy, however, this was too late. In the couple sessions, Judy spoke about the tenderness and loving caresses she experienced in prayer with Jesus. Jesus was always present, always available, always able to understand. Jesus wanted no more from her than her love and devotion. As she praised Jesus, Judy poured scorn and disdain upon Ronald for the years she had felt alone, detailing all the unspoken hurts that had accumulated for years. Ronald was baffled and devastated. So far as he had understood it, they had always had a good marriage.

My work as a marital therapist was brief and futile. From Judy's perspective, Jesus was a perfect man and perfect partner. Ronald tried to make offers she could accept, including an early retirement and a move to a new place to start a fresh life together. Judy acknowledged that Ronald had good qualities and might be sincere, but what he offered was only a shadow of the love she now found from Jesus. As therapist, I tried to come up with questions that would locate some conversational vantage point from which any possibilities other than immediate divorce could be discussed. Did she sense Jesus calling her only into union with him and away from Ronald, or could there be room for both? This question failed to open space for dialogue. She responded by stating her belief: Marriage is a human institution that God provides for people unable to live in union with the Divine. She was confident that Jesus both understood and would forgive her divorce.

When Ronald and Judy canceled future sessions and went on to divorce, I did not feel that I had failed because of their choice of divorce. I was in no position to say that divorce was wrong for them; this was their choice to make. I was very aware, however, that I had failed in one of my primary tasks as a therapist, which was to create the kind of thoughtful, reflective dialogue in which such important questions can be examined collaboratively and from multiple perspectives. I knew also that this failure rested in large part on my inability to bring Judy's primary conversational partner—Jesus—into meaningful participation in our dialogue.

In each of these cases, an aspect of the person's spirituality took him or her out of relationship with others. I considered each case to be a therapeutic failure because the powerful influence of religious beliefs or the voice of God itself did not meaningfully enter the dialogue.

A CLUE FROM HABERMAS

Puzzling over our successes and failures whetted our desire to understand how to create conversations in which the voice of God or spirit could meaningfully participate. In a sense, the questions we were asking were akin to those a German philosopher, Jurgen Habermas, had posed years earlier (Giddens, 1985). Habermas had grown up through the years of the Second World War. He was a scholar who assimilated the best that the German intellectual traditions could provide. During the war, he remained preoccupied with his scholarly work and was largely a bystander to the drama of war unfolding around him. Only during the Nuremburg trials did he begin to grasp the extent of evil committed by a culture that he had trusted. This revelation was traumatic for Habermas. How could it be, he wondered, that a culture so well educated and steeped in intellectual rigor could fall so completely under the sway of the irrational myths of National Socialism? As an intellectual, he felt guilty for what he had not done to stop fascism. What kind of public discourse might have prevented these atrocities from happening? It came to be Habermas's conviction that an absolute standard for judging truth was essential if future human societies were to be protected from recurrences of irrational, emotionally persuasive ideologies, like Nazism. However, Habermas recognized that all traditional sources upon which the authority of truth could be asserted—monarchies, religious institutions, science, societal traditions—had suffered irreversible erosion in the 20th century. There was no authority to which one could appeal. How then could truth be determined?

The solution, thought Habermas, was to define the kind of conversation whose processes could be trusted to protect reason and to generate truth. For Habermas, the important truths of human experience required a reaching of agreement through critical discussion by those involved in the problem. If a standard for judging were to claim validity, then its consequences ought to be satisfactory for all those involved in the discussion. This "ideal speech situation," in which each participant would have an equal and open opportunity to enter into the discussion free of coercion, constituted for Habermas an objective, albeit procedural, standard for truth. This procedure would follow a "discourse ethics" anchored in principles of justice (Habermas, 1990). In such a conversation, it would be expected that all participants should place themselves in the positions of each other and speak from those positions (Giddens, 1985; Habermas, 1990).

A similar theme emerged from the work of Mikhail Bakhtin, Russian literary critic and philosopher whose life nearly spanned both ends of the communist era in Russia. Bakhtin's early career as a gifted teacher and scholar in Moscow in the 1920s was cut short by the Stalinist oppression that descended upon Russian society. Although his life was saved by fleeing the city universities for remote countryside, his works were banned. He suffered the confiscation and disappearance of lengthy book manuscripts by government publishers who never put his words into print. Imprisoned and finally released, Bakhtin lived in obscurity, revealing only as the end of his life neared that copies of lost manuscripts had been hidden in a woodshed. After his students recovered the lost manuscripts, 50 years after they were written, his greatest works were finally published (Holquist, 1993).

Bakhtin's (1986, 1990) brilliant insights into the dialogical character of human life underpin much of our therapeutic work. One central idea, articulated by his life as well as his writings, stands out: Power consists in having a space in the discourse. Few struggles have exemplified this principle so graphically as Bakhtin's struggle to be read and heard among his own people. Opening the possibility for dialogue with another person means helping that person first find a position in which he or she has effective power in the relationship. In therapy that means knowing that one's utterances will be heard, understood, and taken seriously when matters at hand are considered (Shotter, 1933b).

For us, Habermas's and Bakhtin's works were important because they clarified the need for addressing power relationships and issues of justice among the conversational participants in therapy. As philosopher John Shotter (1993b, p. 162) has stated: "To the extent that the changing sea of enablements and constraints within which conversation takes place, is a changing sea of privileges and obligations, of entitlements and sanctions, the changes taking place are of a moral kind: people act with a respect both for their own and the being of the others around them." Therapy from this perspective is not about persuading, seducing, or coercing a person into accepting new ideas or changing behaviors, but about a responsibility for constructing and maintaining a kind of conversation that enables each participant to experience him- or herself as heard, understood, and seriously considered.

The stories of Ron and Judy and of Terry and his partner each illustrate the kind of clinical knowledge—or lack of it—that Shotter has dubbed "knowledge of the third kind." Knowledge of the third kind is a knowledge that cannot be grasped before one has immersed oneself within the therapeutic relationship or conversation. Like an artist's brushstroke or a line of improvisation in jazz, it cannot be planned, predicted, or known before the moment when it is needed. One can, however, provide certain conditions that open a therapist's access to this knowledge. These conditions enable dialogue to be sustained long enough for unexpectable options and possibilities to make themselves evident. Some of these conditions are physiological in kind.

PHYSIOLOGICAL PREREQUISITES FOR DIALOGUE

Through language, one conversational participant can touch the body of another participant from a distance. As conversational participants talk and listen, there is a flow of coordinated bodily activity that links not only the language systems of the participants, but also their autonomic nervous systems, endocrine systems, and postural motor systems (Griffith & Griffith, 1994).

Vanessa gave a down-to-earth description of this sociophysiological reality in Chapter 5. "From your experience with therapy and therapists, what do you think enables someone to speak about spiritual things?" was a question I (Melissa) posed to her, when asking permission to tell the story of the conversation she had with the spirit of her father. "Oh, it's mostly the expression on the therapist's face, I think. Not so much what they say, but a facial expression, of compassion, I suppose." I asked if she would detail the compassion more specifically. "Compassion is the look that says 'I want to know more,' instead of the look that says, 'I'm going to debate you about this.' When I see that look, then I can feel calm."

As a general rule, a participant in a conversation can open him- or herself to the touch of another's words only when it can be assured that pain will not be inflicted. The distinction between dialogue with its openness and reflective listening, and debate with its attacks, defensive parries, and counterattacks is an important one. Cognitively, dialogue is characterized by an inward focus in which the voice of the other can join one's inner voices in a reflective search for new meaning. Debate, however, is characterized by an external, defensive focus on the other that shuts down creativity and novel thinking. Whether the back-and-forth of a conversation evolves into debate or dialogue depends greatly on how the physical bodies of the conversational participants are primed.

An initial task for a therapist is to interact with people in such a manner that all conversational participants begin the session in emotional postures of tranquillity. In our book *The Body Speaks* (Griffith & Griffith, 1994), we detailed in Chapter 4, "Language and Emotional

Postures," some practical methods through which a therapist can help sustain emotional postures of tranquillity during therapy sessions.

THE PUBLIC CONVERSATIONS PROJECT
AND THE DUBLIN TEAM REVISITED

Dialogue about religious beliefs or spiritual practices often seems impossible with someone whose intense convictions or zealous practices appear to violate the relatedness of spirituality. In such situations, we have learned to focus first on the quality of our conversation and relationships with the person, rather than on a discussion about religious or spiritual topics. The first priority is to create a context that can foster dialogue. This means establishing egalitarian power relations among the conversational participants—between therapist and client or patient, or among the members of a family or other group. Then active steps can be taken that foster emotional postures of tranquillity among the participants.

As introduced in Chapter 8, some of the best demonstrations of this approach have been the work of the Public Conversations Project in Cambridge, Massachusetts, and the Dublin Family Therapy Team in Ireland. In the previous chapter, we described their methods in terms of community-building. In many ways these methods might have been the same ones that Habermas or Bakhtin would have prescribed as a way to address systemic evil through dialogue—structuring a setting in which each participant experiences safety, countering efforts by some participants to attack or belittle others, keeping a focus on the telling and listening to personal stories, opening the dialogue into "pockets of uncertainty" within the polarized debate, and articulating experience not yet expressed in language. As one might surmise, the presence of this kind of community inhibits processes of systemic evil.

COUNTERING DESTRUCTIVE ENTITLEMENT
THROUGH RESTORATION OF DIGNITY

The problem of destructive entitlement requires specific attention, in part because its perspective is so often seductive for a therapist who identifies with victims of injustice. The injured person's claim is "I have

been hurt so much that I have the right to hate. . . . " There are many instances when the evidence is compelling that the person suffered harm
that was both unjust and quite real.

Mr. Hussam, for example, was a refugee from a war-torn nation
who was referred for evaluation and treatment of depression. He had
come to the United States hoping to escape from the poverty, violence,
and social disintegration that had befallen his country. The Americans he
had met in his country seemed warm and generous. In the United States,
however, it was difficult to find a job due to his language difficulties and
lack of understanding of American culture. When he did find a job, he
was soon fired. Mr. Hussam had responded angrily toward a customer
whom he felt was treating him rudely. When he confronted the customer,
an argument ensued that escalated into a fist fight. With no investigation
of the incident, Mr. Hussam was fired from his job. He believed that his
dismissal was unfair and tried unsuccessfully for a year to sue his former
employer in a court of law on charges of job discrimination. At the time
I (Griff) evaluated him, his humiliation and outrage were funneled into
hatred of all Americans: "In my country, I knew good Americans. Here
there are only bad Americans. Some days I want to take a gun and blow
all of them off the face of the earth!" It was evident that he felt any act
of violence toward Americans in general would have been justified by
the unfairness with which he had been treated by those who had hurt
him. His rage was tempered only when an empathic Arabic-speaking
psychotherapist heard his story fully, acknowledged the injustices that
had occurred, and helped him to begin taking steps to build a new life.

Destructive entitlement usually must be addressed before there can
exist enough trust in the room for dialogue to emerge. This usually begins with therapist's actions to help restore dignity to the entitled person,
which involves responding to the humiliation that the person experienced. Aaron Lazare (1999) has described humiliation as a social emotion that arises out of the perception that one has been lowered in social
status by the action of the other person. It represents a readying of one's
being to retaliate against the other who had committed the humiliating
act. The prototypical situation is that of the duel: In response to a perceived insult, the injured man demands "satisfaction" from the offender
in a challenge to a duel. They then select weapons and in the violence
that follows, regardless who is killed, the debt of honor is paid and the
social structure restored. Acts of humiliation thus tend to elicit a cycle of

attacks and counterattacks. Lazare has noted that acts of humiliation, even minor ones, are seldom forgotten even after the passage of years. The act that repairs humiliation is typically an apology. Two criteria must be met if an apology is to be effective: The apologizing person must accept responsibility for the act, and he or she must voluntarily accept a degree of humiliation by somehow lowering him- or herself in status vis-à-vis the humiliated person.

Responding to destructive entitlement in a clinical encounter usually requires that the complaint of injustice be acknowledged as valid by those involved, and that a reparative response be made to the injured person. When the relationship is a dyadic one, as between couple partners or between child and parent, this reparation may consist of a negotiated apology. In a family where incest has occurred, for example, or in a couple where there has been an affair, an acceptable apology by the father or couple partner who violated trust often is an essential step before healing can begin in the relationships. In a society where systematic political oppression has occurred, public acts of acknowledgment and apology by those who held power or benefited from exploitation of the weak, while not always sufficient, are essential for initiating healing in the society, as in the work of the Truth and Reconciliation Commission in South Africa or Sorry Day in Australia. With the maturation of the peace movement in the United States, bumper stickers began to change from the word "Peace" on a cheerful pastel background to a simple black and white sign that said, "If you want Peace, Work for Justice." Again and again, this lesson comes home to us in our society, in our own families, and in those who consult us.

Ivan Boszormenyi-Nagy, one of the early pioneers of family therapy, has provided a therapeutic model that implements reparation of humiliation within complex social systems. His approach was distinguished among the early originators of family therapy by his central focus on justice. In Nagy's approach (Boszormenyi-Nagy & Spark, 1973), the interview begins with the therapist first establishing "multilateral partiality" with each person in the group, such that each participant feels that his or her point of view is understood and acknowledged. The therapist then elicits from each person the history of the problem, noting how each may have gained debits or credits in a "family ledger of merits." There then follows a slow, reflective discussion among all the participants as to how those with debits may receive reparation for the losses they have incurred. Nagy aims to provide a serious, thoughtful dialogue in which the valid injuries that a person may have sustained can be publicly acknowledged and steps toward reparation made by those involved. This process extends beyond the usual limits of what can be accomplished in an apology and provides a mechanism through which members of a family or community can respond to an injured or humiliated person when the one who committed the violation may not be available to participate.

Throughout the ages and even now, more often than not, people work out these dilemmas without therapists. As therapists and as fellow men and women, we can listen and learn from those who have suffered injustice and whose spirits have survived. Several years ago, to aid me (Melissa) at a time when my heart was hardening, I kept taped to our bathroom mirror a passage from Alice Walker's (1970) novel *The Third Life of Grange Copeland*. Walker's character, Grange, was an old man who had endured a lifetime of oppression and violence from whites, and who in turn had oppressed and violated women. Grange finally discovered a new life in the purity of his love for Ruth, his granddaughter. Though he did not absolve the whites who injured him, he turned from hating and blaming them and assumed responsibility for his own violence. However, he knew he could never forgive them. In this passage he persuades Ruth to leave their home in Alabama so that her life will not be subject to the oppression, nor her spirit to the numbness he developed toward whites:

> "So that I wouldn't add kindling to a fire that was roasting them, but I wouldn't hear 'em calling me neither."
>
> Ruth chuckled.
>
> "That ain't no feeling to be proud of," Grange said sternly, "not if you going to call yourself human." He leaned forward, looking sadly into the fire.
>
> "When I was a child," he said, "I used to cry if somebody killed an ant. As I look back on it now, I liked feeling that way. I don't want to set here now numb to half the peoples in the world. I feel like something soft and warm an' delicate an' sort of shy has just been burned right out of me."
>
> "Numbness is probably better than hate," said Ruth gently. She had never seen her grandfather so anguished.
>
> "The trouble with numbness," said Grange, as if he'd thought it over for a long time, "is that it spreads to all your organs, mainly the heart. Pretty soon after I don't hear the white folks crying for help, I don't hear the black." He looked at Ruth. "Maybe I don't even hear you." (p. 293)

ADDRESSING THE DESTRUCTIVE CONSEQUENCES OF A SPIRITUALITY OR RELIGION IN THERAPY

When responding to destructive consequences of religious or spiritual experience in a therapy, we are guided by what we have learned from our own successes and failures, from such philosophers as Bakhtin, Habermas, and Wittgenstein, and from courageous family therapy colleagues, such as the Public Conversations Project and the Dublin team, who have worked to bring warring political factions into meaningful dialogue. Some guidelines that the two of us find helpful are the following:

1. The dialogue of therapy should be structured in a sufficiently egalitarian manner that all participants in the conversation feel that they can speak freely and know that they will be heard. Questions that are useful to reflect upon prior to beginning the session include the following:

- What is necessary for dialogue, rather than debate, to occur?
- How must the conversation be organized so that each participant can speak freely?
- How must the conversation be organized so that each participant's words will be taken seriously?

2. A therapist should help structure the sociobiological conditions necessary for dialogue. For there to be emotional postures of tranquillity, participants need to feel an assurance of safety and attitudes of respect, openness, and curiosity from other participants. Toward this end, it is helpful to ask questions both about oneself and about the other.

Some useful questions to ask of oneself follow:

- Why am I having such a strong reaction?
- Am I responding to this person as a person or to this person as representative of a group? If I am responding to the group (i.e., a church denomination, a cult, an ethnic group), how can I particularize this person?
- Am I trying to resolve my own ambivalence about spiritual or religious commitment by pressing my convictions on this person?

Some questions that can be asked about the other person follow:

- How does this person hope to be shaped by these stories?
- What have been some specific stories in this person's life experience such that these beliefs and lifestyle came to be adopted?
- With what person or community does this person's stories connect him or her? What can I learn and appreciate about the life of this community with whom this person is connected?
- From what person or community is this person separated by these stories or beliefs?
- What other positions or stories are sometimes held alongside this one? Is my strong response to this story deafening me to these others?

3. Beginning with the first interview of therapy, a relationship should be established, with each participant treated as someone who is assumed to be worthy and capable of doing good. Usually, only after this step can the problematic belief or action effectively be addressed. Toward the end of meeting the honorable other (Madsen, 1999), in these difficult situations one can ask:

- What can I appreciate about this person's intentions, if not their actions?
- How are this person's beliefs or actions keeping me from seeing him or her as a person?
- Are there any signs that there is some other voice or story within this person that would not hold this belief or express these actions?

This guideline is antithetical to an approach that first challenges the disputed belief or action, then establishes a personal relationship only after the politics have been resolved.

4. The destructive potential in certain sacred metaphors, narratives, beliefs, conversations, rituals, or other religious or spiritual practices is best recognized through a collaborative process with the client or patient. Together we can examine how a particular metaphor or belief bears influence upon the events of daily life. Any usage of symbolic language can be deemed destructive if it generates isolation, helplessness, meaningless, or despair in the person's relationships with others.

5. Psychotherapy can help a person to design counterpractices and to build spiritual communities that oppose the exploitative practices of

malignant narcissism, destructive entitlement, and radical fundamental-ism.

6. Confronting the destructive influence that a specific "spiritual guide"—a pastor, rabbi, priest, or counselor—holds is sometimes neces-sary. Processes of discernment for this situation are similar to those for recognizing a therapist who uses his or her power to abuse. When a spir-itual guide claims authority, one can ask what emotional postures this effects. These questions ask about "the music, not just the words":

- Does this spiritual guide's message convey humility or arrogance? One marker for malignant narcissism is its claim to specialness—a special access to God, special powers, special entitlements.
- Does this person's message convey compassion or scorn? In Christian Scripture, Jesus did not express scorn or contempt, ex-cept toward predators of society who profited by injustice and deceit. No one was scorned for being simply weak or sinful. The same description can be applied to modern spiritual leaders, such as the Mahatma Gandhi and the Dalai Lama. Unfortunately, too many televangelists and spiritual guides on lecture circuits thrive by heaping ridicule on those whom they judge to be falling short.
- Does this person's message express reverence for the spiritual world, or does it use spiritual principles in an attempt to acquire personal power or to manipulate others for personal gain? When I (Griff) was growing up, some people from the community would give testimony at the front of the church each year about how their cows began giving more milk or their hens more eggs after they began tithing their income. This testimony, of course, would be given during pledge week, when the church elicited fi-nancial commitments from its members for the coming fiscal year. This is not too different from various "spiritual experts" today who sell their version of spirituality to clients, church members, or followers by promising money or power as the payback.
- Does this person go too far in taking his or her own idiosyncratic spiritual encounters and generalizing them as the normative model for every other person? Many people have shared, through writing or public speaking, the wisdom gained from their own life crises. Often they give others guidance, help, and hope. But a red flag should be raised whenever such an author or speaker falls into too much enthusiasm for declaring that this is how every

other person's life ought to be organized. The more certainty expressed as to what the spiritual experiences of others ought to be, the more skepticism is deserved.

8. It is useful to collaborate with a person in therapy in identifying and naming the rhetorical devices that predatory spiritual guides employ to achieve their ends. Claiming a position as victim by fabricating facts, relabeling exploitation as "helping," and invoking the authority of God to warrant aggression are only a few of the devices regularly employed by those who exploit in the name of spirituality or religion.

9. When there exists a threat of violence or other danger for someone in the situation, social control, not therapy, is often the appropriate response. Lynn Hoffman (1985) has pointed out that therapy does not begin until safety has been secured for those involved. Spouse battering, child abuse, mutilation of one's body, and threat of suicide often require protective measures, not therapy, as the initial intervention. One particularly poignant story stands in my (Griff) memory as the prototype for situations when it is important that I accept a role as social control agent, instead of a collaborative psychotherapist. A young woman with a psychiatric history of bipolar disorder, or manic–depressive illness, had been admitted to the hospital for surgical removal of a brain tumor. The tumor was benign and its successful removal was fully curative. However, in one of her eyes the nerve fibers enabling a normal blinking reflex were damaged during the surgery. As can happen in such cases, she developed a corneal abrasion and had to be rehospitalized so that ophthalmologists could treat the eye injury. Medically, this was a simple problem, requiring only a 3-day admission to the hospital. However, this woman was insistent about going home. Faced with her doctors' predictions that she could lose her sight in that eye without acute medical treatment, she said, "I don't care. I've got two eyes." When her doctors refused to discharge her she precipitously fled down the hall to the elevators. Hospital security guards intercepted her, and she was placed back in her bed in physical restraints, with arms and legs tied down. She was outraged and began clawing at her eye whenever a hand was released, determined to get rid of the eye if that was what was keeping her in the hospital, quoting the Bible: "If your eye offends you, pluck it out!"

At this point, I (Griff) was asked, as psychiatric consultant, to evaluate her capacity to make decisions about her care. She cursed me and

angrily refused to answer any questions about how this eye was offending her. Suspecting that psychosis was driving her religious zeal, I recommended that she be given antipsychotic medications, but she refused to
take them (as was her legal right in our jurisdiction). One morning, one
of her medical doctors, not understanding either the seriousness of her
psychiatric disorder or our legal obligation to prevent self-harm, released
her from the hospital, feeling that she should have the right to make her
own decisions. Her family, however, brought her back to the hospital
within 24 hours with her eyeball ruptured and mostly pulled out of its
socket. Emergency surgery repaired the injury, and she was again placed
in physical restraints. This time she spoke more openly about the
thoughts that propelled her actions: She had become convinced that
Satan was residing in her eye; hence, she should pluck out the eye and
destroy it. By this time, legal proceedings were finally concluded that
permitted the administration of antipsychotic medications against her
will and her transfer to a psychiatric facility. She was hospitalized there,
treated with medications for mania and psychosis, and subsequently discharged to home. When I later saw her as she was coming to an outpatient neurosurgery appointment, she was thinking clearly and in good
humor about the whole episode. She said her eye was fine and cheerfully
apologized for "for making your life hell" during the hospitalization. I
smiled and told her I was glad her eye was fine.

THE STORY OF LUTCHI AND THELMA

In real life, dilemmas raised by destructive uses of spirituality or religion
are often too complex for any set of guidelines to provide clear solutions. While as therapists we may be convinced that a very vulnerable
person is being endangered and exploited, the person states that he or
she not only chooses this relationship, but that God has guided this
choice. This knotty dilemma is familiar to therapists who work with the
most vulnerable in our society: Shall I choose to intervene in a way that
is disrespectful to the person's autonomy and also risk disconnection in
our relationship, or shall I follow and stay connected, knowing this person is at serious risk? The added strand of spiritual issues only ties the
knot tighter. Many religious traditions revere obedience to spiritual authority and suffering for one's faith. An implicit, if not explicit, audience
is created, perhaps others in the faith, perhaps God. Even when the per-

son has an inkling of being misused, it may be extremely hard to change direction. Exponentially more difficult than the therapist's dilemma is the one of the family and friends who love the vulnerable person, who fear for him or her, who may want to scream, but must stay calmly connected. I (Melissa) learned the most about how to hold these dilemmas and not be held by them, how to stay connected and find a way out of the exploitative situation from one such family member. It was Thelma, the mother of Lutchi. She put into daily practice what I, as a family therapist, have preached for years: Keep the connection, but widen the circle.

Several years ago, Thelma brought Lutchi from their home in Mozambique to the United States with an absolute determination to get good treatment for the psychiatric illness afflicting him. All the strength of her determination was required for the trip, because so many friends and professionals advised against it. She had taken him to psychiatrists in Mozambique and in neighboring South Africa, and he was no better. They treated him briefly but soon urged her to accept that Lutchi had a chronic, disabling mental illness, probably schizophrenia, and that she should proceed with institutionalizing him. "But the boy you are meeting in these quick consultations is not Lutchi!" she told them, "and you cannot make a judgment about him when you don't even know who he really is. He is still here," she insisted, for she could catch glimpses of the child she had known, the Lutchi who had been a pleasant, friendly boy, an excellent student. Then, as a 17-year-old, Lutchi began having difficulties with his school work and disorganization in his thinking. The next year he affiliated with a local Christian church that became increasingly the central focus of his life as his school and social functioning declined. Dark, depressed moods appeared with days of isolation and weeping, alternating with other periods of intense activity when Lutchi would walk the streets at all hours of the night, aggressively proselytizing his religion upon strangers. Thelma knew that something was dreadfully wrong with his mind, and believed that somewhere, someone could help him get well.

Coming to the United States was not a new idea for Thelma. When Mozambique had won its independence from Portugal, she had worked to improve the economic system in her new country by advocacy of giving a fair chance to women. In working toward this goal, she had won a scholarship for a U.S. education and afterwards had returned to contribute to building her new country. Now Lutchi's illness had brought them back to the United States, and, thereby took them away from the sub-

stantial network of family and friends who had been caring for and helping them during the illness. Thelma was steered by friends here to seek
out Griff for psychiatric treatment. Griff determined that Lutchi had the
symptoms of Bipolar I Disorder, with extreme mood swings and psy-
chotic thought disturbance, a serious illness, but quite treatable. We
worked as a team, with Griff acting as Lutchi's physician and me meeting with Thelma and Lutchi in family therapy.

Our family meetings had an open format. Usually only the three of
us met, but sometimes they brought along other people, Mozambican
visitors and American friends. Occasionally we had agreed in advance to
have a particular person join us for a purpose, but more often the arrival
of the guests was a pleasant surprise to me. Lutchi was happy to have
other people in our sessions. Always an inclusive person, he seemed to
enjoy introducing people he cared about to each other. Together we
made the therapy a hospitable environment. Lutchi's illness held the potential to be isolating for both Thelma and himself. It was difficult to explain to other people, and sometimes his symptoms could be misinter-
preted as willful behavior, reflecting badly on both mother and son.
Thelma wanted their friends to participate in the meetings so that they
could better understand the illness and could then become more supportive. This was only one of her ways of widening the circle. She also
made her home open to Lutchi's friends, many of whom were from his
church, an exuberant, warm African American community who accepted him into their group, appreciating and encouraging his musical
talents. When friends were down on their luck, Lutchi would bring them
home, offering shelter and Thelma's home cooking. Their apartment was
sometimes crowded, and often unpredictable, but Thelma remained flexible and interested in getting to know Lutchi's friends. Though she is a
kind person, these were not simply acts of kindness. She realized early
on that along with the many in Lutchi's world of conservative charismatic Christianity who would nurture and support him, there were a
few who could captivate and exploit him. It was not her world, but she
needed its doors to be open to her, so that she could enter when necessary to help Lutchi safely navigate.

I was glad for their friends to join us for another reason: They
helped to balance the power of the therapy relationship. The more community members involved, the more I shifted toward the position of a
visitor, learning their ways rather than vice versa. Because we were primarily treating a medically based problem, Griff and I were in the posi-

tion of experts and had the power commensurate with that position. Along with our expert position, we knew that, both as white people and U.S. citizens, we might unwittingly perpetuate colonizing practices, might fall into knowing better what was right for Thelma and Lutchi and be culturally inappropriate or disrespectful. What we did not fully appreciate was Thelma's keen awareness of this danger. From childhood she had direct experience with colonizers in her country, and in her later years experienced the effects of the lingering colonialist attitudes and racist habits of relating, even when engaging with people of good intent. When our relationship felt solid enough, I told her of my concerns and asked her to be on watch with me, to inform me if ever she sensed this. She explained that she had been on alert since the beginning of their search for treatment, and that they had settled with us because they felt respected, that they would not stay otherwise. Of course, we both knew that I could at any time inadvertently perpetuate these attitudes, but now we would have a means to address it.

Lutchi's treatment progressed well. Though he was not keen on taking medications, he trusted Griff and took the mood stabilizers and antipsychotics as prescribed. They were effective in many ways, including supporting Lutchi's efforts to act with more consideration toward Thelma. His concentration improved, and he enrolled in school and restarted music lessons. He had been waylaid by the ferocity of the symptoms, so the family work focused on his accepting more household responsibilities as Thelma began to grant him more autonomy. For a brief period their lives improved. Thelma said she felt that the son she had known was coming back.

Lutchi agreed that he was better off, but even as his symptoms lessened, his conflicts over taking the medicine intensified. His hope and the word he said he had received from God was that God alone would give him complete healing. His church friends understood his struggle over how to most faithfully deal with his illness. We invited the minister and some of the church members to a therapy session. One guest, Randy, was particularly helpful. He was a gentle man, greatly admired by Lutchi, who would figure significantly in Lutchi's future. Along with the minister, he held a "both/and" philosophy—God and medicines—but some other church members did not. Finally, after Lutchi attended an evangelist's healing service, he decided to stop taking his medications. Within days a manic state and psychosis took over. He frightened people in a restaurant with threats that his bag of food actually contained a bomb. A SWAT team arrived in minu~~~, ~~~ested Lutchi, and took him to jail. He was stunned, but, again relying on his religious foundation, sustained himself by singing hymns in jail, "just like the apostle Paul when the Romans jailed him for proclaiming Jesus." This served him well, for, unlike Paul, Lutchi's captors soon realized he needed to be in a hospital instead of a jail.

Later, Lutchi spoke about a new understanding both of the limitations of his illness and of the tricks it could play on him. He saw the interaction of sin and the illness. He felt that he had given way to the sin of pridefulness—"I want to be special and I want it now, God"—and that pride had let the bipolar illness trick him. After the episode, friends from the church came and apologized to Thelma for not listening to her, thus placing Lutchi in danger. The circle now seemed wide, strong, and wise. The obstacles to Lutchi's recovery were cleared away. His moods stable and mind clear, he began taking steps again toward hobbies, a job, and the promise of a more independent life in the future.

Then without warning a new illness intruded, a neurological movement disorder. In the space of a single day, Lutchi's head, arms, legs, and trunk began twitching and jerking, spontaneously and uncontrollably. It seemed logical to consider these movements to be a medication side-effect, yet their pattern was disturbingly different from that of tardive dyskinesia, a medication-induced disorder familiar to most mental health clinicians. Griff could only tell Lutchi he did not know what was wrong, but would try to help him find someone who did. Over the ensuing weeks, however, the psychiatric and neurological consultants he contacted were unable to diagnose or successfully control the movements. All the treatment trials failed, unless medication doses were raised to such high doses that Lutchi could not stay awake. Indeed, the disorder intensified to tragic proportions. The writhing movements became so incapacitating that Lutchi was unable to attend to his basic needs and, as it progressed, could not sit in a chair or walk, even with an aid. So determined was he to keep going that he resorted to crawling. His knees became scraped and bloodied from crawling, and his head bald in the back from the unceasing twisting and rubbing against walls while bracing himself as he attempted to walk.

One referral led to another, and Lutchi was admitted to a prestigious psychiatric inpatient unit in another state. When the pharmacological treatments were again unsuccessful, the staff became convinced that his problem was psychological in its origins and reinforced by the attention his illness received. They told Thelma that she was too emotionally involved with Lutchi and needed to let him be more independent. Did she really want to help him, they asked her? "Of course, I would do anything to help Lutchi," she responded. Then she would need to join their team, they told her. They were certain they could help Lutchi, but only if she participated. They planned to approach Lutchi with her in order to confront him with their beliefs that he had been fooling them and could stop the movements. They deemed the strongest motivator for Lutchi to be his mother's visits, so their behavioral modification protocol called for Thelma telling him that she would return when she had word that he had improved himself. When he fell, she was not to help him up, and she was not to help him when he struggled with his food.

Thelma wept when she later told me that the hurt and betrayed expression on Lutchi's face, as he saw her standing in his hospital room in line with the experts, would be seared into her memory. The team spokesperson announced to him that they had not been completely honest with him, that they felt that he had much more control than he let on and they were going to act accordingly. Lutchi was amazed, but responded in a remarkably clear way. "How could you think that I would do this on purpose? It must be that you think that way because you yourselves are, as you just said, deceptive. But I am not. This is how it is: People who lie are always suspicious of others, but I, I tell you, am an honest guy." The behavioral program brought only pain and humiliation, and Thelma soon removed Lutchi and brought him home. Never again, she said, would she follow an expert against her better judgment.

Back in our session, Lutchi's writhing body could not stay in the chair, but his mind was clear and focused. He had made meaning of his trial, and had not lost hope, but had transferred it away from medicine. "Perhaps great difficulties are being manifest so that God's glory can be greater when He heals me." He said the doctors' arrogance had made them "intellectual barbarians," and proclaimed that he would see no other doctor than Griff from now on. "But Lutchi," I tried to persuade him, "Griff doesn't know what to do. He wants to help you by finding someone who does know." As we concluded, Thelma begged for Lutchi's forgiveness for believing the experts instead of him and for participating in it all. He granted it, acknowledging that he knew she was trying to do what was best for him; however, he said that it would take time to repair the trust that was broken. The circle of care was weakened now: There was a gap between Lutchi and the hope of future medical aid, but, more importantly, a rift between Thelma and Lutchi. Into this rift entered Sister Jane.

Sister Jane was a semiretired white evangelist with no particular denominational affiliation, who made her living by selling nutritional supplements. Although not a member of Lutchi's church, she had been peripherally involved in his life before the hospitalization. Following that treatment failure, she became central. She persuaded Lutchi that God had appointed her to help him be miraculously healed. In our meetings, I could see the worried expression on Thelma's face as Lutchi exclaimed to me what an unbelievably wonderful woman Sister Jane was. She visited with him for hours every day, conducted prayer and Bible study with him, and even wanted to employ him in her business. Thelma and I raised serious questions with Lutchi about Sister Jane. Thelma went to others in Lutchi's community, ministers and friends, and asked them to help. Some did, but there was no convincing Lutchi that the intensity of his relationship with Sister Jane might not be in his best interest. He felt that she was wonderful, a gift from God. It was clear to Thelma that further objections to Sister Jane would create a breach with Lutchi, so she chose to watch carefully and bite her tongue. This was hard, especially when Sister Jane would give Thelma tips on how to mother Lutchi. Thelma vented in our sessions alone, "Not only is Sister Jane an expert on Lutchi, but now she tells us she is an expert on Africa! She was an evangelist there. I asked her which part of Africa she knew about. 'All of it,' she said. Melissa, can you imagine? All of it!" I cringed with a sense of sick association with all the Sister Janes. Thelma, though, threw back her head and laughed so hard that it overcame my embarrassment about the conduct of white people, and I joined her delight in the absurdity of it all.

The connection between Sister Jane and Lutchi posed an expensive dilemma for Thelma, emotionally and financially. Sister Jane insisted, and Lutchi believed, that dietary supplements, including the ones she sold, would help him, so Thelma purchased them at considerable cost. Thelma feared that Sister Jane was on the brink of directing Lutchi to cease contact with medical people.

Sister Jane had declined my (Melissa's) invitations to our meetings, but Thelma understood that Sister Jane was very important in Lutchi's life and urged us to invite her again. We did so, with the stated purpose of discussing what her role in Lutchi's life and health would be. Sister Jane came, armed with information about her dietary supplements, and told me how God had put Lutchi in her life as her "last great mission." Lutchi, usually gregarious and talkative, was submissive and quiet within Sister Jane's presence, seemingly in awe of her. I asked if there was room for medicine or therapy within her plan, and she said that since Lutchi was already seeing doctors, she would not stand in the way of medical treatment. She had not known Lutchi long, so I led a detailed recollection of what had happened previously when he had ceased all medications, and she nodded.

Later, at home, Thelma reported, Sister Jane told Lutchi she had a word from God that he should indeed quit all medicines and other treatments. Also in this word, God had told Sister Jane to adopt Lutchi, that she was his true spiritual mother and that he should live with her to complete his healing. She would teach him music, manners, and Bible every day, so that when the healing was complete he would be ready to fulfill his special mission in life, for he could carry on the work she had begun. As a 20-year-old, Lutchi was free to make his own decisions. He chose to stay connected with his mother Thelma, but to live with his spiritual mother, Sister Jane. Because he wanted to honor his mother, Thelma, he said, he would continue to take the medicine. Lutchi required assistance with physical mobility, eating, and other tasks of daily life. Thelma did not contest the move, hoping that the work would soon wear Sister Jane out. It did, and Lutchi came back home, though Sister Jane kept up her visits. Due to travel, I did not see Lutchi or Thelma for a few weeks. Much changed during that time.

Several months had now passed since the onset of the movement disorder and, with the possible exception of Lutchi, we had all been coming to terms with the likelihood that he might never be able to control his movements again. Griff bore the burden that it was likely one of the drugs he had prescribed, that Lutchi had not wanted, that had initiated the movement disorder. He was deeply saddened, but could not say what he would do differently if given the situation again, nor what he could do now except be faithful to the relationship and, as long as they wanted, to continue the search for help. Thelma struggled with whether the time for acceptance had come, but felt in her heart that she had not exhausted all means. She persuaded Lutchi to see one more doctor, Dr. Jose Apud. He had been a researcher in the National Institutes of Health and was an expert in unusual movement disorders. He diagnosed Lutchi's problem as tardive dystonia, a rare complication of treatment with antipsychotic medications. Tardive dystonia has a poor prognosis with little known about effective treatments, unlike the more common tardive dyskinesia. Dr. Apud, however, had in mind an experimental regimen that had helped some other patients. With a combination of careful research, hope, and humility, Dr. Apud started Lutchi on the regimen.

After 4 months of treatment, Thelma left me a message that there was some improvement. Lutchi could manage his basic physical needs now, and she was departing for a long-needed trip to Mozambique. Thelma said it was the only way she could make the salary she needed to continue Lutchi's treatment. It was not an easy decision, but she left. Randy had become a close and trusted friend, and he would be staying with Lutchi during her absence. She said she could feel better about leaving if an appointment was made for Lutchi to come and see me soon, as he was eager to do. She mentioned, too, that there was nothing more to worry about with Sister Jane.

When Lutchi arrived at my office, he walked in with a steady gait. He had asked Randy to hang back so he could show me independently how well he was. He sat in the chair, almost still, with only a few un-willed movements remaining. "These will get better, too," he said, "and if they don't, praise God anyway." I was so amazed that I could not speak. I started to cry and could not stop. He started to laugh heartily. And this is how we spent much of the hour.

Immediately afterward I called Griff to share the joy. At home that evening I wrote Thelma a jubilant e-mail, thinking I was breaking the news to her. She thanked me generously, but I now realize that she already knew. Perhaps she just did not want to spoil the surprise for me.

Lutchi continues to do well, and he and Thelma are quite willing to have their story shared with anyone who might benefit. As is obvious from the length of this vignette, it was impossible for me to isolate the thread from their story to discuss only the exploitative potential of religion. One thread seemed to pull out another. Lutchi's movement disorder could not be relayed without the precedent of his psychiatric treatment. Sister Jane could not have bonded so powerfully with Lutchi if the inpatient psychiatric treatment had not created the gap. Her absolute certainty about the cure, cultural disrespect, and recklessness regarding Thelma and Lutchi's relationship was almost a mirror of the attitudes of those doctors who inadvertently paved her way. Most importantly, there is no quick explanation of how therapy, or even family therapy, helped

Lutchi to escape Sister Jane's influence, because therapy alone could not have done so. Therapy did act to support and strengthen the circle that Thelma and Lutchi were creating, and within that circle, in the conversation that follows, Lutchi points to Randy as the one who helped him see that he was being used. Lutchi agreed to make a tape with me for a workshop that Griff and I were teaching to therapists on the harmful potential of religion and spirituality, and Randy accepted our invitation to join us. Here is a segment of that interview:

MELISSA: So I was planning to tell the workshop group about you and Thelma and Randy and your friends, but to especially focus on the story of your experience with Sister Jane. Would that be okay?

LUTCHI: Wait. Don't just tell about her, but about my early immature faith. You should share that, too.

MELISSA: What do you mean? What would you want me to say about that?

LUTCHI: As a zealous, immature Christian—faith without knowledge. Not wanting to take the medicine. I don't mind, really, I would like for you to share that, too. There was a phase where I, like many religious people, was immature and a young believer. I would call spirituality, mature religion. Spirituality is the positive side of religion, and zeal without knowledge the negative side. Zeal without knowledge is religion with just rituals.

MELISSA: Without spirit?

LUTCHI: Without spirit. Like the Pharisees, the Zealots. Not zealots in the positive sense as people on fire for God, but people who are narrow-minded, stubborn, and stiff-necked. We all go through that at some point in our lives. We meet God and God says come, and we run. We want to go ahead of God. We get overexcited. And there are so many doctrines out there, so many people saying so many things, and we don't know. It's normal that we don't. There is a foundation being built, a filter being built in our lives and not yet finished, and we don't know how to filter yet. When someone like Sister Jane comes on the scene, proclaiming that she is appointed by God to help heal you, with so much authority, well, the filter just doesn't always catch it.

MELISSA: Is there a way that therapists can be of help with that?

LUTCHI: I wasn't thinking so much of therapy. I was just thinking of myself, what I have to do.

MELISSA: So, it's pretty much something you have to do alone?

LUTCHI: Oh, no. (*laughing*) Not alone! You know the Holy Spirit is a pretty good therapist. And Randy is a pretty good therapist, too, sometimes. But real therapists, I think they just have to let it go, you know. You have to let me go through that trial. But it's okay, it's okay, because remember trials cause perseverance, and perseverance causes character, and character causes hope, and hope doesn't disappoint. I am wiser now. I know the signs, but the first time you see the signs you ignore them and then you shipwreck.

MELISSA: The signs, you can look back and see signs?

LUTCHI: Yes. Domination and intimidation. And I think I had something in me that was attracting this type of relationship.

MELISSA: So you've done some serious thinking about that. But she was pretty convincing.

LUTCHI: Yeah, very convincing. In fact, I sometimes miss her. It scares me. Not that I am afraid of her curses, but just afraid of being with an unstable person. I know that God will protect me, but, still I will stay away from her. I've got to stay away from her. When she gets familiar with you, she starts treating you like trash.

MELISSA: Lutchi, how did you get free of her influence? One time when I saw you she had so much power, then the next time, I saw you and Randy—no more Jane.

LUTCHI: I didn't have to get shipwrecked, I got someone who could show me and wake me up to it.

MELISSA: Who was that?

LUTCHI: It was Randy, right here! He opened my eyes, showed me how she was using me.

MELISSA: Randy, how did you do that?

RANDY: We just talked.

MELISSA: But, how did you know?

RANDY: I just noticed several times where she kind of ran over us. I just told Lutchi. I'd been holding it in my gut a long time. So I told him, "Lutchi, she is hyperreligious and she is using you. She's intrusive."

MELISSA: How did you spot the using thing?

RANDY: Hey! Don't you know? I've had 11 years of experience working in a Christian bookstore. Lots of nice folks, but I met all types. I've been through it all.

MELISSA: I bet you have, but still I don't know how you spot the users.

RANDY: I just do. I don't know if it's their actions or what they say, or that they just have an air about them.

MELISSA: An air?

LUTCHI: I think Randy has a "user alarm." (*much laughter all around*) And it's a good one!

MELISSA: A user alarm! Wow, what a great thing to have. Do you really, Randy?

RANDY: You know, I do keep my antennae up. And I knew Jane. She was so superior, like, "I listen to God and you don't." And I'm like, "Okay. Next!" I don't even entertain it. I walk circumspectly and can take care of myself, but when I found that Lutchi was involved with her, I said, "Oh, yikes!" So I just started pointing out to Lutchi all of the day-to-day ways she was disrespecting him, and Thelma, and me.

LUTCHI: And once he told me I started connecting things, and then, I just didn't believe her anymore.

As we continued the conversation, I tried to learn more from Lutchi and Randy about the role of a therapist. "Stay connected, but let go," was one message I heard, reminding me of Michael White's (2000a) message, "Be influential, but de-centered." Lutchi commented that it was helpful for a therapist to make a record for a person. In supporting his movement toward accountability, I had recorded in writing, as he dictated, what he had learned were signs to attend to, signs that he was on-track, warning signs, and his plan of what to do if he were about to get offtrack. Most of our talking time was detailing and documenting what Lutchi, Randy, and Thelma had done together. We learned more from Randy about how people can develop good user alarms, and from Lutchi about the both/and of believing the best about people even while assembling a user alarm. It seems the best role for a therapist is to foster individuals' connection to those in their own community where knowledge, connectedness, credibility, and vigilance for exploitation are close at hand.

The other lasting lesson here came from Lutchi's insistence on being accountable. I was prepared to see him as vulnerable, almost a victim, and Sister Jane as a powerful villain, but Lutchi said, "Wait." His foremost desire was to tell the listening workshop therapists about his part in it, his immature ways. His insistence on accountability echoed the story with which we began this chapter. Introduced to the Parker family first by the movie, we, along with the movie makers focused on their sadness and vulnerability. Years later, we read Larry Parker's own account in his book. The tone was strikingly different than the film. His first and last words were about his accountability. If we are to genuinely respect Lutchi, Thelma, Randy, Larry, Alice, Wesley, and the enormous grief they have endured, we must also listen to their lessons just as they tell them. It is in balancing both vulnerability and accountability—theirs, the exploiters, and ours—that we have hope to be helpful when spirituality harms.

NOTES

1. We have continued to search for Larry and Alice Parker but have been unable to locate them. We would be grateful for any information that could be provided. The Parkers chose not to appeal the initial felony judgment of the court. After an exemplary probationary period, however, the judge terminated the sentence, reduced the charge from felony to misdemeanor, and overturned the conviction from "guilty" to "not guilty."
2. The postmodern therapies, including narrative, solution-focused, collaborative language systems, and feminist therapy, are prone to encounter this difficulty due to their commitment to a collaborative relationship that de-emphasizes the therapist's role as expert.

Chapter Ten

Living beyond Medical
and Psychiatric Illnesses

Medical and psychiatric illnesses can violate spiritual ways of being in the world. Most commonly, illness violates spirituality by assaulting the relatedness upon which spirituality rests (Penn, 2001; Weingarten, 1999). *Illness*, as the way that a sick person and family members experience and cope with symptoms and disability, is distinguished by Arthur Kleinman (1988, p. 3) from *disease*, as the biomedical understanding of a patient's condition in medical terms of anatomy and physiology.

It can be argued that disease is neither good nor evil. It simply poses challenges. The presence of disease in a person's body compels a person to begin *relating* to the diseased body, rather than treating self and body as though they were the same. Disability and disfigurement from disease force renegotiations of relationships with family members, friends, and colleagues. The suffering and threat of death that disease brings often prompt renegotiations with one's God, Higher Power, or spiritual world around such questions as Why am I permitted to suffer? Why am I permitted to die?

By responding to these challenges, the experience of illness takes form, not only in the person's life but also in the communal life of family, community, and culture. Whether medical or psychiatric, illness can

258

threaten relationships between the sufferer and other people, the sufferer and his or her heritage and, often, the sufferer and his or her God.

The following three stories illustrate different situations that a therapist may face in helping people draw from their spirituality or religion to counter adversities of illness. I (Griff) entered into each of these situations in the role of hospital consultation psychiatrist. In the first account, my task was to help someone who is experienced in spiritual ways of being to expand their range of use while living with illness. In the second account, it was to respond to someone who has made no obvious use of spiritual resources. In the third, it was to help someone whose religious beliefs or spiritual practices paradoxically hindered coping.

The rheumatoid arthritis that afflicted Ms. Lawson had disfigured her arms and legs and caused her nearly constant pain. Her condition was worsened by complications of being treated for systemic lupus erythematosus with steroids that caused mood shifts. Her internist had requested our consultation due to her concern about Ms. Lawson's depression. In the same sentence in which Ms. Lawson told me about her illness, she introduced herself as a former school teacher and a 20-month-old "born again" Christian. Unsure how best to respond to such a forthright declaration of her identity, I asked her how I might be helpful. My tone must have implied my assumption that she most wanted relief from the pain she suffered. She quickly interrupted to say that relief of suffering was not what she was seeking: "I want to be able to live in a space of joy." After pausing to think about her request, I then asked what obstacles kept her from staying in a space of joy. She told how she struggled not to fall into despair when her pain was intense.

We began discussing how to blunt the impact of the pain on her morale. I asked who in her life she felt understood her situation. She said she had a network of friends and family members, many of whom attended her church. In fact, she was considering moving to an apartment closer to her church community. She shared many of her burdens with a particular friend, and she thought this friend could not reasonably bear more. Her experience of pain, she said, could not be fully understood by any human. I understood her to be saying that she felt only her God could understand and respond to the severity and complexity of her distress.

I asked Ms. Lawson what she experienced inside her body when she was in prayer with God. "I can feel God's arms around me," she replied.

"How do you experience pain differently when God's arms are around you?" I asked. "The pain is still there," she said, "But it's a distraction from the pain. The pain stops mattering." This helped as long as she was able to sustain the experience, but when she lost her focus, the intensity of the pain would return. I wondered if other steps could be taken in addition to this one. I asked specifically about her daily routines, expecting that her answer would reveal something about any spiritual practices or rituals that maintained focus in her life. She said she had been thinking how throughout the previous year each morning she had read her devotional book and Scripture readings, but she was not able to do that now. It had now turned January, and she had not yet obtained a new devotional book for the current year. As we talked, she decided to contact a church member who could obtain a new book for her. She said she would then renew her daily scripture readings that once had helped her cope with pain.

Ms. Lawson's story is one in which her religious beliefs, spiritual community, communion with God in prayer, and daily spiritual practices all worked together to support her resilience against the suffering she experienced from a disease that could not be cured. Her account is contrasted with the following one of Mr. Dillard.

Mr. Dillard requested that I come to see him at his hospital room. He was in his third week of hospitalization during a fourth round of chemotherapy for lymphoma. His oncologist a year earlier had consulted me about Mr. Dillard's depressed mood when taking steroid medications. During that hospital admission, Mr. Dillard was initially hostile to anything referring to psychiatry and only reluctantly agreed to take an antidepressant, although he later acknowledged that it helped his depression. I had not seen him during the ensuing year. During my previous visit he was not visibly sick. On this day he looked like a dying man, with a swollen body, bald head, parched lips, and difficulty keeping his concentration focused. I thought it significant and a bit surprising that he, rather than his doctor, was requesting my visit.

Mr. Dillard was a business executive. It was obvious from both my initial visit and the present one that his work was the driving force in his life. He had inferred that he became anxious when not fully in control of his life circumstances. This was his present complaint—he sensed that this hospital admission was different. He was sicker, both from the illness and the chemotherapy side effects. He suspected that his oncologist was running out of options from which to choose.

The strain was showing on Ms. Dillard. She had moved into the hospital room, sleeping on a cot. All about the room she had placed pictures of their life together, their wedding, vacations, and home. She had made a pretty sign to remind him of the date to reorient him when he became confused.

Ms. Dillard's voice and body were tensed with fatigue and unexpressed feelings. She told how the marriage had been strained even before he had become ill. She had suffered from depression. He criticized her for seeking psychotherapy and taking antidepressants. When Mr. Dillard became ill, however, she had devoted herself to his care, to such an extent that she now felt more nurse than wife. She wanted to speak from her heart to him but felt silenced by his bitter responses.

Mr. Dillard stated explicitly that he could not live with so much out of his control. He did not believe that he was being told the full story about his illness. He needed help dressing, bathing, and eating. He missed his home. He wept as he recounted a realization that struck him the day before, that the only pleasure he could now feel was drinking ice water. He sat in a chair sipping ice water and despairing that his life had come to this. I asked Mr. Dillard what sustained him through his suffering. He responded: "When I can get back to my work and do a couple of pages of it." He told me how, with the assistance of his office employees, he still could stay on top of his job.

At the end of an hour during which I had mostly listened quietly, I said, "There is a lot to sort out. This is not a problem that can be dealt with by an antidepressant medication. You are turning over important questions. During this time of your illness, what is most important in your life?. . . With Julie [Ms. Dillard], what do you most want your marriage to be?" He shook his head, closed his eyes, and ended the conversation.

In contrast to Ms. Lawson, there was a striking absence of anything remotely "spiritual" in Mr. Dillard's responses to illness. Faced with a deteriorating and failing body, he was dying as he had lived, with his primary frame of reference his suffering and his sole striving that of keeping the world around him under control.

If the previous two stories represent two ends of a spectrum of spirituality, there also exists a region in the middle where spiritual beliefs and practices are invoked in responding to illness but act only to accentuate its suffering. Mr. Holloway was lying quietly with his eyes closed as I arrived at his bedside. Earlier in the day he had tried to persuade a friend to bring a gun so he could kill himself. He had become distraught after learning that his left leg needed to be amputated. His surgeon had asked me to assess Mr. Holloway's refusal of the surgery. The surgeon felt that he was suicidal and legally incompetent to make this decision. Due to impending gangrene in his leg, Mr. Holloway would soon die if the diseased leg were not removed.

I explained the reason for my visit: His doctors were worried about his safety and wondered as well if his thinking had become confused by his medications. I inquired about what he understood his doctors to be telling him about his condition and what they recommended. Instead of answering my question, he began telling me how hard it would be for a man who lives alone to take care of himself—mowing the yard, repairing things, getting groceries from his kitchen cabinets—if he has only one leg.

I asked him what would be the alternative if he were not to have the surgery. He said he realized that he was developing gangrene that would spread and could kill him within a matter of hours. Had he stopped considering an amputation as an option to save his life? He nodded. I asked what had been the turning point while deliberating this.

"I prayed like hell. I asked God to take this away . . . but he didn't," Mr. Holloway said bitterly.

"Do you have a sense of what God would want you to do right now?" I asked.

"He wouldn't want me to kill myself," he responded.

"What do you think God understands about your situation?" I asked.

"He knows I've done the best I could," he said, weeping.

"Can you feel God's presence?" I wondered.

He showed no response.

"Is it that you feel you know what God would want you to do, but it is hard to understand what he has in mind, or to trust him right now?" I wondered.

He nodded silently.

"What does God know about you as a person that gives God the confidence that you can bear this?" I asked.

Mr. Holloway thought for a moment, then responded, "The Bible says that God won't give you anything heavier than you can bear."

"Do you have any sense of what God might be experiencing as he witnesses your going through this?" I asked.

He sobbed but made no response in words. Finally he said, "I'll go along with it."

I asked who were other important people in his life, those who understood his suffering and supported him. He then told about telephone calls from his children, who had encouraged him to have the surgery. He began weeping again as he told about his former wife, who called to tell him she still loved him and wanted him to have the surgery. He spoke with appreciation about his family doctor who throughout his illness had been readily available when needed. A few minutes later, his surgeon, who had been waiting nearby, escorted Mr. Holloway down the hall to the surgical suite. He went to surgery with some degree of equanimity.

The story of Mr. Holloway is one in which his religious beliefs and desperate prayers served to set the stage for a sense of betrayal and abandonment by his God. Much that had transpired between Mr. Holloway and his God had remained private. I did not know exactly what words he had spoken to his God or the details of what he had sensed to be God's response. It seemed that he had prayed, and that he had felt bitter rejection on receiving God's response to his prayer, and that any present interaction with God was at an impasse. A shift occurred in our conversation, the process of which I could only partly discern. I could not tell if Mr. Holloway's tears, when he considered God witnessing his suffering, were tears of abandonment or acceptance, but he did recall and accept the appreciation and love of his children, his former wife, and his family doctor, and he was able to proceed with clarity.

ILLNESS VIOLATES THE RELATEDNESS
THAT CONSTITUTES SPIRITUALITY

Illness attacks the relatedness of spirituality along multiple fronts. It fosters despair, isolation, helplessness, meaninglessness, and sorrow, so that efforts to rebuild a relational world easily falter.

The experience of severe illness intrinsically isolates one from other people, even when they make good-hearted efforts to understand. To begin with, no one ever can really know what it is like to live within another's body. We base our empathy with others on extrapolations from those everyday bodily experiences that we all share, such as hunger, sleepiness, fright, and sexual arousal. The bodily experience of severe illness is distant from what is familiar to most of us in everyday life. Of all the aspects of illness, chronic pain among the medical illnesses and psychosis among the psychiatric ones seem to be the most isolating because in each the torment that grasps so tightly is imperceptible to other people.

Disease can transform one's body into an alien and threatening presence. An ill person may be unable to predict when the body will refuse to function, or when it will produce so much pain that engaging in life's activities is impossible. When a sense of trust in one's body is missing, the flow of daily life turns into turbulence.

The presence of a medical or psychiatric disorder makes thinking about the future a struggle of the will. Possibilities are hard to imagine. Distanced from one's dreams, it becomes difficult to feel the presence of one's traditions, heritage, or ancestors, from which meaning and purpose derive.

Severe illness poses questions about a person's relationship with his or her God that are questions of trust and betrayal. Doubts may arise whether a relationship with God had existed in the first place. The experience of C. S. Lewis is a sobering reminder about the duress that serious illness can bring. In *The Problem of Pain* (1962, p. 93), Lewis, one of the main Christian apologists of the 20th century, argued the case that physical pain is necessary as a wake-up call from God: "It is His megaphone to rouse a deaf world." In this book, he argued for the rationality and value of pain as a needed signal, a constant and vital reminder that we are finite beings who must look beyond the material world to eternity. However, years later Lewis himself found these theological arguments to be hollow words as he suffered with his beloved wife, Joy, through her cancer and death. Then he wrote another book, *A Grief Observed* (Lewis, 1976), writing personally and open-heartedly, not so much about answers, but about his struggles and unanswerable questions.

Severe illness strikes a double blow. It stresses a person through physical pain and disability, while disabling some of the most effective mechanisms for coping with stress: communion with others, a capacity to hope, a sense of control over one's destiny, and a sense of purpose in living.

EXISTENTIAL CRISIS STATES, DISEASE, AND ILLNESS

The particular way illness is experienced appears in some cases either to undermine or to strengthen the body's physiological defenses against further progression of the disease. How illness is experienced also shapes in a reflexive manner how disease is transmuted into illness. Certain states of being that we term *existential crisis states* mark points of juncture between mind and body, in that they couple specific dimensions of experience with simultaneous dysfunction in endocrine, immune, autonomic, and postural motor systems. In each of these existential crisis states, the psychosocial and physiological worlds converge (Griffith, 2000, 2001).

Existential crisis states have been discussed philosophically as the boundaries of human existence,[1] and psychologically as sources of anxiety that limit how deeply and fully life can be experienced (Havens, 1972; May et al., 1958; Yalom, 1980). Together they have been described as the state of demoralization, considered to be a universal human response to loss or trauma (Frank & Frank, 1991). What has not been sufficiently appreciated until recently has been the profound impairment of the body's physiological systems accompanying these existential crisis states. Here we focus on this extension of experience into the body, which bears important consequences for health or illness.

Each existential crisis state is itself one half of a couplet of emotional postures: despair versus hope, meaninglessness versus purpose, helplessness versus personal agency, isolation versus communion, resentment versus gratitude, sorrow versus joy (Griffith, 2000, 2001). Despair, meaninglessness, helplessness, isolation, resentment, and sorrow each represent a retreat from purposeful activity, a readiness to quit responding to challenges whether they be mental or physical ones. These are states of breakdown in which coping actions become chaotic and ineffective. As such, they constitute states of vulnerability to illness.

Hope, purpose, agency, communion, gratitude, and joy, on the other hand, represent readiness to move forward with goal-directed actions that care for self and others. They are states of resilience to illness.

There are, of course, other emotional postures in human life than the six pairs we focus upon here. We selected these six because they can be related to different bodies of empirical research on health and illness. For example, there is general acceptance in medical and scientific communities that close and intimate relationships produce measurable salutary effects on the progression of many chronic disorders, both medical and psychiatric (Broadhead et al., 1983; Uchino, Cacioppo, & Kiecolt-Glaser, 1996; Weihs et al., 2001). Ready availability of supportive relationships and secure attachments within those relationships foster resilience, while isolation and insecure attachments foster vulnerability (Fisher & Weihs, 2000; Weihs et al., 2001).

The significance of emotional postures in speeding or retarding progression of cancer can be seen in psychosocial studies of cancer survival. Social isolation is established as a risk factor for early death in cancer studies (Spiegel & Kato, 1996). In breast cancer (Derogatis et al., 1979) and malignant melanoma (Temoshok, 1985) patients with a "fighting spirit," distinguished by their optimism, assertiveness, and determination to fight the cancer, lived longer than those who did not. Negative affectivity, when combined with restriction of emotional expression, has been shown to predict early death from metastatic breast cancer (Weihs et al., 2000). For both breast cancer (Spiegel et al., 1989) and malignant melanoma (Fawzy et. al., 1993), specific group therapies have extended the average survival of participating patients. These group therapies were designed to facilitate hope and communal support within the group, and an assertive, problem-solving attitude toward the illness.

The laboratory research of Janice Kiecolt-Glaser and Ronald Glaser (Anderson, Kiecolt-Glaser, & Glaser, 1994; Kiecolt-Glaser et al., 1987) has suggested some mechanisms through which these effects may occur. They have shown that research subjects who are stressed show a lowering of immune competence, elevations in stress hormones, and hyperarousal of the autonomic nervous system, changes that plausibly could make a person more vulnerable to disease. In a high-stress setting drawn from real life, family caregivers of relatives with Alzheimer's disease who have readily supportive relationships show less heart rate and blood pressure reactivity to stress than those who do not (Uchino, Kiecolt-Glaser, & Cacioppo, 1992). Similarly, caregivers of Alzheimer's patients who have few social supports show diminished competence of their immune systems (Irwin et al., 1992).

There may be many different ways, in addition to the support a religious community provides, that spirituality may affect resilience to disease. Religious beliefs and practices can powerfully counter such health risks as cigarette smoking and alcohol use. They also can influence when and how a person makes use of medical care, as when a patient with cancer chooses to seek healing from a spiritual healer rather than take chemotherapy, or a depressed person refuses referral to a psychiatrist in the belief that religious faith ought to be sufficient. In our clinical work, we have sought ways to engage religious or spiritual experience through any of these avenues in order to bolster resilience against relapse of illness in a vulnerable person. However, it has been the capacity of spirituality and religion to modulate emotional postures that has most engaged our interest.

A spiritual perspective sharpens the focus of therapy on the kinds of relational and emotional processes most likely to influence the course of medical or psychiatric illnesses, for good or bad. It keeps the integrity of important relationships a central theme in the conversations of therapy. It guides a therapist to keep center stage those strategies that can buffer existential crisis states and counter their adverse influences. It establishes as primary objectives of therapy the sustenance of hope, purpose, and self-agency. Through these links religious beliefs, spiritual practices, rituals, and other expressive genres of spiritual experience can play a role in countering illness.

A CLINICAL MODEL FOR RESILIENCE TO ILLNESS

A basic model that organizes our clinical work with those who are medically ill or psychiatrically ill is illustrated in Figure 2. This is a clinical model, meaning that it is conceptually simple enough for a clinician to hold in mind while engaged in a reflective dialogue. Despite this simplicity, it is consistent with a substantial body of medical research, and it can help a therapist to stay focused on processes that are likely to counter progression of illness.[2] There is ample clinical and research evidence that existential crisis states on the left side of Figure 2—despair, helplessness, meaninglessness, isolation, resentment, sorrow—can activate recurrences of illness or accelerate progression of illness for either medically ill or psychiatrically ill patients. Presumably, these adverse effects are mediated through the brain limbic and basal ganglia systems, which in turn regulate endocrine, immune, autonomic, and postural motor systems of the body.

Emotional postures that are their counterparts, on the right side of Figure 2—hope, agency, purpose, communion, gratitude, joy—are protective against exacerbations or recurrences of medical and psychiatric illnesses for the same set of reasons. We propose that spiritual ways of

Medical Illnesses

States of Vulnerability	States of Resilience
Despair	Hope
Helplessness	Agency
Meaninglessness	Purpose
Isolation	Communion
Resentment	Gratitude
Sorrow	Joy

Axis I Psychiatric Disorders

FIGURE 2. Existential crisis states that render a person vulnerable or resilient to illness.

being, whether expressed as beliefs, prayer, ritual, participation in community, or through other genres, physiologically influence these systems of the body by buffering existential crisis states.

This model also guides how pharmacotherapy and psychotherapy can be integrated in treating psychiatric symptoms. States of vulnerability in the left column of Figure 2 can trigger relapse for most Axis I psychiatric disorders, whether schizophrenia, bipolar disorder, obsessive–compulsive disorder, panic disorder, or depression. Either medicines or psychosocial interventions can help shield the person from these existential crisis states. Antidepressant, anxiolytic, and antipsychotic medications all shift information processing within the nervous system so that hope, agency, purpose, communion, gratitude, and joy are easier to maintain. These medications make it easier to sustain these emotional postures with less effort. We will expand this discussion of medications in promoting resilience in a later section of this chapter.

UNSPEAKABLE DILEMMAS AS PATHOLOGICAL SOCIAL CONTEXTS

In our previously published work (Griffith & Griffith, 1994; Griffith et al., 1998), we described *unspeakable dilemmas* as social contexts frequently associated with unexplained physical symptoms and other symptoms of somatization. Somatization is the appearance or exacerbation of bodily symptoms—fatigue, pain, dizziness, blackouts, seizures—that are related to psychological or social stress. In somatization, the occurrences, or the severity, of bodily symptoms are not understandable through known physiological mechanisms of diseases.

An unspeakable dilemma is a relational bind in which a person experiences a forced choice for which (1) it can be expected that all options for escaping the dilemma will result in intolerable distress, and (2) meaningful dialogue about the dilemma cannot be safely discussed among those involved in the situation, such that (3) the person minimizes or tries to hide the distress. Some unspeakable dilemmas arise from the fear of violence, as with a child who has been sexually abused, who cannot bear the abuse yet fears harm if she or he speaks openly, or an employee who cannot bear the maltreatment inflicted by a boss yet fears being fired if objections are treated as insolence. Other unspeakable dilemmas arise when open dialogue is silenced by shame or guilt, as with a son who hates playing on his sports team but feels too ashamed to let his father know, or a man who hates working in a family business but does not want to hurt his family members by letting them know. Although we were interested in the relationship between unspeakable dilemmas and somatization, what stood out in our clinical interviews was that unspeakable dilemmas were particularly potent social contexts for generating despair, meaninglessness, isolation, and sorrow. Moreover, the added imperative to minimize or hide the distress appeared to amplify its severity. Finally, we noted that other literatures in psychosomatic medicine suggested that an unspeakable dilemma is as unhealthy for medical disorders as for somatoform ones. A broad research literature on inhibition of emotional expression has established its deleterious effects on many medical and psychophysiological disorders (Traue & Pennebaker, 1993).

Weingarten and Worthen (1997) have described how intimacy between a medically ill person and others is critically dependent upon that person speaking openly and fully from his or her experience while sensing that those listening understand and appreciate the significance of what is said. Conversely, conversation can paradoxically heighten a sense of isolation when it lacks this openness, understanding, and appreciation. As Penn (2001, p. 34) has noted: "To say how it really is with you, to be able to express your deep feelings around illness to those you love, produces physical relief and frees others to respond in kind."

This dependence of intimacy with others upon the quality of their witnessing and responding appears to apply as well to relationships with spiritual beings. It has been notable from our interviews with medically ill patients that a relationship with a personal God can intensify an unspeakable dilemma. The man introduced in Chapter 9 believed that homosexuality was evil in God's judgment, even though he could not find it possible to live as a heterosexual. He understood his God as demanding that he be heterosexual, yet he carried within him an equally absolute sense of "who I am" that was gay. There was no conversation in which he could discuss this dilemma, neither with his family of origin nor with his partner, who otherwise shared his intimate thoughts and feelings. The entrapment and isolation that this dilemma posed for him was amplified by his conviction that it must also remain secret. It is difficult to imagine more adverse circumstances for coping physically, psychologically, and spiritually with AIDS.

As another illustration, I (Griff) treated a woman at late midlife who was depressed and disabled from Crohn's disease. She said: "My career has been my life for 30 years. . . . I have ignored my family. . . . I gave everything to that company. . . . I have died inside. . . . I am dead spiritually. . . . And what has driven it has been my fear that they would say, 'You're not good enough.' " Both she and her internist recognized that stress from her 60-hour-a-week job was a factor that exacerbated her cramping, diarrhea, and vomiting to such an extent that it was beyond medical control. In addition, she was stressed by her awareness that she had placed her job before her God in importance, making it, in a sense, an idol. The distress she felt in her body was unbearable, yet she did not dare let her boss and coworkers know its extent lest she risk being laid off. She felt so distant from her God that she could not pray. The shame surrounding this dilemma was such that she only revealed the extent when it could be discussed in therapy.

When an unspeakable dilemma involves religious issues, it often is the case that a perceived expectation from God conflicts with some other imperative. Due to this conflict, God may be felt to be an emotionally distant, scornful, or indifferent presence. This scorn or indifference can generate emotions of desperation that place either physical or mental health at risk. Direct engagement of the person–God relationship in such cases often can help render the unspeakable dilemma either resolvable or, at the least, speakable.

LISTENING FOR COMPLEXITY
OF SPIRITUAL EXPERIENCE

When individuals with medical or psychiatric symptoms contact a clinician, they are usually seeking treatment for illness, not a discussion of spiritual issues. Any talk of spiritual or religious life occurs in the context of treatment for the illness. What matters then is that a clinician know how to listen within this conversation for clues that point to ways in which the person's spiritual or religious life can be drawn upon to counter the adverse effects of illness. We have described this kind of listening as "multichannel listening," alert for any of the expressive forms in which spiritual or religious experience may be represented. This approach can be summarized in the following questions on which the clinician reflects while listening during the interview:

- Does the person use idioms when speaking about illness that point to spiritual or religious experience?
- What metaphors or other tropes are used to map the relationship between person, illness, and spiritual life?
- Are there rituals that matter? Have they been interrupted by the illness? Could accommodations be made to renew and continue them?
- What are spiritual practices that are followed? Are caregivers aware of the schedule, dietary, or privacy needs to support these practices? Are our therapy meetings planned with respect for these practices?
- Does the canon of spiritual stories include those of devastating disease as well as stories of healing?
- Are there religious beliefs that imbue suffering with redemptive meaning? Are there beliefs that implicate suffering as punishment?
- How does illness alter—intensify or interrupt—the flow of conversation (prayer, meditation) with God or the numinous?
- Does this person have a spiritual community? Is he or she being remembered, spoken of in his or her absence, prayed for? In what ways does the community protect against the adversity of illness? Is treatment supported and harmonious with community faith practices, or does it clash with the community, separating the person from needed support?

Answers to these questions often point to openings for a productive dia-logue about the role of spiritual experience in countering illness.

THE SPECIFIC IMPORTANCE
OF ILLNESS NARRATIVES

More than any other form of expression, narratives provide portals through which a therapist can enter another's experience of illness to en-able that person to feel heard and understood (Frank, 1995, 1998; Penn, 2001). It is particularly important to listen for stories that are told by the ill person and those with whom he or she converses.

Tellings and retellings of stories can either sustain or dissipate exis-tential crisis states. This depends not only on the content of the story, but also on the audience and the response to the story. Several questions that come into play are the following:

• *Is this type of illness familiar to those who listen?* Weingarten and Worthen (1997) have described how to listeners' ears certain illness narratives are more understandable than others. Illnesses that are experi-enced broadly within the culture—breast cancer, epilepsy, heart dis-ease—are more understandable than those that occur rarely. The exis-tence of a culturewide shared experience of illness fosters or hinders possibilities for communion with others.

• *Can stories of the illness be comfortably spoken about among those involved in the ill person's life?* The silencing that ensues when talk about the illness risks shame, blame, stigma, or political or economic re-prisal amplifies the severity of despair, isolation, and other states of vul-nerability. Examples include HIV and other sexually transmitted dis-eases, tuberculosis and other feared contagions, genetic diseases that raise a question of blame for transmission, and work-related injuries where employment, disability, and compensation are at stake.

• *Is the illness narrative coherent or chaotic?* A narrative that makes sense out of one's experience of illness gives meaning to suffering and points to ways in which the person can influence the course of ill-ness. Disorganized, chaotic narratives foster meaninglessness and help-lessness (Frank, 1995, 1998).

• *Does the progression of the illness narrative, from beginning to end, generate such states of resilience as hope, communion with others, or purpose, or does it engender their opposites?* Engaging in a specific narrative is a way of committing oneself to a particular version of reality. Entering into a particular illness narrative shapes what words are used to think about the illness and to talk about it with other people. It shapes how one relates both to self and others around the illness. It influences how the past is reflected upon, how the present is enacted, and how the future is planned. An illness narrative in its telling and retelling moves the ill person from a starting place to a different place. It is important whether this shift is toward, or away from, such states of resilience as hope, purpose, and communion with others.

When family members and other significant people are included, therapy can become a setting for needed conversations that otherwise could not have occurred involving these narratives of illness. The conversations of therapy can also consider what other ways of telling the story of illness might be more generative of hope, purpose, communion with others, and other states of resilience.

QUESTIONS TO ASK

Our therapy with ill persons is more about attentive listening than asking the perfect question. Often shared cultural experiences guide the clinician to ask appropriate, comfortable, or even expected questions, such as those concerning religious beliefs, communities, or prayer life. At other times these can close the conversation, either because they are overly familiar and lead to banalities or because they are too unusual and lead to a disconnection. The two of us find existential questions, like those discussed in the third chapter, to be the most fruitful ones for opening conversation about spirituality and illness. These are questions about experiences in living that are both profound in their meaning and universally experienced when coping with serious illness. They are not limited to any specific spiritual tradition or its language. These include the following:

- What sustains you through this illness?
- What gives you hope when coping with this illness is most difficult?
- Who truly understands what you are experiencing with this illness?

- How do you find comfort in your suffering? How do you find some moments of joy despite being ill?
- For what are you most deeply grateful?
- How does your life matter? What is your best sense as to what your life is about and how this illness fits in it?

Responses to these questions suggest whether the person resides more in the left column or right column of Figure 2, which then suggests additional questions. An opening is usually created by existential questions that then permit more direct and specific questions to be asked.

In these inquiries, one listens carefully for what the customary genres are for the person's particular spiritual expression—whether it be stories, beliefs, practices, community, or other forms of expression. Knowing which ones are customary leads to specific lines of questions or specific therapeutic interventions, as we have illustrated throughout the chapters of this text. In the following case illustrations, we will show how this process of inquiry and intervention can be conducted with persons suffering from either medical or psychiatric illnesses.

INTERVIEWING THAT PROMOTES
RESILIENCE TO MEDICAL ILLNESS

It is helpful to keep in mind all three avenues through which beliefs, practices, and other expressions of spiritual experience could conceivably influence the course or severity of illness:

- By influencing how the ill person adheres to recommended treatments;
- By influencing health practices—diet, exercise, and use of tobacco, alcohol, or recreational drugs.
- By altering physiological states and the underlying disease process through modulation of existential crisis states.

Which of these influences is significant depends in part upon the natural course of the particular illness. The influence of beliefs or practices in promoting hope may help a patient with epilepsy, diabetes, or end-stage renal disease to adhere to his or her treatment program, because despair in these illnesses is often manifested by taking medications erratically or ignoring prescribed guidelines for diet. When a disease course is largely dictated by the state of the immune system, as in chronic fatigue syndrome, asthma, or some cancers, despair and other existential states of vulnerability may effect more rapid progression. In such degenerative diseases as Alzheimer's disease or amyotropic lateral sclerosis, optimal care is dependent on flexibility of roles and responsibilities among family members and friends, which may be influenced by beliefs, practices, and community. While the underlying disease may continue to progress, these beliefs and practices may help sustain meaning, purpose, and a cohesive organization for the family in ways that protect against a premature and unnecessary decline.

Spirituality and religion provide for many people the knowledge and skills needed to sustain resilience against debilitating or painful medical diseases. For example, Mr. O'Carrol was an elderly man hospitalized for congestive heart failure. My (Griff) psychiatric consultation was requested to see whether anything could be recommended that would help him cope with his severe, progressive heart disease that had rendered him bedridden for many weeks. Mr. O'Carrol explained that he had been out of prison for 5 years after incarceration for embezzling money. His crime had created such a scandal within his large, extended family that he was shunned by them. Only one cousin had remained supportive of him. Shortly after his release from prison, his heart disease worsened and became a progressive disability. He was unable to work and was presently homeless, living in a residence supported by a church that provided shelter for persons who were both homeless and medically ill.

Noting the adversities he had experienced, I asked what had sustained him through these recent years. "My faith in God," he replied. I asked whether this faith was mainly an idea within his mind or whether it was also something that he experienced in his feelings. He responded that it was the latter. "I pray to God and to Mary." He told how he came from an Irish family with a strong Catholic heritage. He had never left or forgotten the Church despite shame about his personal failures. I asked what words he prayed to God. "That my body will stay strong . . . that my sins will be forgiven . . . that I have paid my debt to society." "Do you sense that your prayer is heard by God?" I asked. "Yes, I do." he replied. "What do you sense is God's response to your prayer?" "That he will take care of me," he replied.

Mr. O'Carrol's beliefs and his personal, immediate sense of God's presence helped sustain purpose, communion, and hope when all else—his family, his social status, his body—had fallen away. Despite the severity of disease, he was mostly living within the right column emotional postures of Figure 2, supported by his religious beliefs and experience of God.

We could tell many stories of persons with whom we have talked who have sustained resilience in the face of illness. As the following vignettes will illustrate, they have employed an array of spiritual and religious resources.

COPING WITH CHRONIC PAIN

Chronic pain is a hallmark for numerous medical illnesses. Usually acute pain from surgery, infections, or deep flesh wounds can be alleviated with narcotics and other analgesic medications. However, pain from a chronic medical illness, such as degenerative spine disease, arthritis, or chronic pancreatitis, often cannot be adequately relieved by narcotics without an unacceptable risk of addiction. Other analgesics, physical therapy, and such adjunctive measures as acupuncture and transcutaneous nerve stimulators are then tried, but often also fail to bring enough relief. Even when a decision is made, as a last resort, to provide narcotics on a continuous basis through liquid morphine or a fentanyl skin patch, the pain often is only blunted rather than removed.

The consequences of unremitting chronic pain are often tragic. Chronic pain can devastate one's personality, reducing the sufferer to one who whimpers in self-absorbed despair, bitterness, and self-pity (Good et al., 1992; Scarry, 1985; Strong, 1999). Chronic pain, because it cannot be witnessed by others, can be profoundly isolating—that which is felt to be the most real for a person in pain is entirely unreal to others with whom he or she must engage in conversations and relationships. Chronic pain robs life of joy and meaning. It generates a helplessness that alternates between resignation and anger toward the healthcare professionals who have been unable to bring relief. For many in pain, religious and spiritual resources are a necessity for coping.

For example, Ms. Towson told how she had suffered for 20 years with physical pain that began with an automobile accident. Since then, her cervical and lumbar disks had degenerated, and she had numerous spine surgeries. As she described what the pain had taken from her life, I

(Griff) wondered how she imagined her future. She shook her head—"Nothing but pain." I asked whether it was more that she felt the pain would be unbearable or whether she could not bear what it had taken from her. "Both," she said. I asked whether there was anyone who understood her well enough that she could talk openly about her experience. "My pastor," she replied. What did her pastor tell her? "To let God do his will in me." Did she feel that God took her side, or that God was not involved, or that God was causing the pain? She said she believed that God was always on her side. Did she feel God's presence to be far away, or a short distance away, or close at hand? Right now, she felt God to be far away. I wondered what kept her from feeling the close presence of God. "The pain," she responded. Was there any person whose presence she felt to be close at hand? She told how her sister understood. She could tell her sister about everything, because her sister herself had suffered so much.

"When you feel the presence of your sister, what do you feel inside your body? Where do you feel it?" I asked.

She described a "warmth" that she felt in her heart.

"When you feel this warmth, what changes in your relationship with the pain?" I asked.

"I don't have to pay it attention," she responded.

"Have there ever been times when you experienced this 'warmth' from God's presence as well?" I then asked.

She concurred that there indeed had been such times, but recently she had become so depressed that she had given up focusing upon God. Therefore, we planned an approach for managing her pain that would integrate a variety of different components: optimizing her pain medications, adding an antidepressant, and increasing physical therapy. Alongside these medical treatments, she would also practice opening her awareness to the felt presence of her sister and to God's felt presence, so that the accompanying "warmth" could come more often and more easily.

PROMOTING RESILIENCE
TO PSYCHIATRIC ILLNESSES

The decade of the 1990s was dubbed the "Decade of the Brain" in American psychiatry for its focus on the role that neurophysiological mechanisms play in mental disorders. Brain imaging and an array of new psychotropic medications helped foster a view of psychiatric disorders as brain disorders, rather than a consequence of moral failure, bad parenting, or maladaptive learning, as past generations of clinicians had viewed them. By the end of the decade, however, a more complex picture was emerging (Reiss et al., 2000): A genetic vulnerability, or a structural brain lesion, may be a necessary precondition before a serious psychiatric disorder can occur. However, such biological factors alone appear to be insufficient in producing serious illness until activated by psychosocial factors found in the family, social, or cultural contexts in which a person lives. Moreover, these symptom-generating interactions between biological factors and family, social, and cultural factors are dynamic, shifting, and changing over the life span of the person. For such disorders as schizophrenia and bipolar disorder, innovative psychosocial therapies during recent decades have advanced the effectiveness of their treatment as much as has the development of new medications (Hogarty et al., 1986, 1991; McFarlane et al., 1995). These therapies in large part buffer the existential states of vulnerability in Figure 2.

Mr. Prospero was a 40-year-old man who came to the clinic with symptoms of severe depression. He had a diagnosis of bipolar disorder. Over the past 15 years, he had many episodes of depression and two episodes of mania, during one of which he had made a suicide attempt. He had lived on Social Security Insurance disability payments, unable to work. He was taking a cocktail of mood-stabilizing drugs each day— Zyprexa, Depakote, Klonopin—plus an antidepressant, Serzone. Although this pharmacological regimen kept his moods relatively stable, his sense of well-being would nose dive when he became caught up in anxiety and "negative thinking." In particular, perceived criticism, whether from himself or other people, would send his mood plummeting, despite his medications. Marital conflicts almost always brought a relapse of depression. Clearly he needed an "emotionally cool," low-stress lifestyle.

Mr. Prospero became involved with the Catholic church and the Salvation Army as a volunteer. The beliefs they taught proved to be a good antidote for the destabilizing effects of his anxiety and guilt; he could put his trust in God's hands and stop expecting so much from himself. He went through a ritual religious cleansing. He began praying that the arguments with his wife could end, asking: "Dear Jesus, please give me patience with Irma." He worked to recall gratitude for times when she helped him when he had been sick. He prayed to be able to understand her rather than to judge her. He rebuked "bad thoughts" that invited depression by quoting Scripture: "I can do all things through Christ Jesus who strengtheneth me" (Phillipians 4:13, RSV).

Eight weeks later Mr. Prospero still looked well. The conflicts with Ms. Prospero had diminished. He had navigated the bureaucratic process of obtaining subsidized housing and was in the process of moving. His sleep patterns, appetite, and energy were satisfactory. "When I can put the anxieties aside, I can stay in control," he said.

Four months later Mr. Prospero was successfully completing work assignments as a volunteer in a child care program. This had been the first time in 8 years that he had worked. This volunteer work led to employment supervising and teaching children at a local Catholic school. He was managing his anxieties without decompensating: "I just roll it over to the Lord and take one day at a time." Now he was considering adding a job coaching children's athletic teams.

With serious psychiatric disorders medications are usually essential, yet their benefits are often disappointing unless accompanied by changes in relationships, lifestyle, and habits of thinking that shield a vulnerable brain from physiological arousal through despair, isolation, helplessness, and sorrow. Patients require careful modulation of sleep/wake cycle, diet, exercise, and life stressors in order to stay free of mood or thought symptoms. While there are many ways to achieve these aims, the use of prayer, beliefs, community, and such spiritual practices as chanting or quoting scripture are methods that in unique ways can sustain states of resilience.

COUNTERING THE EFFECTS
OF PSYCHOLOGICAL TRAUMA

Emotional numbness, intrusive memories, nightmares, and constant edginess and vigilance can be long-term sequelae of psychological trauma, after a person has been suddenly threatened with bodily harm in circumstances wherein self-protection would be futile. Such symptoms occur in natural disasters, such as earthquakes, floods, or tornadoes. More commonly, they are due to predatory violence or the violence of hatred— assaults, rapes, or political torture. The violence of trauma can immobilize the usual methods with which a person copes with the stresses of life. Reliance on religious and spiritual resources can become essential for coping and recovery (Gaby et al., 2000).

Ms. Lynne Smith was a woman at midlife who had entered psychotherapy with one of our psychiatry residents, Dr. Alfredo Soto, for posttraumatic symptoms after a long history of abuse by men. I (Griff) first met her in a consultation as she and Dr. Soto were concluding their psychotherapy. Dr. Soto was completing his residency training and moving across the country, which necessitated ending their psychotherapy. He was concerned that the therapy be terminated in a manner that would not risk retraumatizing her, because the therapy had opened fresh memories of abuse that were still difficult for her to bear emotionally. He also wondered whether there were ways that her religious faith could be incorporated into the therapy so that it could support the therapeutic changes she had made. He provided the following account of her life:

Ms. Smith had grown up as the second oldest of 11 children. She and her older sister were full siblings, and the younger children halfsiblings. Her stepfather was an alcoholic who regularly abused his wife and children. Ms. Smith remembered how he would line up the children by age for each to receive a beating. She would pray that he would be too tired to beat her when her turn came. One of her worst memories was her step-father following her with a belt, forcing her to open the cabinets and unload dead rats from rat traps. This led to repetitive nightmares and a phobia of rats that has continued to plague her ever since.

One particular incident changed the course of her life when she was 11 and her older sister was 13. Their stepfather was unusually violent. When he began beating her youngest brother, his wife tried to stop him, which prompted him to start beating her. Ms. Smith tried to interfere, and she and her older sister became his targets. That evening, as the stepfather lay on his couch sleeping off his intoxication, Ms. Smith's sister planned to murder him. Ms. Smith's role was to hold the basket into which the step-father's head would roll. Just as the plan was about to unfold, however, it was interrupted by their mother. Ms. Smith's sister was sent to live with relatives, and Ms. Smith stepped into her sister's role of protector for the younger siblings. Understanding this, she would regularly take blame for circumstances that were not her fault so that she, instead of the younger children, would be punished.

At age 18, Ms. Smith was thrown out of the home by her stepfather after an argument. She was befriended by a minister and soon married him. However, she quickly discovered that this was "jumping out of the frying pan into the fire." Although not physically abusive, her new husband was more verbally abusive than her stepfather had been. He had multiple affairs with other women. Eventually she left him.

Subsequent years were better ones, during which she worked productively and enjoyed parenting her children. In fact, it was not traumatic memories of her earlier life but physical illness years later that brought Ms. Smith to a psychotherapist. At midlife, she developed breast cancer. She recovered, but then developed fibromyalgia and lumbar disc disease, which necessitated her leaving work due to disability from chronic pain. Symptoms of depression upon losing her ability to work led to treatment with antidepressant medications and referral for psychotherapy.

The context for the consultation was an interview that was conducted in a Department of Psychiatry teaching conference in the presence of Dr. Soto and other psychiatry residents, psychotherapy trainees, and faculty. As Ms. Smith entered the room for the consultation, I wondered to myself whether it would be possible to have an open, reflective conversation: Given the betrayals and abuse she had suffered from men, was it fair to ask her to discuss such intimate aspects of her life in this public setting with a man she had never before met? Could I, as a white Southern male, ask her, an African American woman, to extend enough trust for us to talk about serious matters? From Dr. Soto's account, she had experienced a significant remission of symptoms during her therapy with him, and I was concerned that the interview not undermine what had been accomplished.

After discussing with her the rationale and context of the interview, I suggested she answer only those questions she comfortably could discuss in this setting. I indicated some of what I had understood from my previous conversation with Dr. Soto. From this account, it sounded as though her childhood years had been very hard ones to live through. Was that how it was? She nodded and detailed a story of a whipping that she had received from her stepfather. I asked her what would be an appropriate title for her life story if she were to imagine it as a book with different chapters. She paused, then answered, "My Victories and My Trials." I noted how this title focused equally on both the victories and the trials of her story. I asked whether I was understanding this correctly: Was it her commitment to look even-handedly at both what had been wonderful and what had been awful in her life? She stated an emphatic, "Yes," and described how difficult her therapy had been with Dr. Soto, in that painful and frightening memories often came flooding back during the hours immediately after her psychotherapy sessions, yet she felt committed to facing the memories. For example, she had tried through the years to avoid thinking about her fear of rats, but those memories came back in graphic detail as she and Dr. Soto had talked through the history of her life. It had helped, she said, that she had learned to feel safe with Dr. Soto, whom she now considered "family."

I asked her what had sustained her through the awful times. She reflected, then answered, "My belief in God. My belief that God would take care of me. My belief that everything has a purpose. The most important thing was that I learned not to hate, even when someone hurts you. I learned this from my mother."

I guessed that she must have faced a choice at some point whether to be guided by her mother's response of not hating, or to rebel against it. "As my sisters did . . . " she mused.

"Was there a turning point, a watershed, when you made a decision not to hate?" I asked.

"When I was about 5 years old. . . . I was watching how my mother responded. . . . I then started reading everything I could get my hands on. . . . I read the Bible. . . . I prayed."

I asked where, as she looked back on the worst times with her stepfather, she now saw God's presence in those situations? "When my stepfather didn't kill me. . . . That's how I know God was there," she responded. She went on to tell how years later, as an elderly man, her stepfather came to her and all the other children to ask their forgiveness. The anger she once had felt toward him was tempered. After learning from her mother that he had been a neglected, abused child himself, she practiced viewing him in that light and blaming the abuse he had suffered as the main source of his violence toward her. Her anger dissipated with this change in frame of meaning.

I noted that she earlier had mentioned "Everything has a purpose" as an important belief for her. I assumed this meant that she believed God intended that her therapy with Dr. Soto should take place, and that there were certain things that ought to be accomplished in it. What was her sense of this?

"To free me from the past," she replied. She described how she suffered from symptoms that she now realized were posttraumatic symptoms, such illusions as seeing blood on the curtains, hearing the cry of a baby, and nightmares. These symptoms had diminished during the therapy as she and Dr. Soto had talked about her story, and she had faced her fears.

I asked questions about the mechanism of change: What had contributed to her symptoms diminishing? She believed that change had occurred through coming to face her fears, confronting them rather than fleeing from them. The therapy had been not been easy. However, she felt that this stepwise process of confronting fears was the path that God wanted her to take.

She told how throughout her life she had been looking for someone who would rescue her. Now she was realizing that there never would be such a person, only God. This was particularly important for her to realize at this time, because she was newly engaged to be married.

I wondered what God might have in mind for her future: If the therapy with Dr. Soto were one chapter in her book, what chapters would come next? She told how she had become a gospel singer and was recording a compact disc. She was in fact writing a book about her life. She believed that God wanted her to share with others the story of what he had accomplished in her life. She felt more relaxed and shook my hand warmly in concluding the interview.

What responses could be made to Dr. Soto's two consultation questions in light of this interview? I first reflected on the striking difference between Ms. Smith's story and one that might have been told according to commonplace assumptions about the impact of physical abuse on child development, alcoholism in the home, and physical and sexual assaults on women. Ms. Smith's life stood as a challenge to these assumptions. While it was true that she suffered from some dissociative symptoms and phobic fears as sequelae of abuse, she had not been disabled by them. Her life had been rich in relationships, parenting, and work.

Posttraumatic stress symptoms arise through exposure to life events that simultaneously impose intense terror and helplessness. Ms. Smith said that her belief in God, praying, reading the Bible, and, later, her practice of viewing her stepfather in the light of compassion sustained her. In addition, her metaphor of "trials and tribulations" provided a frame of meaning that helped her experience violence and loss as challenges rather than tragedy. Terror and helplessness seemed to have been buffered by her telling of her life story as a balanced and progressive narrative, rather than a regressive or chaotic one, in which there was purposeful, incremental movement over time away from sorrow and danger in the past, to comfort and safety in a future with God.

I offered two suggestions to Dr. Soto that they might consider for the therapy. First, because he had asked initially how Ms. Smith's religious beliefs might be included in the therapy, I suggested expanding one of the themes of our interview: What is the place of this therapy within God's larger plan for your life? What does God hope that we can accomplish here? Such questions shift the figure and ground from what psychotherapists often are accustomed to. Rather than framing the therapy as the primary process of change in a person's life, it is assumed that there is a larger, more expansive process within which the therapy plays an important, but limited and specific, role. The initial task of therapy is discerning this role.

Second, Dr. Soto had expressed concern that his sessions with Ms. Smith had unintendedly reawakened memories of past abuse. The emotional impact of these memories had not yet been fully dealt with. He worried that ending therapy prematurely might act as yet another trauma in her life. I recommended that the therapy ending not be defined as "termination," as has been traditional within psychodynamic psychotherapy, with implications of finality and a focus on grieving the loss of the relationship with the therapist. I suggested rather that the therapy be viewed as another "chapter" in a larger book of her life. The subsequent sessions could then be focused on discerning what should be in the next chapter: What were the next steps that needed to be taken, how, where, with whom? His good-bye need not signal extinguishing the felt presence of him in Ms. Smith's life, or she in his. She had even said she considered him "family." Perhaps he now would be another part of her sustaining spiritual community that included people near and far, those present and those departed.

"HOLDING THE MYSTERY" IN RELATION TO THE DILEMMAS OF ILLNESS

Ms. Thomas was a woman in her 40s who suffered with a medical illness that had relapsed while she was traveling constantly, trying to care for her dying mother who lived in another state. She brought to her session with me notes she had written, but was unable to read them and handed them to me. She wanted to know why so many people have to suffer unnecessarily. Why had her mother, who had only brought goodness into the world, suffered so much in her dying? Wherever she looked, there were people suffering for no purpose. If God exists, why does God permit this? She felt hatred for God at times when she pondered these questions.

I asked Ms. Thomas whether she could feel God's presence. She said she struggled to feel God's presence, but most of the time could not. When she felt emotionally numb, in particular, she could not feel God's presence. Ironically, she could both feel the world and God's presence more clearly when her body hurt. She prayed for pain. I told her that I was moved by her desire to feel God's presence to the extent that she would choose to live with pain if that were to be the price of it.

"To feel God's presence is to be comforted. That is what I want more than anything else," she said.

"Do I understand this correctly?" I asked. "That the question that you ask—'How can suffering be so present in the world if God is actively involved it and does care for us?'—has not only failed to bring forth answers that would resolve the dilemma, but that asking it so persistently also has made it harder for you to feel God's presence?"

She responded affirmatively.

"Suppose you were to hold the questions in abeyance," I continued, "and focus instead upon holding this as a mystery—experiencing the presence of this mystery—rather than trying to dispel it or to avoid it. There is a long tradition of this among Christians and in other religions." She was aware of this tradition. There were other aspects of her faith tradition that she approached with reverence and accepted as mystery.

She agreed to try this approach. When she returned for the next session, she related how she had worked to let go of the constant questioning—"Why is suffering permitted? If God exists, why doesn't God help us?"—to listen in silence and to experience her life in relation to the mystery of suffering. "I am finding God more easily and am happier. I can recognize more things as blessings," she said. "I am staying more in my body, without numbness."

INCORPORATING PHARMACOLOGY
INTO A SPIRITUAL FRAME FOR THERAPY

The notion that religious beliefs or spiritual practices should suffice for healing can itself prompt a crisis when serious illness occurs. Some people wonder, "To show my faith in God's ability to heal, should I refuse medical or psychiatric medications?" or "Should one accept medications for medical diseases afflicting the body, but refuse those given for psychiatric disorders?" or "If a medication helps a medical or psychiatric condition, is there still a role for religious beliefs or spiritual practices?"

Ms. Singer originally had sought psychotherapy to aid her coping with multiple sclerosis. Formerly simple tasks in her workplace were now formidable due to the fatigue, weakness, and loss of coordination that her illness had brought. We had spent several productive sessions on strategies for optimizing use of her limited energy, thereby limiting the control illness held over her daily life.

On this day, however, she was upset and demoralized for a different reason. "I'm tired of the anger." She described different episodes when she became irritable in situations where she should not have been so angry. Irritants so minor that they ought to be ignored instead enraged her. She spent a lot of time on the verge of tears. She did not know "what to do with it." She likened her experience to "raw flesh without skin" after a burn, where anything that touches it hurts, even a cool breeze. It was not that she did not feel entitled to be angry; she felt she had good reasons to be angry given the burdens that multiple sclerosis had brought into her life. But she also knew of many other people whose fates were even worse, and how fortunate by comparison was her life.

As in a previous session, I asked whether we should consider using medications to attune her body so that it would be less reactive. It was my impression that she was describing mood lability—not a pervasive state of depression but strong, unanticipated emotional reactions to life events that ought not to have prompted such dramatic responses. About half of patients with multiple sclerosis have mood problems, which appear when brain systems regulating mood are injured by the disease. In addition, she was taking a medication intended to prevent future exacerbations of the multiple sclerosis. This drug, however, tended to bring up-and-down swings in her moods. I told her I thought it likely that a mood-stabilizing medication would offer a "higher floor and lower ceiling" for the swings she was experiencing in her moods.

She did not want to take a mood stabilizer. Her neurologist had prescribed the antidepressant amitriptyline when she had depressive symptoms shortly after diagnosis with multiple sclerosis. Ms. Singer remembered how she had relaxed, slept well, and gained a better sense of well-being. She remembered feeling more at peace than did her family members around her, who were upset and concerned about her illness. However, she felt that the mood of well-being was "artificial." It did not feel like an authentic part of her self and her experience, so she stopped taking the amitriptyline.

Spiritually, she said she believed that there ought to be a way to transcend such anger, to open herself fully to her experience and to find something beyond it. Her spiritual life was sustained by practices of meditation and intentional positive thinking. As an adult, Ms. Singer had chosen not to be a part of any organized religious group, but she was still influenced by the Christian Science teachings from her childhood. These teachings stressed the importance of recognizing the nonreality of emotions. She felt that her correct path was to seek an observing distance from her strong emotions, so that she could then stay sensitive to and empathic with the suffering of other people.

I wondered what ought to happen when "the other" was her own body in its suffering. That is, I was concerned that her ideas about spirituality resembled a nonembodied spirituality. Where in her reality was there guidance for how a spirit ought to live within its biological body? When the question was posed in this manner, she commented that she had in fact struggled with this issue in other contexts. She compared her dilemma to that of the conflict in Christianity over how to reconcile sexuality and spirituality. She recalled her astonishment upon reading about the Heaven's Gate cult members who tried to circumvent this problem through self-castration, so they could live more nearly like disembodied beings. She also had thoughts about the Catholic church, and the manner in which it addressed sexuality among its priests. She thought that the structure of the Catholic church in which priests and nuns do not marry was right in the ideal but wrong in the real world.

I noted that her present dilemma raised an even more complex question than the one for priests and marriage. For her the question was not whether but in what way she would include her body in her spirituality. Currently, the illness was intruding its unwanted presence into her relatedness with other people. Due to changes it had wrought in her brain systems regulating emotion, neither she nor others found her to be quite the person she knew herself to be, or desired to be. Would she try to recalibrate these brain systems with medications? This decision was a burden for her—an ethical choice unknown to those living in past ages, one's accountability for choosing, within limits, one's embodied self.

In the end, Ms. Singer reluctantly chose to take a low dose of sertraline, an antidepressant. It provided some of the hoped-for effects. Emotional responses to life events came neither so quickly nor so intensely. She more easily could reflect before acting. Her capacity to experience and express feelings was not compromised by the medication. Even as she acknowledged the benefits, however, the conflict with her beliefs continued to nag her. Eventually she decided to discontinue the medication.

Experiences with such patients as Ms. Singer led the two of us to seek a more systematic way to assess collaboratively with individuals how a medication may influence the religious or spiritual domain of their lives. The framework we have developed is divided into three parts:

- Opening a dialogue in which the pros and cons of medication use can be discussed in an even handed manner;
- Dealing with conflicts over medication use that arise when religious beliefs, spiritual practices, or stigma from one's religious or spiritual community mitigates against use of medications; and
- Evaluating how a trial of a medication is influencing religious or spiritual experiences.

In opening a dialogue about possible use of a psychotropic medication, it is important to offer a rationale broad enough to encompass both psychotherapy and medications (Griffith et al., 1991). Some people accept a recommended psychotropic medication or a referral for psychiatric consultation as matter of factly as a medical treatment for arthritis or high blood pressure. For others, such as Ms. Singer, taking a psychotropic medication is so loaded with special meaning that much conversation is called for before it can even be considered. Although therapists of every discipline are involved in such conversations, people who consult psychiatrists have already entertained the possibility of, and often are ready to employ, medications in their treatment. People who consult me (Melissa) have generally not considered utilizing medications and may feel surprised or pathologized when I suggest a psychopharmacological consultation. I have talked with other therapists who have had the same experience, and I offer their suggestions and mine for ways to open a dialogue that broaches the topic of psychotropic medications in a tentative manner, leaving space for the person to express beliefs or concerns about taking medication, including those that touch on spiritual or religious themes:

- I am worried that your body cannot give you the support you need to deal with the difficult problem you are facing. Have you had any concerns of your own about how your body is going to support you? I'm hoping that the physician can help to take a look at this with you (W. McKenzie, personal communication, 1999).

- How different might your days be if you were able to sleep at night? It may be tough to continue in this difficult struggle if you are sleep-deprived and fatigued all the time. There are many ways to address sleep problems. Medication is one of them. You may like to try it along with other ways, or you might want to try other ways first. How would you want to plan this?

- In addition to working on these fears in therapy and practicing relaxation at home, medication may help to tone down your body's state of arousal. What would you think about getting an opinion on that so that you could have it available?

- Here are some kinds of symptoms that medications have helped with [list examples]. What would indicate to you that you might wish to have a consultation to discuss the possibility of taking medicine?

- I am suggesting that you seek an opinion from a psychopharmacologist. After that you will still need to evaluate whether and how you will make use of any recommendation you receive.

After the question of medication has been raised, it is then important to listen closely for problematic meanings that medication may hold. Sometimes taking a medicine may hold the undesired meaning of linking a person's identity to another family member who took this medicine. Concerns embedded in religious beliefs, spiritual practices, or attitudes of the spiritual community commonly exist but often are not expressed explicitly. Some groups, such as Alcoholics Anonymous (some meeting groups and not others), EST and the Forum, and the Church of Scientology, are vocal in excluding psychopharmacology from a role in the care of mental health. Questions that can help articulate ambivalence from religious or spiritual life include the following:

- Does the idea of taking a medication for [depression, anxiety, etc.] fit well with your basic beliefs or is it at odds with them?
- Would it be a problem if members of your [church, AA meeting, prayer group, etc.] knew you were taking an antidepressant?
- If you were to discuss the question of medication in prayer with

God at a moment when sensed the God's close presence, how do you imagine God would respond?

Ambivalence about taking a psychotropic medication in the first place can be a different process than ambivalence about continuing it after its effects are known. A medical recommendation to continue a psychotropic medication will rest on the documentation that symptoms have remitted while the degree of side effects is acceptable. However, this symptom assessment does not address the question of meaning of the medication, which for some people, as with Ms. Singer, is the determinant for its use.

We have addressed the more common concern, that a person's religious community may disapprove of psychotropic medications, but I (Melissa) have also encountered, more than once, just the opposite. The community may open possibilities for inclusion of this form of treatment alongside spiritual and other therapeutic work. One experience stands out in my mind because of the relief and gratitude it brought to me. Griff and I had been traveling for a few weeks. I had known when we left that it was bad timing in Sandy's life for me to be away. The severe depression with which Sandy was struggling was isolating her and dogging her with thoughts of self-blame and self-harm. She had recently begun a trial of antidepressants, although she had not told the prescribing physician the full extent of her despair. Before I left, she had mentioned that she had told no one except her God and me how bad things really were. I told her that I appreciated her courage in telling the full truth to me, but also I was troubled that telling no one else might support the isolating ways of the depression. I wondered if there was anyone else with whom she could talk during my long time away. She thought not, at least for now.

I hoped that when we met again the medicine would have taken effect, creating possibilities for better conversations both inside and outside of therapy. I left her with telephone numbers for an on-call colleague, whom I suspected she would never call, and numbers where she could reach me, at least on the weekdays.

Sandy did call. She had been unable to reach me over the weekend, but caught up with me on a Monday. She was telling me how the depression had been relentlessly bearing down on her, "and one of the things I've been thinking is that, if I'm really relying on God, I would not be taking these medications."

"No, Sandy. No, wait!" was my immediate response. While not

very therapeutic or conversational, I spoke out of my sense of alarm, of being far away on the phone, and of knowing the seriousness of the depression.

"No, you wait," she rightly interrupted me. "Let me tell you. When I was really feeling suicidal last weekend, and I could not get a hold of you, I was watching TV and saw my childhood pastor on The Methodist Hour. I knew he had really cared about me, so I called him long-distance. He was very helpful. He said it was very special to him that I had called. I told him what was going on and I mentioned this conflict about medication. We didn't talk about it much, but when he prayed with me, during his prayer, I heard him say, 'Thank you, God, for medications for really difficult struggles.' That made me feel a lot better and settled the conflict for me."

Hearing this from Sandy was rather humbling to me. One could say she had begun a process of "re-membering" (White, 2000b) herself in the midst of these difficult times. I got on board with her in this work when I returned, and soon she was forming what promised to be the nucleus of an understanding and appreciative spiritual community. She felt that the medicine was working in concert with God, that it opened possibilities for relatedness to others, especially for being able to consider and gradually to believe in others' appreciation of her.

The following questions have been useful ones to use in evaluating the outcome after a trial on a psychotropic medication. These questions survey how the medication may have influenced a person's capacity for relatedness to others, to self, to God, and to one's body:

- Does use of the medicine open new possibilities for dialogue and relationship with others?
- Does the medication alter the relationship between person and the world, such that the person comes to experience the world as near and the illness distant (Sacks, 1990)?
- Does the medication influence relationship to oneself so that the person feels more the person he or she desires to be?
- Does use of medication help or hinder access to spiritual experience—a capacity to meditate, to pray, or to experience the presence of God?

The optimal experience of taking a psychotropic medication has been aptly described as "an awakening" by Oliver Sacks (1990, p. 241): "The patient ceases to feel the presence of illness and the absence of the world, and comes to feel the absence of his illness and the full presence of the world. He becomes, in D. H. Lawrence's words, 'a man in his wholeness wholly attending.' " In kitchen table terms, as a woman put it to me (Melissa), "When I get the medicines, and finally get them straight—it's true I don't feel my feelings as much, whether good, bad, or whatever—but I do feel my children, my friends, my workmates. The anxiety and bipolar symptoms take up all my time when they are running loose. I feel a lot then, but it takes all my attention just to take care of myself. It's like it makes me selfish, but I'm know I'm not selfish. With the meds, I can live in tune with what I really care about."

COPING WITH AMBIGUITY OR UNCERTAINTY

Sometimes the facts concerning an illness cannot be determined. This ambiguity amplifies the adverse impacts of existential states of vulnerability. Pauline Boss (1990, 1999) in her research studies of ambiguous loss in Alzheimer's disease, has underscored the extent to which ambiguity and uncertainty magnify suffering and hinder coping with illnesses, whether medical or psychiatric (Boss, 1999; Boss et al., 1990). Ambiguity in illness occurs when a diagnosis cannot be established, when a prognosis is uncertain, or when a particular illness is so unusual that there is no shared understanding in the surrounding culture to guide how others should relate to the ill person (Weingarten & Worthen, 1997). Ambiguity immobilizes efforts by people and their families to cope with the circumstances of illness. Because that which is ambiguous cannot be clearly communicated to others, it fosters a felt sense of isolation and limits how much well-meaning friends, family members, and a community can help. In order to escape the frustration of ambiguity, families sometimes make detrimental judgments in caring for ill family members, as when a family either totally reorganizes its life around this ill member or extrudes the ill member from the family (Boss, 1999). Over time ambiguity about the illness invites hopelessness and despair. When the identity, character, or prognosis of an illness is uncertain, and when there is little shared understanding about the illness in the school, workplace, and other life settings, then spiritual or religious resources often play a vital role in combating the destructive processes of ambiguity.

The summer before her 40th birthday, Ms. Lewis began experiencing a disturbing set of symptoms within her body—hoarseness and sore throats, tender lymph nodes, painful muscle spasms over her face and shoulders, and numbness and weakness in her legs. A decade earlier a similar poorly defined but chronic illness had occurred that lingered for several years, then disappeared. She had been diagnosed with fibromyalgia by her primary care physician.

The symptoms began during a year of fatigue and stress when she had cared for a chronically ill parent, grieved a death, and undertook a major job transition. In the beginning, she noticed tingling and numbness in her hands and feet. Over the next few months, she had repeated sore throats and cough symptoms. As fatigue, weakness, and muscle stiffness and pains increased, she became unable to work.

By the time I (Griff) first met Ms. Lewis, she was terrified that there might exist an undiscovered disease that her internist had been unable to diagnose. As time passed, her internist's lab tests continued to produce negative results on tests for other serious diseases. However, her uneasiness persisted.

Ms. Lewis engaged in a therapy that integrated the antidepressant doxepin with a psychotherapy focused on heightened awareness of the state of her body, managing stress by careful pacing of her daily activities, and cognitive strategies for countering anxiety and depression. Over a 2-month period her anxiety and depressive symptoms steadily diminished, and the quality of her sleep improved. She successfully returned to work on a part-time basis. Although physical symptoms of her illness—muscle stiffness, muscle aches, fatigue—were persisting, progress was being made.

I was puzzled when she arrived at the 10th therapy session looking troubled and demoralized. I assumed she must have experienced a recurrence of symptoms. However, this was not the case. A review of her symptoms indicated that, if anything, she was continuing to improve. I finally spoke about my confusion and asked what was so distressing her. "First," she replied, "the pain is still present, even though it is improved from months ago. That makes me think that there still is something wrong, something that hasn't been explained. Second, I keep thinking, what if it comes back?"

"Is it the uncertainty that is difficult?' I asked.

Ms. Lewis nodded.

"Suppose the tests were to come back negative," I asked, "Or only mildly abnormal, in a pattern that points to no particular diagnosis? Or to a diagnosis of fibromyalgia, with all its ambiguities? After all, this pattern of symptoms—fatigue, sore lymph nodes, muscle stiffness and pain—fits what is usually termed fibromyalgia. Would it be better if it had a specific name like fibromyalgia, even if that name did not imply a specific way to treat your symptoms?"

"Yes," she responded. "It would make a great difference, just to have a name for it."

We clarified that her anxiety stemmed mostly from two thoughts that persistently haunted her: (1) "I don't know what this is," and (2) "What if it comes back?" I then asked how she experienced each of these thoughts: When she began dwelling upon each of them, what changes did she note in how she experienced her body differently? She described how they together fostered a sense of foreboding and darkness, as if living on the fault line in an earthquake zone, with her body in a tense, vigilant posture.

"What would you want to be your relationship with these two thoughts?" I asked. "When they drift into your mind, what should be your relationship with them?" I explained that such thoughts can be considered in two different ways. First, they can be posed as scientific questions: What is the correct diagnosis? Will it recur? In her case, the use of medical investigations to resolve such questions had reached a dead end. The tests and examinations had been conducted, yet the questions remained unanswered. A second approach, however, would be to assume that these questions, unanswered by science, will continue to dwell in her mind and her body, so that somehow she must learn how to live alongside them. Considered in this way, the focus would shift to the question: What should be her relationship with these thoughts in the days ahead?

From this point on in the therapy, we agreed to name "ambiguity" itself as a source of distress, alongside her physical pain, fatigue, and frustration from living with work and lifestyle limitations. Over the ensuing year a variety of strategies were utilized in order to neutralize the detrimental effects from ambiguity:

• *Deconstructing the fear.* The fear that ambiguity introduced had at its core a dread sense that "there is something awfully wrong." This idea proved to be embedded in powerful stories of her two parents' deaths. She remembered how her father, a brilliant man, "became a vegetable" from Parkinson's disease, lying in bed with legs bent, "absolutely, totally helpless." "Will I be alone like that?" she asked herself. She also remembered her mother's slow deterioration from Alzheimer's disease. "I don't want to be cut off from my husband and children. I saw my mother go through that." After clarifying that these nihilistic images were an important source of her fears of dying, she became more able to confront the fear more directly, including discussion of what would constitute a "good death" when that time came.

• *Relying on a spiritual community.* She worked to share more openly the story of her illness with a trusted circle of friends at church. Always one who had cared for others, she sought to become able to accept their support comfortably and graciously. Her friends prayed for her. This awareness that others were praying for her was a potent antidote for anxiety that came up at vulnerable moments. As she reflected one day, "It has been hard for me to pray. When I get scared, it's hard for me to pray although I know it shouldn't be. . . . I'd never done this before, but I couldn't pray so I called for the prayer group at church to pray for me. I asked that they pray my anxiety would go away. Today I feel less anxious. . . . It was hard to do. It was my pride."

• *Countering the isolation of ambiguity.* The ambiguity of her illness was not only a problem for her, but for other people who knew she was at home and unable to work, but for reasons they could not understand. Ms. Lewis feared other people would assume the problem was "all in my head." Unable to predict when she would have "good days" and "bad days," she hesitated to make social commitments at all, not wanting to burden others with cancelled lunches or changed travel plans. In situations where she needed to make some explanation for her fatigue or limited work schedule, she felt at a loss about what to say. It was helpful for the two of us to compose together a few sentences of prepared explanation that she could say to other people: "I had a viral illness that left me disabled for 2 years. I'm better now, but haven't yet tried out this busy a schedule. If I tire and need to rest, I will do that, so you don't need to worry about me."

• *Reading Scripture, prayer, and meditation.* She developed consistent spiritual practices, one of which was reading from the Psalms in the Bible during a daily devotional time. In the repetitive speaking of the words, she could feel more clearly the presence of God.

• *Revision of religious beliefs.* As her illness persisted, Ms. Lewis struggled with the question: Why does God permit such suffering in the world? She asked it not only about her medical illness, but about the life situations of people throughout the world who also seemed to suffer needlessly. This question had stirred her anger toward God and brought emotional distancing and detachment from him. In the therapy, she sought ways to feel more openly the immediate presence of God, rather than to reason about and to analyze ideas about him. This became an important aspect of her Scripture readings and daily meditation. Eventually, she acknowledged, "I feel more of God's presence than I had before. It is a "giving over" of this illness. . . . I'm not in control. . . . God is all there is . . . I've got to turn this over to God no matter what happens. I've just got to try to know that . . . to know God is there. I'm going to believe that. There is a sense of release with that belief." This shift represented her relying less on abstract theological beliefs, and relying more on belief as a kind of knowledge that presents itself only from inside a felt relationship and dialogue.

• *Articulating her religious beliefs in language evocative of hope and intimacy with God.* As discussed in Chapter 3, an important step was selecting which metaphors for God brought forth emotional postures of tranquillity. It became important for Ms. Lewis to image God as "the Good Shepherd," rather than "Father" or "Judge."

By the end of a year in therapy, Ms. Lewis's illness was no less ambiguous than it had been, in terms of medical diagnosis and prognosis. She continued to have a weak leg, numbness, stiff muscles, painful muscles, difficulty with her voice, and fatigue. Fibromyalgia was still the presumed diagnosis, as a vague medical concept with an etiology not yet established, debate over its diagnostic criteria, and an unclear prognosis and treatment. However, the illness was less central in her life. She had become more able to become attuned to signals from her body in pacing her level of activity. She had progressed in a program of aerobic exercise. With this program and her medication, she was able to work on nearly a full-time basis. Her anxiety about the questions "What is wrong with me? What if it comes back?" was now more distant in her experience. When asked to compare how she was dealing with the residual anxiety, she named the following measures as ones that after a year she still relied upon to maintain her equanimity:

1. Reasoning with myself—"I've been through this before, and I've always gotten better."

2. Using imagery during prayer—Image God as the Good Shepherd, which "also evokes my mother's presence. . . . I feel comforted."
3. Engaging in daily Bible study, meditation, and prayer.
4. Keeping my focus on God's work and his "greater plan."
5. Asking God in prayer, "Help me get through this," which then led to, "What can I do?" She described she found one answer in her volunteer pastoral care, through which she helped others.

In the context of our earlier discussion of existential crisis states as vulnerability factors in illness, it is evident how each of Ms. Lewis's different measures targets a particular existential crisis: the first counters despair; the second counters isolation; the third counters helplessness; the fourth counters meaninglessness; and the fifth counters a composite of each of them.

During this year of psychotherapy, Ms. Lewis's disease persisted both in its physical effects and its ambiguity. Despite this she became a resilient person as she experienced her illness. While her religious beliefs, spiritual practices, and community were only some of the components in her program of recovery, their roles were vital.

INTERWEAVING THE THERAPEUTIC DISCOURSES OF BODY, MIND, AND SPIRIT

The last half of the 20th century has witnessed the synthesis of a broad array of medications that relieve anxiety, depression, and other forms of distress by altering brain physiology. Likewise, a remarkable elaboration of individual and family psychotherapies has taken place. More recently, clinical methods have appeared that are designed to draw from the spiritual and religious resources that individuals bring to therapy. Can each of these three strands be woven into therapy in a manner that is seamless?

The two of us consider emotional postures to be points of union between body, mind, and spirit, where clinical methods organized within each of these domains bring to bear their influences upon healing. A subset set of emotional postures, the existential crisis states, have been shown by both clinical observation and empirical research to exacerbate or protect against recurrences of medical or psychiatric illnesses. Perhaps what matters most from spiritual practices, psychotherapy, or psychopharmacology are the contributions each can make to help the salutary emotional postures of hope, communion, personal agency, purpose, gratitude, and joy to persist and endure in the daily lives of people who struggle with illness.

THE PLACE OF SPIRITUALITY IN ILLNESS

The experience of illness—medical or psychiatric—is the experience of a whole person living in the perpetual awareness that one is not whole. Coping with illness entails negotiation with a disease that has intruded to steal one's innocent awareness of wholeness. Spirituality in its manifold expressions can bolster the connectedness between an ill person and other people—those living now, those who have come before, and those who come after. It can restore relatedness between an ill person and his or her God or other spiritual beings. It can bring peace to a warring relationship with one's diseased body.

Psychoimmunologists and psychoendocrinologists may yet show that spiritual beliefs and practices help cure at least some diseases through physiological effects that at present can only be conjectured. Short of that, spirituality provides human beings with a repertoire of methods to keep disease in its proper place, yielding no more influence to it in the living of one's life than one is biologically obligated to. Too little has been drawn from this repertoire when psychotherapy has been offered to ill people as an applied science.

*   *   *

While writing this book, in our therapy offices and in our world, we have witnessed both the life-giving connections and the murderous divisions created by religion and spirituality.

We have witnessed senseless schisms within families, as between once-close sisters, when one declared herself to be the bearer of the Truth and her sister to be ignorant of it. In our own church body, there have been divisions between those who will and those who will not accept the ministry of clerics who are lesbian or gay. Internationally, we have witnessed our Kosovar colleagues working against the devastation wrought when nationalism is imbued with religious identity.

It seems that the destructiveness occurs when religion is more about group identity than connections that join all people. In the former case it is employed to create a closed club, to draw lines that define and devalue others. In this book we have written about conversations individuals have described as meaningful, mystical, and moving. We also have been inspired by these conversations, but we want to heed the pointed questions that White (2000a) poses, "If we say, as therapists, that we are moved by the people who consult us, what is the movement? From where to where? What real steps will be put in motion?" This debt we owe to those who have inspired us, to promote in our work and be in our lives the neighbors Mrs. Regina Spiegel[3] could count on.

Thelma[4] once told us that her mother taught her to always keep in her kitchen food that would be acceptable both to Muslims and to Christians. This way, she could provide hospitality to whomever came. "We must not let our differences divide us," Thelma said, "if we do, Mozambique will not survive." We want our therapy offices to be like Thelma's kitchen. We have so much yet to learn about how to be hospitable to all our guests. We will continue to learn from the people who consult us and from our colleagues. We hope that this book will introduce us to new teachers. This book is merely a start—some ingredients, some methods, some principles. We offer it not as a cuisine complete, but as an invitation to a potluck supper.

NOTES

1. H. J. Blackham (1952, p. 52), in presenting the existentialist philosophy of Karl Jaspers, writes:

> Ingredient in the concrete particular situation of every self are the inescapable limitations inherent in the human condition, such as death, suffering, conflict, fault. Human life in the world is riddled with the dreadful insecurity and irremediability of these universal limits. But it is not the taking note of them as objective facts that brings home their full fatality; it is only in the irreplaceable bitterness of personal experience of them in the pursuits in which we are engaged that personal existence may learn to accept them as definitive and at the same time find that they are not deadends but frontiers where being-in-itself is to be encountered.

2. With this model we are not discussing what brings about the onset of a disease, but rather our attempts to alter its rate of progression or risk for relapse. It is not yet clear to what extent these factors may place a person at risk for initial onset of disease, even though many adherents to alternative and complementary medicine have strong convictions that these factors are causal. There is good evidence that these factors can alter rate of progression of many diseases.

3. Mrs. Regina Spiegel, please see Chapter 1, page 12.

4. Thelma, please see Chapter 9, page 246.

References

Andersen, B. L., Kiecolt-Glaser, J. K., & Glaser, R. (1994). A biobehavioral model of cancer stress and disease course. *American Psychologist* 49: 389–404.

Andersen, T. (1987). The reflecting team: Dialogue and meta-dialogue in clinical work. *Family Process* 26: 415–428.

Andersen, T. (1991). *The Reflecting Team: Dialogues and Dialogues about the Dialogues.* New York: Norton.

Anderson, H. (1997). *Conversation, Language, and Possibilities.* New York: Basic Books.

Anderson, H., & Goolishian, H. (1986). Systems consultation with agencies dealing with domestic violence. In L. C. Wynne, S. H. McDaniel, & T. T. Weber (Eds.), *Systems Consultation: A New Perspective for Family Therapy* (pp. 284–299). New York: Guilford Press.

Bakhtin, M. (1986). *Speech Genres and Other Late Essays* (V. W. McGee, Trans.). Austin: University of Texas Press.

Bakhtin, M. (1990). *Art and Answerability* (M. Holquist & V. Liapunov, Trans.). Austin, TX: University of Texas Press.

Becker, C., Chasin, L., Chasin, R., Herzig, M., & Roth, S. (1995). From stuck debate to new conversation on controversial issues: A report from the Public Conversations Project. *Journal of Feminist Family Therapy* 7: 143–167. (Also in Weingarten, K. (Ed.). (1995). *Cultural Resistance: Challenging Beliefs about Men, Women, and Therapy.* New York: Haworth Press.)

Becker, E. (1986). *When the War Was Over.* New York: Simon & Schuster.

Blackham, H. J. (1952). *Six Existentialist Thinkers.* New York: Harper Torchbooks.

Blatner, A. (1994). Psychodramatic methods in family therapy. In C. E. Schaefer & L. J. Carey (Eds.), *Family Play Therapy*. Northvale, NJ: Aronson.

Boss, P. (1999). *Ambiguous Loss*. Cambridge, MA: Harvard University Press.

Boss, P., Caron, W., Horbal, J., & Mortimer, J. (1990). Predictors of depression in caregivers of dementia patients: Boundary ambiguity and mastery. *Family Process* 29: 245–254.

Boszormenyi-Nagy, I., & Spark, G. (1973). *Invisible Loyalties: Reciprocity in Intergenerational Family Therapy*. New York: Harper & Row.

Braten, S. (1987). Paradigms of autonomy: Dialogical or monological? In G. Geubner (Ed.), *Autopoesis in Law and Society*. Hawthorne, NY: de Gruyter.

Broadhead, W. B., Kaplan, B. H., James, S. A., Wagner, E. H., Schoenbach, V. J., Grimson, R., Heyden, S., Tibblin, G., & Gehlbach, S. H. (1983). The epidemiologic evidence for a relationship between social support and health. *American Journal of Epidemiology* 117: 521–537.

Bruner, E. M., & Gorfain, P. (1984). Dialogic narration and the paradoxes of Masada. In E. M. Bruner (Ed.), *Text, Play, and Story: The Construction and Reconstruction of Self and Society*. Prospect Heights, IL: Waveland Press.

Bruner, J. (1986). *Actual Minds, Possible Worlds*. Cambridge, MA: Harvard University Press.

Buber, M. (1958). *I and Thou* (2nd ed.). New York: Macmillan.

Bultmann, R. (1960). *Existence and Faith* (S. M. Ogden, Trans.). New York: World.

Butler, M. H., Gardner, B. C., & Bird, M. H. (1998). Not just a time-out: Change dynamics of prayer for religious couples in conflict situations. *Family Process* 37: 451–478.

Combs, G., & Freedman, J. (1990). *Symbol, Story and Ceremony: Using Metaphor in Individual and Family Therapy*. New York: Norton.

Csordas, T. J. (1994). *The Sacred Self: A Cultural Phenomenology of Charismatic Healing*. Berkeley: University of California Press.

Davies, B., & Harre, R. (1990). Positioning: The discursive production of selves. *Journal for the Theory of Social Behaviour* 20: 1.

Derogatis, L. R., Abeloff, M. D., & Melisaratos, N. (1979). Psychological coping mechanisms and survival time in metastatic breast cancer. *Journal of the American Medical Association* 242: 1504–1508.

Dostoevsky, F. (1990). *The Brothers Karamazov* (R. Pervear & L. Volokhonsky, Trans.). New York: Alfred A. Knopf.

Dostoevsky, F. (1992). *Crime and Punishment* (R. Pevear & L. Volokhonsky, Trans.). New York: Vintage Books.

Durham, D., & Fernandez, J. W. (1991). Tropical dominions: The figurative struggle over domains of belonging and apartness in Africa. In J. W. Fernandez (Ed.), *Beyond Metaphor: The Theory of Tropes in Anthropology*. Stanford, CA: Stanford University Press.

Epston, D. (1989). *Collected Papers*. Adelaide, South Australia: Dulwich Centre Publications.

Epston, D. (1993). Internalizing discourses versus externalizing discourses. In S. Gilligan & R. Price (Eds.), *Therapeutic Conversations*. New York: Norton.

Epston, D., & White, M. (1990). Consulting your consultants: The documentation of alternative knowledges. *Dulwich Centre Newsletter* 4: 25–35.

Epston, D., & White, M. (Eds). (1992). *Experience, Contradiction, Narrative, and Imagination*. Adelaide, South Australia: Dulwich Centre Publications.

Epston, D., White, M., & Murray, K. (1992). A proposal for a re-authoring therapy: Rose's revisioning of her life and a commentary. In S. McNamee & K. J. Gergen (Eds.), *Therapy as Social Construction*. Newbury Park, CA: Sage.

Family Centre, The. (1990). Social justice and family therapy. *The Dulwich Centre Newsletter* 1, 7.

Faulkner, W. (1978). Tomorrow. In *Knight's Gambit*. New York: Vintage Books.

Fawzy, F. I., Fawzy, N. W., Hyun, C. S., Elashoff, R., Guthrie, D., Fahey, J. L., & Morton, D. L. (1993). Malignant melanoma: Effects of an early structured psychiatric intervention, coping, and affective state on recurrence and survival 6 years later. *Archives of General Psychiatry* 50: 681–689.

Fernandez, J. W. (1986). *Persuasions and Performances: The Play of Tropes in Culture*. Bloomington: Indiana University Press.

Fernandez, J. W. (Ed.). (1991). *Beyond Metaphor: The Theory of Tropes in Anthropology*. Stanford, CA: Stanford University Press.

Fisher, L., & Weihs, K. L. (2000). Can addressing family relationships improve outcomes in chronic disease? *Journal of Family Practice* 49: 561–566.

Foucault, M. (1980). *Power/Knowledge: Selected Interviews and Other Writings, 1972–1977*. New York: Pantheon Books.

Frank, A. W. (1995). *The Wounded Storyteller: Body, Illness, and Ethics*. Chicago: University of Chicago Press.

Frank, A. W. (1998). Just listening: Narrative and deep illness. *Families, Systems, and Health* 16: 197–212.

Frank, J. D., & Frank, J. B. (1991). *Persuasion and Healing: A Comparative Study of Psychotherapy* (3rd ed.). Baltimore: Johns Hopkins University Press.

Freedman, J., & Combs, G. (1995). *Narrative Therapy: The Social Construction of Preferred Realities*. New York: Norton.

Freeman, J., Epston, D., & Lobovits, D. (1997). *Playful Approaches to Serious Problems: Narrative Therapy with Children and Their Families*. New York: Norton.

Friedman, E. H. (1985). *Generation to Generation: Family Process in Church and Synagogue*. New York: Guilford Press.

Friedman, S. (Ed.) (1993). *The New Language of Change*. New York: Guilford Press.

Friedman, S. (Ed.). (1995). *The Reflecting Team in Action: Collaborative Practice in Family Therapy*. New York: Guilford Press.

Friedrich, P. (1991). Polytropy. In J. W. Fernandez (Ed.), *Beyond Metaphor: The Theory of Tropes in Anthropology*. Stanford, CA: Stanford University Press.

Fullilove, M. (1996). Psychiatric implications of displacement: Contributions from the psychology of place. *American Journal of Psychiatry* 153: 1516–1523.

Gaby, L., Griffith, J. L., Griffith, M. E., & Okawa, J. (2000a, May). *Spirituality and Resilience to Trauma in Political Torture-Survivors*. Paper presented at the 153rd Annual Meeting of the American Psychiatric Association, Chicago.

Gaby, L., Griffith, J. L., Griffith, M. E., & Okawa, J. (2000b, October). *Narratives of Spirituality and Coping with Severe Trauma*. Paper presented at the 52nd Institute on Psychiatric Services, Philadelphia.

Geertz, C. (1986). Making experiences, authoring lives. In V. Turner & E. Bruner (Eds.), *The Anthropology of Experience*. Chicago: University of Illinois Press.

Gergen, K., & Gergen, M. (1985). Narratives of the self. In T. R. Sarbin & K. E. Scheibe (Eds.), *Studies in Social Identity*. Westport, CT: Praeger.

Giddens, A. (1985). Jürgen Habermas. In Q. Skinner (Ed.), *Return of Grand Theory in the Human Sciences*. New York: Cambridge University Press.

Gilligan, S., & Price, R. (Eds.). (1993). *Therapeutic Conversations*. New York: Norton.

Goldhaber Research Associations. (1996, Summer). Religious belief in America: A new poll. *Free Inquiry*, pp. 34–40.

Good, M.-J. D., Brodwin, P. E., Good, B. J., & Kleinman, A. (1992). *Pain as Human Experience*. Berkeley: University of California Press.

Goodman, E. (1992, May 31). A demilitarized zone in the abortion war. *The Boston Globe*, p. 79.

Griffith, J. L. (1986). Employing the God–family relationship in therapy with religious families. *Family Process* 25: 609–618.

Griffith, J. L. (2000, May). *Brief Psychotherapy in Consultation–Liaison Psychiatry*. Pape presented at the symposium "Innovative Therapies in Consultation–Liaison Psychiatry," at the 153rd Annual Meeting of the American Psychiatric Association, Chicago.

Griffith, J. L. (2001, May). Brief psychotherapy at the bedside. In F. Fernandez, E. H. Cassem, & J. L. Griffith, *Innovative therapeutics in consultation–liaison psychiatry*. Presentation at the 154th Annual Meeting of the American Psychiatric Association, New Orleans, LA.

Griffith, J. L., & Griffith, M. E. (1990). Mind–body problems in family therapy: Contrasting first- and second-order cybernetics approaches. *Family Process* 29: 13–28.

Griffith, J. L., & Griffith, M. E. (1992a). Owning one's epistemological stance in therapy. *Dulwich Centre Newsletter* 1: 11–20.

Griffith, J. L., & Griffith, M. E. (1992b). Therapeutic change in religious families—Working with the God-construct. In L. Burton (Ed.), *Religion and the Family*. Binghamton, NY: Haworth Press.

Griffith, J. L., & Griffith, M. E. (1994). *The Body Speaks: Therapeutic Dialogues for Mind/Body Problems*. New York: Basic Books.

Griffith, J. L., Griffith, M. E., Meydrech, E., Grantham, D., & Bearden, S. (1991). A model for psychiatric consultation in systemic therapy. *Journal of Marital and Family Therapy* 17: 291–294.

Griffith, J. L., Griffith, M. E., Rains, J., Polles, A., Tingle, C., Krejmas, N., & Mittal, D. (1995, October). *Analysis of Intrapersonal Self–God Communi-*

cations Utilizing Structural Analysis of Social Behavior (SASB). Paper presented at the Annual Meeting of the Society for the Scientific Study of Religion, St. Louis, MO.

Griffith, J. L., Griffith, M. E., Rains, J., Tingle, C., Krejmas, N., Mittal, D., & Polles, A. (1992, November). *Quality of Relationship between Self and a Personal God: Its Narrative History and Relationship to Individual and Family Variables*. Paper presented at the American Family Therapy Academy/George Washington University Research Conference at Captiva Island, FL.

Griffith, J. L., Griffith, M. E., & Slovik, L. S. (1989). Mind–body patterns of symptom generation. *Family Process* 28: 137–152.

Griffith, J. L., Polles, A., & Griffith, M. E. (1998). Pseudoseizures, families, & unspeakable dilemmas. *Psychosomatics* 39: 144–153.

Griffith, M. E. (1995a). Opening therapy to conversations with a personal God. *Journal of Feminist Family Therapy* 7: 123–139. (Also in Weingarten, K. (Ed.). (1995). *Challenging Beliefs about Men, Women, and Therapy*. Binghamton, NY: Haworth Press.)

Griffith, M. E. (1995b). Stories of the South, stories of suffering, stories of God. *Family Systems Medicine* 13: 3–9.

Griffith, M. E., & Griffith, J. L. (1997, February). *Body, mind, and spirit*. Workshop presented at the Salesmanship Club for Youth and Families, Dallas, TX.

Habermas, J. (1990). *Moral Consciousness and Communicative Action*. Cambridge, MA: MIT Press.

Havens, L. L. (1972). The development of existential psychiatry (Karl Jaspers, E. Minkowski, and Otto Binswanger). *Journal of Nervous and Mental Disease* 154: 309–331.

Higgins, A., & Block, R. (1999, June 24). Holy war: From ruins of Kosovo, Serbian Church's role raises hard questions. *The Wall Street Journal*, p. 1.

Hillesum, E. (1984). *An Interrupted Life: The Diaries of Etty Hillesum 1941–1943* (A. J. Pomerans, Trans.). New York: Panetheon.

Hillesum, E. (1987). *Letters from Westerbork*. London: Jonathan Cape.

Hoffman, L. (1985). Toward a "second order" family systems therapy. *Family Systems Medicine* 3: 381–396.

Hogarty, G. E., Anderson, C. M., Reiss, D. J., Kornblith, S. J., Greenwald, D. P., Javna, C. P., Madonia, M. J., & EPICS Research Group. (1986). Family psychoeducation, social skills training, and maintenance chemotherapy in the aftercare treatment of schizophrenia: I. One-year effects of a controlled study on relapse and expressed emotion. *Archives of General Psychiatry* 43: 633–642.

Hogarty, G. E., Anderson, C. M., Reiss, D. J., Kornblith, S. J., Greenwald, D. P., Ulrich, R. F., Carter, M., & EPICS Research Group. (1991). Family psychoeducation, social skills training, and maintenance chemotherapy in the aftercare treatment of schizophrenia: II. Two-year effects of a controlled study on relapse and adjustment. *Archives of General Psychiatry* 48: 340–347.

Holquist, M. (1993). Foreword. In M. M. Bakhtin, V. Liapunov, & M. Holquist (Eds.), *Toward a Philosophy of the Act* (V. Liapunov, Trans.). Austin: University of Texas Press.

Hoyt, M. F. (Ed.). (1996). *Constructive Therapies* (Vol. 2). New York: Guilford Press.

Imber-Black, E., & Roberts, J. (1992). *Rituals for Our Times: Celebrating, Healing, and Changing Our Lives and Our Relationships.* New York: HarperPerennial.

Irwin, M., Brown, M., Patterson, T., Hauger, R., Mascovich, A., & Grant, I. (1992). Neuropeptide Y and natural killer activity: Findings in depression and Alzheimer caregiver stress. *FASEB Journal 5*: 3100–3107.

James, W. (1994). *The Varieties of Religious Experience.* New York: Modern Library.

Kahle, P. A. (1997). *The Influence of the Person of the Therapist on the Integration of Spirituality and Psychotherapy.* Unpublished doctoral dissertation, Texas Woman's University College of Arts and Sciences, Denton.

Kernberg, O. F. (1975). *Borderline Conditions and Pathological Narcissism.* Northvale, NJ: Aronson.

Ketchin, S. (1994). *The Christ-Haunted Landscape: Faith and Doubt in Southern Fiction.* Jackson: University of Mississippi Press.

Kiecolt-Glaser, J. K., Fisher, J. K., Ogrock, P., Stout, J. C., Speicher, C. E., & Glaser, R. C. (1987). Marital quality, marital disruption, and immune function. *Psychosomatic Medicine 49*: 13–34.

King, M. L. (1963, August 28). *I Have a Dream.* Washington, DC: U.S. Government Printing Office. (88th Cong., 109(12) Cong Rec. 16241-16242)

Kirmayer, L. (1994, October 14). *Plenary Presentation for "Two Ways of Knowing: Advancing the Dialogue between Family Researchers and Family Therapists."* American Family Therapy Academy Clinical/Research Conference, Captiva Island, FL.

Klein, G. (1990). *The Atheist and the Holy City: Encounters and Reflections.* Cambridge, MA: MIT Press.

Kleinman, A.M. (1988). *The Illness Narratives: Suffering, Healing, and the Human Condition.* New York: Basic Books.

Lakoff, G., & Johnson, M. (1980). *Metaphors We Live By.* Chicago: University of Chicago Press.

Landau, J. (1981). Link therapy as a family therapy technique for transitional extended families. *Psychotherapeia 7*: 4.

Landau-Stanton, J. (1990). Issues and methods of treatment for families in cultural transition. In M. P. Mirkin (Ed.), *The Social and Political Contexts of Family Therapy.* Boston: Allyn & Bacon.

Lazare, A. (1999, March). *Shame and Humiliation in Training and Life.* Keynote address to the 28th Annual Meeting of the American Association of Directors of Psychiatric Residency Training, Santa Monica, CA.

Lewis, C. S. (1962). *The Problem of Pain.* New York: Macmillan.

Lewis, C. S. (1976). *A Grief Observed.* New York: Bantam Books.

Lovinger, R. L. (1984). *Working with Religious Issues in Therapy.* Northvale, NJ: Aronson.

Maclean, N. (1976). *A River Runs through It, and Other Stories*. Chicago: University of Chicago Press.

Madanes, C. (1984). *Behind the One-Way Mirror: Advances in the Practice of Strategic Therapy*. San Francisco: Jossey-Bass.

Madigan, S., & Law, I. (Eds.). (1998). *Praxis: Situating Discourse, Feminism and Politics in Narrative Therapies*. Vancouver, British Columbia: Cardigan Press.

Madsen, W. C. (1999). *Collaborative Therapy with Multi-Stressed Families: From Old Problems to New Futures*. New York: Guilford Press.

Mair, M. (1988). Psychology as storytelling. *International Journal of Personal Construct Psychology* 1: 125–138.

Malcolm, N. (1999). *Kosovo: A Short History*. New York: New York University Press.

Malcolm X. (1966). *Autobiography of Malcolm X*. New York: Grove.

Matlins, S. M., & Magida, A. J. (Eds.). (1999a). *How to Be a Perfect Stranger: Volume I. A Guide to Etiquette in Other People's Religious Ceremonies*. Woodstock, VT: Skylight Paths.

Matlins, S. M., & Magida, A. J. (Eds.). (1999b). *How to Be a Perfect Stranger: Volume II. A Guide to Etiquette in Other People's Religious Ceremonies*. Woodstock, VT: Skylight Paths.

Maturana, H., & Varela, F. J. (1992). *The Tree of Knowledge: The Biological Roots of Human Understanding*. Boston: Shambhala.

May, R., Angel, E., & Ellenberger, H. (Eds.). (1958). *Existence: A New Dimension in Psychiatry and Psychology*. New York: Basic Books.

McCarthy, I. C., & Byrne, N. O. (1988). Mis-taken love: Conversations on the problem of incest in an Irish context. *Family Process* 27: 181–199.

McCarthy, I. C., & Byrne, N. O. (1998, May 14–16). *Fifth Province Approach: From Monologue to Dialogue*. Workshop presented at the Therapeutic Conversations IV Conference, Toronto, Ontario, Canada.

McFarlane, W. R., Link, B., Dushay, R., Marchal, J., & Crilly, J. (1995). Psychoeducational multiple family groups: Four-year relapse outcome in schizophrenia. *Family Process* 34: 127–144.

McGoldrick, J. (1999, March/April). In the beginning is the word: Interview with James and Melissa Griffith. *Common Boundary* 17(2): 15–20.

McNamee, S., & Gergen, K. J. (Eds.). (1992). *Therapy as Social Construction*. Newbury Park, CA: Sage.

Meissner, W. W. (1984). *Psychoanalysis and Religious Experience*. New Haven, CT: Yale University Press.

Merton, E. (Ed.). (1965). *Gandhi on Non-Violence*. New York: New Directions.

Monk, G., Winslade, J., Crocket, K., & Epston, D. (1997). *Narrative Therapy in Practice: The Archaeology of Hope*. San Francisco: Jossey-Bass.

Monk, R. (1990). *Ludwig Wittgenstein: The Duty of Genius*. New York: Penguin Books.

Moore, S. F., & Myerhoff, B. G. (Eds.). (1977). *Secular Ritual*. Assen, Austria: Van Gorcum.

Moreno, Z. T. (1965). Psychodramatic rules, techniques and adjunctive methods. *Group Psychotherapy* 18, 73–86.

Myerhoff, B. (1982). Life history among the elderly: Performance, visibility and remembering. In J. Ruby (Ed.), *A Crack in the Mirror: Reflexive Perspectives in Anthropology*. Philadelphia: University of Pennsylvania Press.

Myerhoff, B. (1986). Life not death in Venice: Its second life. In V. Turner & E. Bruner (Eds.), *The Anthropology of Experience*. Chicago: University of Illinois Press.

Noss, J. B. (1963). *Man's Religions* (3rd ed.). New York: Macmillan.

Nouwen, H. (1972). *The Wounded Healer*. Garden City, NY: Image Books.

Palazzoli, M. S., Boscolo, L., Cecchin, G., & Prata, G. (1978). *Paradox and Counter-Paradox*. New York: Aronson.

Parker, L. (1980). *We Let Our Son Die: A Parent's Search for Truth*. Irvine, CA: Harvest House.

Parry, A., & Doan, R. E. (1994). *Story Re-visions: Narrative Therapy in the Postmodern World*. New York: Guilford Press.

Penn, P. (1991, September/October). Letters to ourselves. *The Networker*, pp. 2–4.

Penn, P. (2001). Chronic illness: Trauma, language, and writing: Breaking the silence. *Family Process* 40: 33–52.

Polkinghorne, D. E. (1988). *Narrative Knowing and the Human Sciences*. Albany: State University of New York Press.

Polles, A., Rains, J., Tingle, C., Krejmas, N., Griffith, J., Griffith, M. E., & Mittal, D. (1994, October). *Characterizing God–Self Relationships*. Paper presented at the 1993 Annual Meeting of the Society for the Scientific Study of Religion, Raleigh, NC.

Quinn, N. (1991). The cultural basis of metaphor. In J. W. Fernandez (Ed.), *Beyond Metaphor: The Theory of Tropes in Anthropology*. Stanford, CA: Stanford University Press.

Reiss, D., Neiderhise, J. M., Hetherington, E. M., & Plomin, R. (2000). *The Relationship Code: Deciphering Genetic and Social Influences on Adolescent Development*. Cambridge, MA: Harvard University Press.

Rizzuto, A.-M. (1979). *The Birth of the Living God: A Psychoanalytic Study*. Chicago: University of Chicago Press.

Robins, R. S., & Post, J. M. (1997). *Political Paranoia: The Psychopolitics of Hatred*. New Haven, CT: Yale University Press.

Roth, S. R., Chasin, L., Chasin, R., Becker, C., & Herzig, M. (1992). From debate to dialogue: A facilitating role for family therapists in the public forum. *Dulwich Centre Newsletter* 2: 41–48.

Roth, S., & Epston, D. (1996). Developing externalizing conversations: An exercise. *Journal of Systemic Therapies* 15: 5–12.

Sacks, O. (1990). *Awakenings*. New York: HarperPerennial.

Scarry, E. (1985). *The Body in Pain*. New York: Oxford University Press.

Seivers, J. (1995). *To Help God: Reflections on the Life and Thought of Etty Hillesum* [Online]. Available: http://www.magma.ca/~fjduggan/sidic/95n3a3.htm

Shotter, J. (1993a). *Conversational Realities: Constructing Life Through Language*. Thousand Oaks, CA: Sage.

Shotter, J. (1993b). *Cultural Politics of Everyday Life: Social Constructionism,*

Rhetoric, and Knowing of the Third Kind. Toronto: University of Toronto Press.

Shotter, J., & Katz, A. M. (1996). Articulating a practice from within the practice itself: Establishing formative dialogues by the use of 'a social poetics.' *Concepts and Transformations* 1(2/3): 213–237.

Smith, C., & Nylund, D. (Eds.). (1997). *Narrative Therapies with Children and Adolescents.* New York: Guilford Press.

Smith, H. (2000, November 30). *Morning Edition: Interview with Huston Smith* [Radio broadcast]. Washington, DC: National Public Radio.

Spiegel, D., Bloom, J. R., Kraemer, H. C., & Gottheil, E. (1989). Effect of psychosocial treatment on survival of patients with metastatic breast cancer. *Lancet* 2: 888–991.

Spiegel, D., & Kato, P. M. (1996). Psychosocial influences on cancer incidence and progression. *Harvard Reviews in Psychiatry* 4: 10–26.

Strong, T. (1999). Macro- and micro-conversations in conspiring with chronic pain. *Journal of Systemic Therapies* 18: 37–50.

Temoshok, L. (1985). Biopsychosocial studies on cutaneous malignant melanoma: Psychosocial factors associated with prognostic indicators, progression, psychophysiology, and tumor-host-response. *Social Science and Medicine* 20: 833–840.

Thilly, F., & Wood, L. (1957). *A History of Philosophy* (3rd ed.). New York: Holt, Rinehart & Winston.

Tingle, C. V., Griffith, J. L., Griffith, M. E., Rains, J., Mittal, D., & Krejmas, N. (1993, May). *God–person relationships: Their Character and Relation to Individual and Family System Variables.* Paper presented at the 146th Annual Meeting of the American Psychiatric Association, San Francisco.

Tomm, K. (1989). Externalizing the problem and internalizing personal agency. *Journal of Strategic and Systemic Therapies* 8: 54–59.

Traue, H. C., & Pennebaker, J. W. (1993). *Emotion, Inhibition, and Health.* Seattle, WA: Hogrefe & Huber.

Turner, T. (1991). "We are parrots," "Twins are birds": Play of tropes as operational structure. In J. W. Fernandez (Ed.), *Beyond Metaphor: The Theory of Tropes in Anthropology.* Stanford, CA: Stanford University Press.

Turner, V. (1969). *The Ritual Process: Structure and Anti-Structure.* Ithaca, NY: Cornell University Press.

Turner, V. (1974). *Dramas, Fields, and Metaphors: Symbolic Action in Human Society.* Ithaca, NY: Cornell University Press.

Turner, V. (1982). *From Ritual to Theatre: The Human Seriousness of Play.* Baltimore, MD: PAJ Publications/Johns Hopkins University Press.

Tyler, S. A. (1978). *The Said and the Unsaid.* New York: Academic Press.

Uchino, B., Cacioppo, J., & Kiecolt-Glaser, J. K. (1996). The relationship between social support and psychological processes: A review with emphasis on underlying mechanisms and implications for health. *Psychological Bulletin* 119: 488–531.

Uchino, B. N., Kiecolt-Glaser, J. K., & Cacioppo, J. T. (1992). Age and social support: Effects on cardiovascular functioning in caregivers of relatives with Alzheimer's disease. *Journal of Personality and Social Psychology* 63: 839–846.

Van Gennep, A. N. (1909). *The Rites of Passage* (M. B. Vizedom & G. L. Caffee, Trans.). London: Routledge & Kegan Paul.

Vygotsky, L. S. (1978). *Mind in Society: The Development of Higher Psychological Processes*. Cambridge, MA: Harvard University Press.

Vygotsky, L. S. (1986). *Thought and Language*. Cambridge, MA: MIT Press.

Waldegrave, C. T. (1990). Just Therapy. *Dulwich Centre Newsletter* 1: 5–46.

Walker, A. (1970). *The Third Life of Grange Copeland*. New York: Simon & Schuster.

Walsh, F. (Ed.). (1999). *Spiritual Resources in Family Therapy*. New York: Guilford Press.

Watkins, M. (1986). *Invisible Guests: The Development of Imaginal Dialogues*. Hillsdale, NJ: Analytic Press.

Weihs, K. L., Enright, T. M., Simmens, S. J., & Reiss, D. (2000). Negative affectivity, restriction of emotions, and site of metastases predict mortality in recurrent breast cancer. *Journal of Psychosomatic Research* 49: 59–68.

Weihs, K. L., Fisher, L., & Baird, M. A. (2001). *Family and Health Report* (Produced for the Committee on Health and Behavior: Research Practice and Policy, Institute of Medicine). Washington, DC: National Academy of Sciences.

Weine, S. W. (1999). *When History is Nightmare*. New Brunswick, NJ: Rutgers University Press.

Weingarten, K. (1994). *The Mother's Voice: Strengthening Intimacy in Families*. New York: Harcourt Brace.

Weingarten, K. (1995a). Introduction: Attending to absence. *Journal of Feminist Family Therapy* 7: 1–5. (Also in K. Weingarten (Ed.). (1995). *Cultural Resistance: Challenging Beliefs about Men, Women, and Therapy*. New York: Haworth Press.

Weingarten, K. (1995b). Radical listening: Challenging cultural beliefs for and about mothers. *Journal of Feminist Family Therapy* 7: 7–22. (Also in K. Weingarten (Ed.). (1995). *Cultural Resistance: Challenging Beliefs about Men, Women, and Therapy*. New York: Haworth Press.)

Weingarten, K. (1999). *Doing Hope: A Memoir of Unreliable Bodies*. Unpublished manuscript. (Available from author, 82 Homer Street, New Centre, MA 02159)

Weingarten, K. (2000). Witnessing, Wonder, and Hope. *Family Process* 39: 389–402.

Weingarten, K., & Worthen, M. E. W. (1997). A narrative approach to understanding the illness experiences of a mother and a daughter. *Family, Systems and Health* 15: 41–54.

White, M. (1988, Winter). The process of questioning: A therapy of literary merit? *Dulwich Centre Newsletter*, pp. 8–14.

White, M. (1989a). The externalizing of the problem and the re-authoring of lives and relationships. In *Selected Papers*. Adelaide, South Australia: Dulwich Centre Publications.

White, M. (1989b). *Selected Papers*. Adelaide, South Australia: Dulwich Centre Publications.

White, M. (1990). Consultation interviews and accountability. *Dulwich Centre Newsletter* 4: 36–40.

White, M. (1993). Deconstruction and therapy. In S. Gilligan & R. Price (Eds.), *Therapeutic Conversations*. New York: Norton.

White, M. (1995a). *Re-Authoring Lives: Interviews and Essays*. Adelaide, South Australia: Dulwich Centre Publications.

White, M. (1995b). Reflecting-team work as definitional ceremony. In M. White, *Re-Authoring Lives: Interviews and Essays*. Adelaide, South Australia: Dulwich Centre Publications.

White, M. (1997). *Narratives of Therapists' Lives*. Adelaide, South Australia: Dulwich Centre Publications.

White, M. (2000a, March 27–31). *Michael White Intensive Workshop* Evanston, IL: Evanston Family Therapy Center.

White, M. (2000b). Reflecting-team work as definitional ceremony revisited. In *Reflections on Narrative Practices: Essays and Interviews*. Adelaide, South Australia: Dulwich Centre Publications.

White, M., & Epston, D. (1990). *Narrative Means to Therapeutic Ends*. New York: Norton.

Winnicott, D. W. (1975). Transitional objects and transitional phenomena. In *Through Paediatrics to Psycho-Analysis*. New York: Basic Books.

Wittgenstein, L. (1922). *Tractutus Logico-Philosophicus*. New York: Routledge.

Wittgenstein, L. (1958). *Philosophical Investigations* (3rd ed.). New York: Macmillan.

Wright, L. M., Watson, W. L., & Bell, J. M. (1996). *Beliefs: The Heart of Healing in Families and Illness*. New York: Basic Books.

Yalom, I. D. (1980). *Existential Psychotherapy*. New York: Basic Books.

Zimmerman, J. L., & Dickerson, V. C. (1996). *If Problems Talked: Narrative Therapy in Action*. New York: Guilford Press.

Index